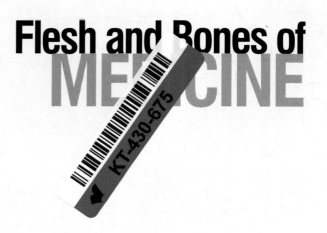

Flesh and Bones of

MEDICINE

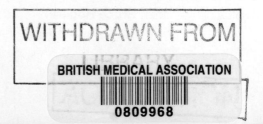

Commissioning Editor: **Timothy Horne**
Development Editor: **Barbara Simmons**
Project Manager: **Frances Affleck**
Designer: **Stewart Larking**
Illustration Manager: **Bruce Hogarth**

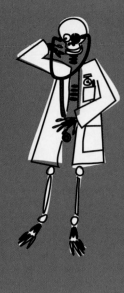

Flesh and Bones of
MEDICINE

Graeme P Currie MBChB, DCH, Pg Dip MEd, MD, FRCP(Edin)
Consultant General and Respiratory Physician
Aberdeen Royal Infirmary, Aberdeen, UK

Graham Douglas BSc(Hons), FRCP (Edin)
Consultant Physician
Aberdeen Royal Infirmary, Aberdeen, UK

Illustrations by Cactus

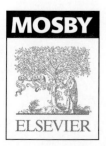

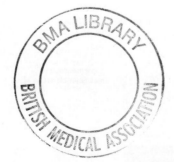

Edinburgh London New York Oxford Philadelphia St Louis Sydney Toronto 2011

ISBN 9780723434382

British Library Cataloguing in Publication Data
A catalogue record for this book is available from the British Library

Library of Congress Cataloging in Publication Data
A catalog record for this book is available from the Library of Congress

Notices
Knowledge and best practice in this field are constantly changing. As new research and experience broaden our understanding, changes in research methods, professional practices, or medical treatment may become necessary.

Practitioners and researchers must always rely on their own experience and knowledge in evaluating and using any information, methods, compounds, or experiments described herein. In using such information or methods they should be mindful of their own safety and the safety of others, including parties for whom they have a professional responsibility.

With respect to any drug or pharmaceutical products identified, readers are advised to check the most current information provided (i) on procedures featured or (ii) by the manufacturer of each product to be administered, to verify the recommended dose or formula, the method and duration of administration, and contraindications. It is the responsibility of practitioners, relying on their own experience and knowledge of their patients, to make diagnoses, to determine dosages and the best treatment for each individual patient, and to take all appropriate safety precautions.

To the fullest extent of the law, neither the Publisher nor the authors, contributors, or editors, assume any liability for any injury and/or damage to persons or property as a matter of products liability, negligence or otherwise, or from any use or operation of any methods, products, instructions, or ideas contained in the material herein.

Printed in China

The publisher's policy is to use **paper manufactured from sustainable forests**

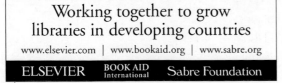

Working together to grow libraries in developing countries

www.elsevier.com | www.bookaid.org | www.sabre.org

ELSEVIER   BOOK AID International   Sabre Foundation

your source for books, journals and multimedia in the health sciences

www.elsevierhealth.com

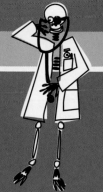

Contents

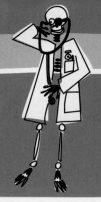

Contributors

Neil Basu MRCP
Honorary Consultant in Rheumatology
Aberdeen Royal Infirmary, Aberdeen

John Bevan MD FRCP(Edin)
Honorary Professor and Consultant Endocrinologist
Aberdeen Royal Infirmary, Aberdeen

Carol Brunton MD MRCP
Consultant Renal Physician
Aberdeen Royal Infirmary, Aberdeen

Graeme Currie DCH Pg Dip MEd MD FRCP(Edin)
Consultant Respiratory and General Physician
Aberdeen Royal Infirmary, Aberdeen

Chris Derry BSc PhD MRCP
Specialist Registrar in Neurology
Aberdeen Royal Infirmary, Aberdeen

Graham Douglas BSc(Hons) FRCP(Edin)
Consultant Physician
Aberdeen Royal Infirmary, Aberdeen

Douglas Elder MRCP
Specialist Registrar in Cardiology
Ninewells Hospital, Dundee

Sian Finlay BMSc PhD MRCP
Consultant in Acute Medicine
Dumfries and Galloway Royal Infirmary, Dumfries

Andrew Fraser MRCP
Consultant Gastroenterologist
Aberdeen Royal Infirmary, Aberdeen

Andrew Gavin MD MRCP
Specialist Registrar in Cardiology
Royal Infirmary of Edinburgh, Edinburgh

Lindsay McLeman BScMedSci MRCP
Specialist Registrar in Gastroenterology
Aberdeen Royal Infirmary, Aberdeen

Sajjan Mittal MD MRCP FRCPath
Consultant Haematologist
Northampton General Hospital, Northampton

Sam Philip MD MRCP
Consultant Diabetologist and Endocrinologist
Aberdeen Royal Infirmary, Aberdeen

Vinod Kumar MRCP
Consultant Rheumatologist
Ninewells Hospital, Dundee

Henry Watson MD FRCP(Edin) FRCPath
Consultant Haematologist
Aberdeen Royal Infirmary, Aberdeen

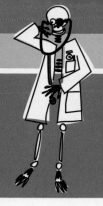

Acknowledgements

The authors would like to thank Drs Alan Denison and Maggie Brookes, Consultant Radiologists at Aberdeen Royal Infirmary, for providing some of the images and Dr Steven Close, Consultant in Acute Medicine, Aberdeen Royal Infirmary, for his contribution towards the Electrolyte Disturbance and Poisoning chapter.

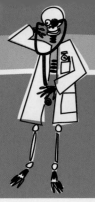

Abbreviations

ACE angiotensin-converting enzyme

AIDS acquired immunodeficiency syndrome

ALT alanine aminotransaminase (alanine aminotransferase)

ARF acute renal failure (also known as acute kidney injury)

AST aspartate aminotransaminase (aspartate aminotransferase)

CNS central nervous system

CRP C-reactive protein

CSF cerebrospinal fluid

CT computed tomography

ECG electrocardiograph

ESR erythrocyte sedimentation rate

FBC full blood count

GI gastrointestinal

HIV human immunodeficiency virus

Ig immunoglobulin

i.m. intramuscular

i.v. intravenous

LDH lactate dehydrogenase

MRI magnetic resonance imaging

NSAID non-steroidal anti-inflammatory drug

PCR polymerase chain reaction

PET positron emission tomography

SARS severe acute respiratory distress syndrome

s.c. subcutaneous

U&Es urea and electrolytes

WHO World Health Organization

Infection

Graham Douglas

The big picture

Infection remains the main cause of morbidity and mortality worldwide, particularly in underdeveloped countries, where it is associated with overcrowding and poverty (Table 1.1). Since 1900, the incidence of infectious disease in developed countries has fallen dramatically, through improved nutrition, better sanitation and housing, immunization and antimicrobial chemotherapy. New infections are always emerging, however, for example severe acute respiratory distress syndrome (SARS), *Escherichia coli* O157, avian H5N1 influenza and the human immunodeficiency virus (HIV) (Fig. 1.1). There are also new concerns about the deliberate release of infectious agents (e.g. smallpox or anthrax) by terrorist groups.

Mortality

Infectious disease causes nearly 25% of all human deaths. In underdeveloped countries, up to 40% of children die of infectious disease before they reach 5 years of age.

Infectious agents

Agents fall into four major classes:

- **prions**: protein molecules with the ability to change an endogenous protein, e.g. the prion linked to variant Creutzfeldt–Jakob disease (vCJD)
- **viruses**: contain protein and nucleic acid (RNA or DNA) and replicate using host cellular apparatus, e.g. chickenpox (DNA virus) and influenza (RNA virus)

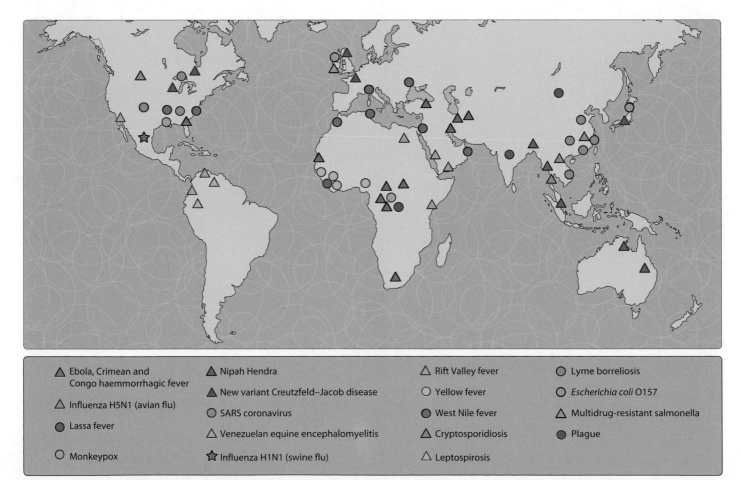

Fig. 1.1 Emerging infections across the world.

- **bacteria**: contain both DNA and RNA enclosed by a cell membrane, have fully autonomous reproduction and are not usually dependent on host cells; bacteria are classified as Gram positive or Gram negative, according to staining characteristics, e.g. *Streptococcus pneumoniae* (Gram positive) a cause of pneumonia and *Salmonella enteritidis* (Gram negative) a cause of acute diarrhoea
- **eukaryotes**: single-celled organisms with subcellular apparatus, for example *Entamoeba histolytica* (the cause of the diarrhoeal disease amoebiasis) *Candida albicans* (the cause of the fungal infection candidiasis) and multicellular worms and flukes.

Host–organism interaction

All of us are colonized by a huge number of microorganisms (10^{14}) with which we coexist. Some are **symbiotic**, when both the organism and the human benefit, while others are **commensals**, living with us without causing harm. It seems probable that most human illness is caused by an infectious agent or the host response to it. For instance, many peptic ulcers are linked with *Helicobacter pylori*, and cervical cancer is associated with papillomavirus.

Source and spread of infection

Infection may arise from the patient's skin, nasopharynx or bowel (endogenous) or from outside sources (exogenous), often an infected person or an asymptomatic carrier. Carriers are usually healthy and may harbour the organism in the throat (e.g. meningococci, causing meningitis), bowel (e.g. salmonellae) or blood (e.g. hepatitis B or C). Animals also can be a source of many infections that are transmitted directly to humans (zoonoses).

Routes of transmission include:

- **endogenous infection**: skin commensal gaining access to subcutaneous tissue and causing soft tissue infection (e.g. erysipelas on the face), or colonic bacteria entering the female urinary tract (e.g. *E. coli* urinary infection)
- **airborne spread**: the usual cause of respiratory tract infection, when secretions are coughed, sneezed or exhaled, e.g. *Legionella* pneumonia and influenza
- **faecal–oral spread**: transmission from hand to mouth, usually with poor personal hygiene or inadequate access to clean water and safe sewage disposal, e.g. acute diarrhoea caused by salmonellae or shigellae
- **vector-borne disease**: spread is often by insects and can be animal to humans (e.g. Lyme disease from deer via tick bites) or human to human (e.g. malaria from mosquito bites)
- **blood-to-blood transmission**: mother to fetus, intravenous drug users sharing equipment, or blood or blood product transfusion, e.g. hepatitis C and hepatitis B
- **sexual transmission**: e.g. syphilis, gonorrhoea
- **direct person-to-person spread**: skin infections (e.g. scabies) or head lice.

The **incubation period** is the time between invasion by the agent and the appearance of features of infection. The **period of infectivity** is the time that the patient is infectious to others.

Immunization

Immunization (Table 1.2) can be either:

- **passive**: preformed antibody for short-term immunity
- **active**: live attenuated or inactivated organism, to achieve long-lasting immunity. Live vaccines should not be given to the immunocompromised.

Table 1.1 WORLDWIDE MORTALITY FROM INFECTION

Disease	Estimated deaths in 2002–3
HIV/AIDS	5 million
Acute lower respiratory infection	3.8 million
Tuberculosis	2.5 million
Diarrhoeal disease	1.8 million
Malaria	1.2 million
Measles	760 thousand
Whooping cough	301 thousand
Tetanus	292 thousand
Meningitis	175 thousand

Table 1.2 EXAMPLES OF VACCINES

Type	Infection
Passive immunoglobulin	Hepatitis B, tetanus, rabies, varicella–zoster
Inactivated organisms	Influenza, hepatitis A, cholera, Japanese encephalitis, rabies
Live attenuated	Measles, mumps, rubella, varicella–zoster, typhoid (oral), BCG for tuberculosis
Subunit vaccines	Hib (*Haemophilus influenza* type b), pneumococcus, meningococcus C, hepatitis B
Toxoid vaccines	Diphtheria, tetanus

High-return facts

1 **Skin and soft tissue infection** is common and affects all age groups; these infections are usually caused by group A streptococci. The various forms—erysipelas, cellulitis and impetigo—have distinctive features. Necrotizing fasciitis, although uncommon, is life threatening. Infection of surgical wounds is becoming less common through the availability of antibiotic prophylaxis, but trauma wounds and bites are commonly infected. Intravenous drug users are prone to skin and soft tissue infection.

2 **Food poisoning** is caused by organisms that produce preformed toxins, causing vomiting and abdominal cramps within a few hours of ingestion. Common organisms include *Bacillus cereus* and *Staphylococcus aureus*. **Gastroenteritis** is spread by the faecal–oral route and causes acute diarrhoea starting 12–48 h after ingestion of the organism. In the UK, the commonest proven bacterial cause is *Campylobacter* sp., while enterotoxigenic *Escherichia coli* (ETEC) is the commonest cause in returning travellers. Norovirus is spread by faecal–oral and respiratory routes, causing outbreaks of acute nausea, vomiting and diarrhoea. Management is with fluid and electrolyte replacement and antibiotics are rarely necessary. *E. coli* O157:H7 causes acute bloodstained diarrhoea and can progress to haemolytic uraemic syndrome and thrombotic thrombocytopenic purpura.

3 **Influenza A virus** has surface proteins that can change, producing a modified virus to which the population has little immunity; consequently, influenza occurs in epidemics, usually in winter. After an incubation period of 2–4 days, acute fever develops associated with cough, fatigue and breathlessness. Influenza vaccination is recommended for those who are at greater risk from infection or who have healthcare roles. **Avian influenza A** (H5N1) has caused outbreaks of influenza in poultry in a number of countries, with some human cases reported from contact with infected birds. **Swine influenza A** is caused by the H1N1 strain and leads to a typical influenza illness. Those with chronic illness, taking immunosuppressant drugs, with morbid obesity or in the last trimester of pregnancy are at greatest risk of complications.

4 **Herpes viruses** are relatively large DNA viruses. Herpes simplex virus (HSV) type I produces stomatitis, cold sores and rarely encephalitis. HSV-2 is sexually transmitted and causes genital herpes. Herpes varicella–zoster virus causes chickenpox as a primary infection and later shingles as reactivation. Shingles occurs in 50% of the population before the age of 85. Aciclovir can be used to treat HSV and varicella–zoster infections. Epstein–Barr virus causes acute glandular fever, with sore throat, generalized lymphadenopathy and atypical mononuclear cells on peripheral blood film. IgM antibodies against the virus confirms the diagnosis. Postviral fatigue is common. **Severe acute respiratory syndrome** (**SARS**) began in southern China in 2002 and is caused by an RNA coronavirus. Incubation period is 2–10 days, following which there is an influenza-like illness with fever progressing to acute pneumonia.

5 **Bacterial meningitis**, although rare, can be life threatening. The main causes are meningococci and pneumococci. Early features include leg pain, cold extremities and mottled skin. Later signs include headache, fever, neck stiffness, photophobia and a non-blanching purpuric rash in meningococcaemia. As soon as the diagnosis is considered, high-dose i.v. benzylpenicillin must be given. Lumbar puncture can be dangerous in the presence of raised intracranial pressure or rash. **Viral meningitis** is usually caused by enteroviruses and can present with similar symptoms to bacterial meningitis but is usually less severe and only requires supportive therapy.

6 **Brain abscesses** may be secondary to infection in an adjacent site or to bacteraemia. Imaging of the brain is required for diagnosis. The abscess should be drained. **Viral encephalitis** is often caused by arthropod-borne viruses and is becoming increasingly recognized across the world. Herpes simplex type 1 is another cause.

7 **Syphilis** is caused by the spirochaete *Treponema pallidum*. Primary syphilis causes a painless anogenital ulcer (chancre). Without treatment, secondary syphilis occurs after 8 weeks—with painless mouth ulcers, lymphadenopathy and anogenital warty lesions. Some patients can develop tertiary complications many years later, including abnormal gait, dementia and aneurysm of the ascending aorta. Treponemal immunoassays are used for screening. Treatment usually includes high-dose intramuscular penicillin. **Gonorrhoea** is caused by *Neisseria gonorrhoeae* and is transmitted sexually. Men develop urethral discharge, while most women are asymptomatic. Treatment consists of a single intramuscular dose of antibiotic.

8 **Human immunodeficiency virus** (**HIV**) infection affects almost 40 million people worldwide. Transmission is mainly through sexual contact, but other routes include parenteral (blood, blood products or injection drug use) or vertical, from mother to fetus. An influenza-like seroconversion illness can occur 6 weeks after exposure. Thereafter, if viraemia is not checked, CD4 lymphocyte count declines, eventually causing immunodeficiency. This is often heralded by opportunistic infections (e.g. oral or oesophageal candidiasis, *Pneumocystis jirovecii* pneumonia or malignancies). AIDS is confirmed by the presence of IgG HIV antibodies and an AIDS-defining illness. Treatment of HIV involves long-term viral suppression, with three or more antiretroviral drugs. Prophylaxis may be required against specific opportunistic infections.

9 **Malaria** is caused by the protozoan parasite *Plasmodium*, which is transmitted in the bite of the female *Anopheles* mosquito. There are four species of *Plasmodium* causing malaria but that caused by *P. falciparum* is the most serious. Malaria presents with high fever after a visit to or residence in an endemic area. Diagnosis is confirmed by microscopy of blood films. Travellers to countries where malaria is endemic should protect themselves against mosquito bites and take appropriate prophylaxis.

10 **Typhoid** is caused by *Salmonella typhi* and is transmitted by the faecal–oral route. After an incubation period of 10–14 days, fever develops associated with headache and abdominal discomfort. Diagnosis is usually made on blood culture and the treatment is intravenous ciprofloxacin. Typhoid must always be considered in any

returned traveller with a fever when malaria has been excluded. **Dengue** is a viral infection transmitted by mosquitoes. It is common in southeast Asia and in the Indian subcontinent. Fever begins 5–8 days after a bite and is associated with headache, retro-orbital pain and intense myalgia. Diagnosis is confirmed by the presence of specific IgM antibodies; treatment is supportive.

11 **Worm infestation** is very common in developing countries. Nematode worms include threadworms, which are common in children and cause intense perianal itching. Hookworms parasitize the small intestine and produce blood eosinophilia and anaemia. Filarial worms live in tissues (e.g. lymphatics or the eye). Trematodes (flatworms) cause schistosomiasis, which is common worldwide and causes haematuria, blood-stained diarrhoea or abdominal symptoms. Cestodes (tapeworms) include *Taenia* spp., which are acquired by eating undercooked meat, and *Echinococcus granulosus*, which is transmitted from dogs by the faecal–oral route and leads to cysts of hydatid disease.

12 **Lyme disease** spreads to humans from deer through the bite of a tick carrying the spirochaete *Borrelia burgdorferi*. The initial symptom is a typical rash, followed months later by secondary disorders. Postinfective fatigue is common. **Toxoplasmosis** is caused by the protozoan parasite *Toxoplasma gondii* transmitted through contact with cats. Symptoms are fever, myalgia and lymphadenopathy. Most infections do not require treatment except in the immunocompromised and in pregnancy.

13 **Healthcare-acquired infections** (HAIs) are becoming increasingly common and now affect 10% of hospital admissions. Common situations include line-associated infection, hospital-acquired pneumonia, surgical wound infection, urinary catheter infection and antibiotic-associated diarrhoea. HAIs often involve multidrug-resistant organisms, for example methicillin-resistant *Staphylococcus aureus* (MRSA), *Clostridium difficile* and extended-spectrum beta-lactamase-resistant Enterobacteriaceae (ESBL), which makes their treatment and eradication difficult. HAIs can be prevented by good personal hygiene, particularly hand washing, and more appropriate use of antibiotics.

1. Skin and soft tissue infection

Questions
- Which groups of patients are more at risk of soft tissue infection?
- What organisms are commonly involved?

Epidemiology

Infections of the skin and underlying soft tissues are common and affect all age groups. This is now the commonest reason for admission to an infectious disease unit.

Pathogenesis

The skin acts as a barrier between the host and the environment and is colonized by various microorganisms, which may invade and cause infection. Predisposing factors for skin and soft tissue infection include:

- diabetes mellitus
- chronic lymphoedema
- peripheral vascular disease
- steroid treatment
- malnutrition
- some immunodeficiency states
- nasal carriage of *Staphylococcus aureus.*

Erysipelas is a superficial infection of the dermis accompanied by lymphatic involvement. It is usually caused by group A streptococci, occurs most commonly on the face and has a typical well-demarcated edge (Fig. 3.1.1).

Cellulitis is a spreading inflammation of the deep dermis and subcutaneous fat. Common pathogens are group A streptococci and *S. aureus*. Rarely, other beta-haemolytic streptococci, Gram-negative bacteria and fungi cause cellulitis.

Impetigo is an infection of the epidermis, usually caused by *S. aureus*. It is most common in hot, humid conditions and is associated with poor hygiene. Children are usually affected, with lesions occurring on the face and hands.

Ulceration is complete loss of the epidermis and part of the dermis; when present on the lower leg (Fig. 3.1.2) it is often associated with vascular disease.

Clinical features

The patient is usually otherwise well, although some disorders (e.g. diabetes mellitus) can predispose to recurrent soft tissue infection. The onset of symptoms is often abrupt with typical features of acute inflammation over the infected area: pain, redness and swelling (oedema).

The skin lesions often have distinct characteristics:

- **erysipelas** is a spreading raised red rash with a well-demarcated edge
- **cellulitis** causes a spreading red tender area of inflammation; it usually affects the legs and can be associated with thrombophlebitis, draining lymphangitis, regional lymphadenopathy and fever
- **impetigo** produces small vesicles, usually on the face, which rupture and crust with a golden-yellow scab.

If infection reaches the systemic circulation, the patient may present with signs of bacteraemia or septicaemia with hypotension, oliguria and shock.

Investigations

The diagnosis is usually easily made on examination, but blood cultures and swabs from areas of discharge are always important in identifying the infecting organism. Occasionally, ultrasound scan of the area can define a subcutaneous abscess and isotope bone scan may reveal underlying osteomyelitis.

Management

In the majority of patients the organism is either group A streptococci or *S. aureus* and, therefore, first-line antibiotic therapy is usually a penicillin, which covers these organisms. If the patient is systemically unwell, initial intravenous (i.v.) antibiotics may be necessary.

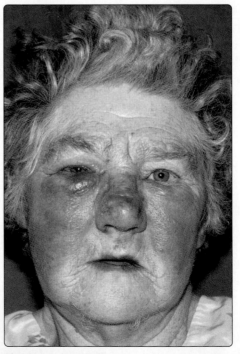

Fig. 3.1.1 Erysipelas.

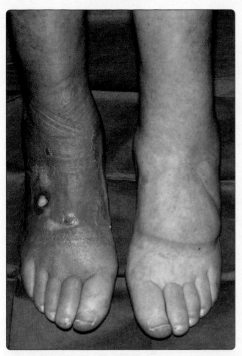

Fig. 3.1.2 Ulceration of dorsum of right foot.

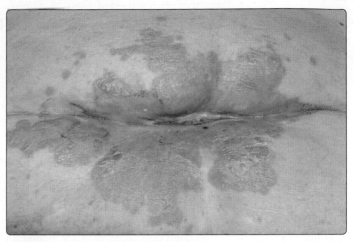

Fig. 3.1.3 Surgical wound infection.

Soft tissue infection in intravenous drug users

Intravenous drug users often infect injection sites, most commonly with *S. aureus*. Cellulitis or abscesses are common and in this situation soft-tissue infection may be associated with bacteraemia, osteomyelitis, septic pulmonary emboli and right-sided bacterial endocarditis. Intravenous antibiotics and surgical drainage or debridement may be required.

Necrotizing fasciitis

Necrotizing fasciitis is an uncommon severe infection of subcutaneous tissue that results in progressive destruction of fascia and fat. Predisposing factors include diabetes mellitus, alcoholism and intravenous drug use. There are two clinical types:

- type 1: mixed infection with Gram-negative organisms and anaerobes, often following surgery
- type 2: pure growth of *Streptococcus pyogenes*, Lancefield group A.

Both types are associated with septicaemia, profound toxaemia and multisystem failure. Onset is rapid, often arising from an apparently minor breach in the skin. Full-thickness gangrene rapidly develops, resembling a thermal burn. The patient becomes systemically unwell with high fever, signs of shock and marked leukocytosis. Management requires urgent and extensive surgical debridement with appropriate i.v. antibiotic therapy against streptococci, anaerobic and Gram-negative organisms. Patients often require intensive care, and mortality in this situation is high.

Surgical wound infection

The prevalence of surgical wound infection has decreased greatly with the use of antibiotic prophylaxis. Wound infections can be divided into superficial and deep, the most common pathogens being *S. aureus*, coagulase-negative staphylococci, enterococci, *Escherichia coli*, candida and anaerobes. Most superficial surgical wound infections present within days of operation, with fever and localized pain, swelling, redness and a purulent discharge or wound dehiscence (Fig. 3.1.3). Ultrasound may be required to identify deeper surgical wound infection. Management involves incision and drainage, debridement of any necrotic tissue, removal of any foreign bodies and local wound care. Most incisional surgical wound infections are left open and allowed to heal by secondary intention.

Bite wounds

Domestic pets are the usual cause of bites and 3–18% of dog wounds and 28–80% of cat wounds become infected. Many organisms can be isolated from bites, most notably *Pasteurella multocida*. The wound should be carefully assessed for damage to underlying joints, muscles and tendons. Treatment includes wound irrigation, debridement, elevation of the affected part and, if appropriate, tetanus and rabies immunization.

2. Food poisoning and gastroenteritis

Questions
- What causes food poisoning and gastroenteritis?
- What are the symptoms and management of food poisoning?

Food poisoning describes an acute illness caused by organisms that produce preformed toxins, resulting in vomiting and abdominal cramps within a few hours of ingestion. Gastroenteritis is when diarrhoea is the more prominent symptom, occurring 12–48 h after ingestion of the infecting organism.

Epidemiology

Acute gastroenteritis is a major cause of morbidity and mortality worldwide, with infants and young children at particular risk. The World Health Organization (WHO) estimates that there are > 1000 million cases of acute diarrhoea each year in developing countries, with 3–4 million deaths. Even in developed countries, diarrhoea remains an important problem, with 38 million cases annually in the USA.

Pathogenesis

The majority of episodes can be directly linked to an infectious agent spread by the faecal–oral route, transmitted either on contaminated hands or in food or water (Fig. 3.2.1). Measures such as the provision of clean water, appropriate disposal of human and animal sewage and simple principles of food hygiene are all very effective means of preventing these infections.

Some organisms (*Bacillus cereus* and *Staphylococcus aureus*) produce **exotoxins**, which have effects on the stomach and small bowel, causing mucosal inflammation and symptoms of food poisoning. Others (salmonellae and enterotoxigenic and enteropathogenic *Escherichia coli*) secrete **enterotoxins**, which cause a syndrome of watery diarrhoea without fever; in this case stool samples usually do not contain blood or mucus. Other organisms (enteroinvasive *E. coli* (ETEC) and *Shigella*, *Campylobacter* and *Yersinia* spp.) can invade the intestinal mucosa (**enteroinvasive**), causing fever, lower abdominal pain, tenesmus and diarrhoea with bleeding and fever (dysentery).

E.coli O157:H7 causes acute blood-stained diarrhoea and the infection can progress to the haemolytic uraemic syndrome (HUS) in some patients. Haemolytic anaemia and thrombocytopenia develop approximately 6 days after the onset of diarrhoea and can progress to acute renal failure. This infection

has become a leading cause for dialysis in children. Thrombotic thrombocytopenia is another rarer complication.

In the UK, *Campylobacter* sp. is the commonest proven bacterial cause of diarrhoea while ETEC is the most frequent cause of acute diarrhoea in a returning traveller. Common causes of traveller's diarrhoea include:

- ETEC 30–70%
- *Salmonella* spp. 10–20%
- *Shigella* spp. 5–15%
- *Campylobacter* spp. 5–15%
- viral pathogens 0–10%
- *Giardia intestinalis* 3%.

Viruses can also cause acute diarrhoea and vomiting, for example norovirus in adults and rotavirus in young children.

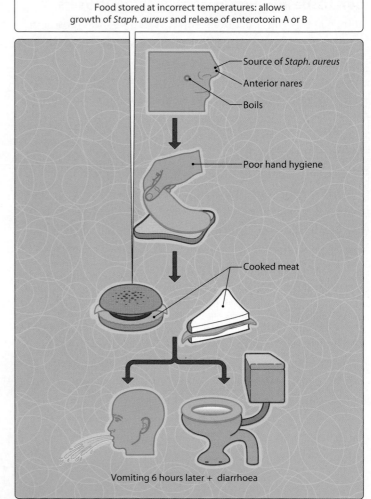

Food stored at incorrect temperatures: allows growth of *Staph. aureus* and release of enterotoxin A or B

Source of *Staph. aureus*
Anterior nares
Boils
Poor hand hygiene
Cooked meat
Vomiting 6 hours later + diarrhoea

Fig. 3.2.1 Staphylococcal food poisoning.

Clinical features

Vomiting or diarrhoea with abdominal pain and tenesmus develop acutely. Fever and bloody diarrhoea suggest an invasive, dysenteric process.

Dehydration can be assessed by skin turgor and by lying and standing blood pressure. Urinary output and ongoing stool losses should be carefully recorded.

Investigations

If the symptoms are severe and persistent:

- stool should be inspected for blood, and culture performed wherever possible
- blood cultures can be helpful in those with fever; a bacterial cause is identified in 15–50% of diarrhoeal episodes
- urea and electrolytes (U&Es) and serum creatinine are important for assessing dehydration.

Management

All patients with acute, potentially infective diarrhoea should be appropriately isolated to minimize person-to-person spread. Fluid replacement is by far the most important aspect in management of both food poisoning and gastroenteritis and can be life saving (Fig. 3.2.2). Many clinicians significantly underestimate the potential for serious dehydration produced by relatively mild gastroenteritis. The normal daily fluid intake in an adult is 1–2 litres; the infective and toxic processes in the gut disturb or reverse the resorptive power of the small and large intestine, resulting in marked dehydration. Fluid lost in diarrhoea is isotonic, requiring replacement of electrolytes.

Oral Rehydration Solution contains a source of carbohydrate, either starch or sugar, with electrolytes. It can be just as effective as i.v. fluid replacement even in fairly severe diarrhoea.

Antibiotics in non-specific gastroenteritis can shorten symptoms by only 1 day in an illness usually lasting 1–3 days. They can also prolong stool carriage of salmonellae, and resistance to ciprofloxacin occurs in 10–30% of infections with *Salmonella* and *Campylobacter* spp. Antibiotics are, therefore, not recommended for acute gastroenteritis unless there is systemic or metastatic infection.

Antidiarrhoeal and antimotility agents should be avoided as these may prolong the illness and make bacteraemia more likely.

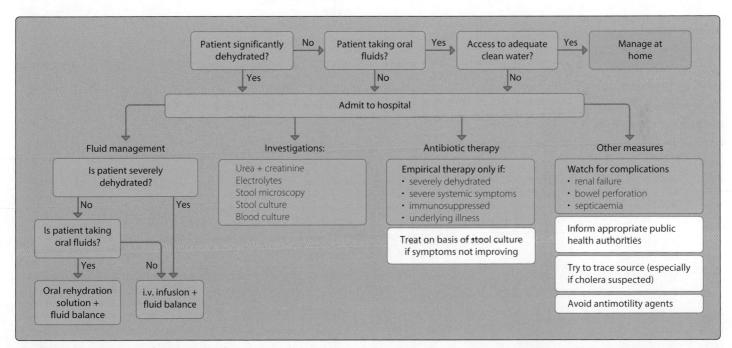

Fig. 3.2.2 Management of gastroenteritis.

3. Influenza

Questions
- What are the clinical features of influenza?
- How can influenza be prevented?

Influenza

Epidemiology

Influenza A virus is labile and minor changes in surface proteins (haemagglutinin (H) and neuraminidase (N)) occur from season to season (antigenic drift) (Fig. 3.3.1). Major changes (antigenic shift) occur when 'new' haemagglutinins arise, resulting in modified viruses against which the population has little immunity. Influenza B viruses have antigenic changes less frequently.

Influenza epidemics occur in October–March in the northern hemisphere and May–September in the southern hemisphere. Infection starts in children and then spreads.

Pathogenesis

Influenza viruses are single-stranded, segmented RNA viruses. Two forms cause most clinical illness: A and B. Influenza C only gives rise to acute pharyngitis.

Clinical features

Incubation period is 2–4 days (range, 1–7). The illness typically presents with abrupt onset of fever, which may reach 41°C. The peak occurs within 24h and lasts typically for 3 days. Any cough is generally dry, and sputum production is more likely in those with chronic lung disease. Cough, weakness and fatigue persist for 1–4 weeks and sometimes up to 6 weeks. There are a range of symptoms associated with influenza, with varying occurrence:

- cough: 85%
- malaise: 80%
- chills: 70%
- headache: 65%
- anorexia: 60%
- coryzal (cold) symptoms: 60%
- myalgia: 53%
- sore throat: 50%.

The patient typically has hot and moist skin, flushed face, injected eyes and redness around the nose and pharynx; 10% will have tender cervical lymphadenopathy and 10% wheezing or lung crackles.

Investigations

Diagnosis is usually clinical. Those with more severe illness require chest X-ray to exclude influenzal or bacterial pneumonia. Renal function and C-reactive protein (CRP) can be helpful. Diagnosis is confirmed by acute and convalescent serology, taken at least 7 days apart, to identify a rise in IgG antibodies or nasopharyngeal swabs for viral polymerase chain reaction (PCR) analysis.

Management

Patients with uncomplicated influenza should be expected to make a full recovery and can be managed at home with symptomatic management, information about natural history and advice as to when to reconsult. Those with new or worsening symptoms—particularly shortness of breath or recurring fever—should be examined for influenza-related pneumonia. Previously well adults with uncomplicated influenza do not require antibiotics. Antibiotics should be considered for those with worsening symptoms or signs of pneumonia.

Prevention

Influenza vaccine is prepared each year using viruses similar to those considered most likely to be circulating in the forthcoming winter (Fig. 3.3.2). The viruses are grown in the allantoic cavity of chick embryos and, therefore, the vaccine is contraindicated in those with egg allergy. It is chemically inactivated and unable to cause infection. Current vaccines are trivalent, containing two type A and one type B subtype viruses. The vaccine is given by intramuscular (i.m.) injection and the main side-effect is local discomfort. In the UK, influenza vaccination is recommended for all those with chronic lung, heart or renal disease,

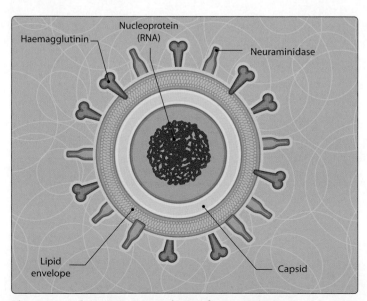

Fig. 3.3.1 Influenza A virus and its surface proteins.

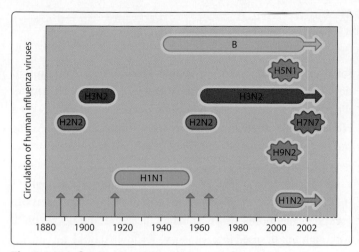

Fig. 3.3.2 Influenza A pandemics, arrows show peaks.

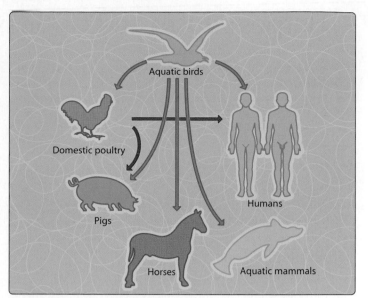

Fig. 3.3.3 Hosts of influenza A virus.

immunosuppression, diabetes mellitus, all those aged 65 years or older, those in long-stay residential care and healthcare workers.

Avian influenza A (H5N1)

The highly pathogenic influenza A virus subtype H5N1 virus has been causing global concern as a potential pandemic threat. It is often referred to as 'bird flu' or 'avian influenza' even though it is only one subtype of avian influenza.

Although H5N1 has killed millions of aquatic birds and poultry in a growing number of countries throughout Asia, Europe and Africa, fewer than 300 humans in 12 countries have died from H5N1 since 2003. Human infections have occurred in children and young adults in direct contact with diseased poultry, of whom 50% have died, usually of an acute overwhelming pneumonia. Coexistence of human flu viruses and avian flu viruses (especially H5N1) may provide an opportunity for genetic material to be exchanged between species, creating a new virulent influenza strain that is easily transmissible and lethal to humans (Fig. 3.3.3). However, the current A/H5N1 virus does not transmit easily from human to human.

Swine influenza A/H1N1

The H1N1 viral strain implicated in the 2009 flu pandemic among humans is often called 'swine flu' because many of the genes in the virus are similar to influenza viruses found in North American swine. It is, however, a wholly human disease. In June 2009, the WHO declared a global pandemic after the virus had spread to two continents.

Clinical features

The symptoms of swine flu are those of typical influenza, including an abrupt fever of > 38°C, occurring after an incubation period of 2–4 days. Other symptoms include cough, sore throat, body aches, chills and fatigue, and some patients report nausea

and diarrhoea. In most healthy individuals, it causes an unpleasant illness lasting 3–5 days but for those in at-risk groups complications are more likely. These include patients with:

- chronic heart, lung, liver, renal and neurological disease
- diabetes mellitus
- those receiving immunosuppressant drugs including biological agents
- HIV infection
- morbid obesity (body mass index > 40)
- in the last trimester of pregnancy.

Investigations

H1N1 swine flu is confirmed by PCR of nasopharyngeal or throat swabs. All patients with persistent symptoms after 4 days should have a chest radiograph.

Management

Treatment involves rest, increased fluid intake and paracetamol to lower temperature. Drugs that inhibit the viral surface protein neuraminidase (Fig 3.3.1)—oseltamivir (tablets) and zanamivir (inhaled powder)—may shorten the illness and length of infectivity by 24 hours. However, oseltamivir commonly causes nausea, vomiting and diarrhoea. Those patients requiring hospital admission often have secondary bacterial pneumonia, and approximately 20% of these patients require additional ventilatory support in intensive care or a high-dependency unit.

Prevention

Transmission of the virus can be reduced by covering the nose and mouth when coughing or sneezing and by frequent hand washing. A specific vaccine against H1N1 swine flu is available.

4. Herpes viruses and coronavirus

Questions
- How many types of herpes virus are there and what illnesses do they produce?
- How did severe acute respiratory syndrome emerge and how is it spread?

Herpes viruses are DNA viruses producing diverse illnesses and establishing latency with later reactivation.

Herpes simplex virus

There are two types of herpes simplex virus (HSV). **HSV-1** is spread readily within families by salivary contact. Primary infection can cause stomatitis but is usually asymptomatic. Reactivation can occur during stress or menstruation, and a 'cold sore' (herpes labialis) is a typical finding in pneumococcal pneumonia. Rarely HSV-1 can cause severe encephalitis. Aciclovir, topical, oral or i.v., is usually effective. **HSV-2** is the main cause of genital herpes and is transmitted by sexual contact.

Herpes varicella–zoster virus

Herpes varicella–zoster virus (VZV) causes varicella (chickenpox) as the primary infection (Fig. 3.4.1) and later zoster (shingles) as reactivation (Fig. 3.4.2).

Chickenpox is the most common notifiable infectious disease in children. After incubation of 14–21 days (median, 15) malaise, sore throat and rhinitis occur. A characteristic vesicular eruption develops on the upper trunk and axillae, spreading in a centripetal distribution to affect head, hands and feet. Vesicles appear on a reddened base, often grouped in crops. Within 12 h, they become infected and develop into pustules, which break down and crust. Fever is common in the first 4 days, and secondary viraemia may cause pneumonia or, more rarely, encephalitis. Management is supportive, but in patients with severe immunosuppression, varicella pneumonia or encephalitis, aciclovir should be used. Although not licensed in pregnancy, aciclovir should be considered for pregnant women who develop chickenpox.

Shingles results from reactivation of VZV latent in dorsal root ganglia. Approximately 50% of the population have had shingles by 85 years of age, but most only experience one attack. Prodromal pain occurs in the dermatome affected, followed by the typical herpetic vesicular rash. Post-herpetic neuralgia is common in patients > 50 years with severe pain at presentation. Shingles can affect any dermatome, (e.g. the cornea, ophthalmic zoster, causing corneal ulceration and the sacral area, causing urinary retention and faecal incontinence) but usually occurs over the thoracic and lumbar dermatomes. Aciclovir, famciclovir or valaciclovir are all effective and good pain control is important.

Cytomegalovirus

Cytomegalovirus (CMV) causes pneumonitis, retinitis and enteritis in immunocompromised patients. Congenital CMV infection can cause learning difficulties and hearing loss. Intravenous ganciclovir can be effective.

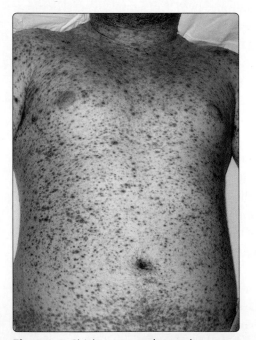

Fig. 3.4.1 Chickenpox on the trunk.

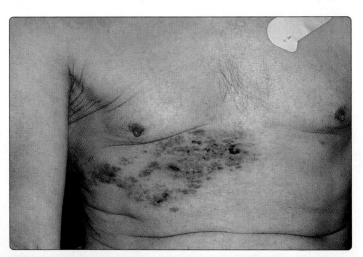

Fig. 3.4.2 Herpes zoster (shingles) of right T_8 affecting right T_6 dermatome.

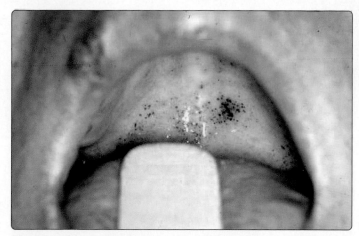

Fig. 3.4.3 Palatal petechiae in glandular fever.

Human herpes viruses

Human herpes virus (HHV) 6 and 7 cause roseola infantum in infants and occasionally encephalopathy and bone marrow suppression in the immunocompromised. HHV-8 causes Kaposi's sarcoma in patients infected with the human immunodeficiency virus (HIV).

Epstein–Barr virus

Epstein–Barr virus (EBV) is present in saliva and is spread by droplet infection, kissing or blood transfusion. There is a good correlation between sexual maturity and the resulting illness, **glandular fever**.

Glandular fever is an acute self-limiting febrile illness with sore throat (Fig. 3.4.3), tonsillitis, generalized lymphadenopathy and atypical mononuclear cells on peripheral blood film (**infectious mononucleosis**). Incubation period is 30–45 days. A widespread macular papular rash induced by penicillin esters (e.g. amoxicillin) occasionally occurs. Periorbital oedema occurs in up to 30% and petechial haemorrhages are characteristic on the hard and soft palate. Splenomegaly occurs in up to 75% and liver function abnormalities are common. Non-specific heterophile antibodies cross-reacting with other animal species can be found in 80% by week 3, producing a positive Monospot test. Acute infection is confirmed by the presence of EBV IgM antibodies.

Management is largely symptomatic, with paracetamol for fever and/or aspirin gargles for sore throat. Rarely, if pharyngeal oedema is severe, i.v. hydrocortisone may be necessary. The illness usually resolves spontaneously, but approximately 10% have a chronic relapsing form, producing symptoms of 'chronic fatigue syndrome'.

SARS-Co-V and severe acute respiratory syndrome
Epidemiology

The severe acute respiratory syndrome (SARS) epidemic began in Guangdong Province of China in 2002. Between 2002 and

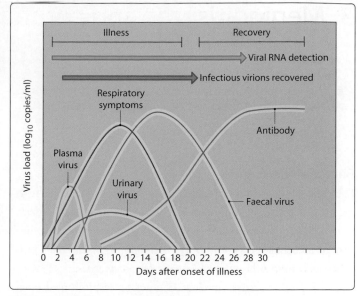

Fig. 3.4.4 SARS coronavirus infection.

2003, 8096 patients were infected, of whom 774 died. Mortality in severely affected countries ranged from 7 to 17%.

Pathogenesis

SARS is caused by the RNA virus SARS-Co-V. Coronaviruses isolated from civet cats and other game animals in China have sequence homology with SARS-Co-V, suggesting that humans might have acquired infection from these animals. SARS-Co-V appears to spread from human to human, mainly by droplet transmission, but viral RNA is also detectable in stool, which may contribute to its spread.

Clinical features

Incubation period for SARS ranges from 2 to 10 days. Thereafter, there is an influenza-like illness with fever, rigors, myalgia, malaise, headache, dry cough and diarrhoea (Fig. 3.4.4). Most patients develop pneumonia during the second week.

Investigations

History of contact in an infected area within the previous 10 days, with radiographic deterioration and systemic symptoms are the mainstay of the acute diagnosis of SARS.

Viral RNA can be detected by reverse transcriptase PCR in nasopharyngeal aspirate, stool and urine. Viral culture is of lower yield than PCR. Detection of a fourfold rise in SARS-Co-V IgG is regarded as the gold standard for diagnosis.

Management

Treatment of SARS is supportive. Most patients will require intensive care and mechanical ventilation; steroids may be helpful. The antiviral agents ribavirin and lopinavir/ritonavir have been used.

5. Meningitis

Questions
- What are the early and the late signs of bacterial meningitis?
- How should suspected bacterial meningitis be managed?

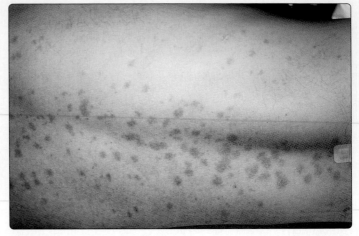

Fig. 3.5.1 Meningococcal rash.

Bacterial meningitis

Bacterial meningitis has an annual incidence of 2–3/100 000, with peaks in infants and adolescence. The main causes are *Neisseria meningitidis* (meningococcus) and *Streptococcus pneumoniae* (pneumococcus), less commonly *Haemophilus influenzae* type b (Hib; in young children) and *Listeria monocytogenes*.

Transmission occurs via close contact or respiratory droplet spread. The bacterium adheres to mucosal membranes in the throat, invades the epithelium and enters the bloodstream. Defects in complement activation increase susceptibility to meningococci, while splenic dysfunction (e.g. in sickle cell disease and postsplenectomy) is associated with pneumococcal meningitis. T cell defects increase the risk of *L. monocytogenes* meningitis.

Pneumococcus is the most common pathogen invading defects in the mucocutaneous barrier (e.g. basal skull fracture or middle or inner ear fistulae). Penetrating cranial trauma and infections of cerebrospinal fluid (CSF) shunts may result in staphylococcal meningitis, particularly with coagulase-negative species.

Clinical features

The early signs of bacterial meningitis include leg pain, cold hands and feet and pale or mottled skin. The classic headache, fever, neck stiffness and photophobia occur relatively late, after 13–22 h, and in 30% neck stiffness may be absent. Raised intracranial pressure is a serious complication and is recognized by:

- reduced or fluctuating consciousness level (common)
- hypertension and relative bradycardia
- unequal, dilated or poorly reactive pupils
- focal neurological signs (e.g. cranial nerve palsies, nystagmus, ataxia)
- abnormal posturing
- seizures: in up to 30%
- papilloedema: a late sign.

In meningococcal septicaemia, a non-blanching purpuric rash (Fig. 3.5.1) occurs starting over pressure areas. Photophobia and neck stiffness are common and Kernig's sign may be positive.

Investigations

Initial priority is to give i.v. antibiotics and to resuscitate the patient. Blood cultures should be taken immediately prior to i.v. antibiotics. Head CT is important; however, i.v. antibiotics must never be delayed.

Gram stain of fine-needle aspirate from a purpuric skin lesion may confirm meningococci and culture of throat swab can often be helpful even after antibiotics have been given.

Confirmation of bacterial meningitis requires examination of CSF (Table 3.5.1). Lumbar puncture can be dangerous in the presence of raised intracranial pressure (Fig. 3.5.2). Gram stain of CSF is positive in more than 40% but is less commonly positive in meningitis secondary to neurosurgery. Antigens from meningococci, pneumococci and Hib capsule may be detected in CSF or blood.

Management

Antibiotics i.v. should be given as soon as bacterial meningitis is considered. High-dose benzylpenicillin is usually effective against meningococcus, but the cephalosporin ceftriaxone is usually given in hospital to cover penicillin-resistant pneumococci. When the bacterial pathogen is unknown, high-dose i.v. amoxicillin should be added to cover *Listeria* spp. Antibiotic therapy i.v. is continued for 7 days. In altered consciousness or central nervous system (CNS) signs, early high-dose steroid (dexamethasone) may improve outcome.

Prevention

Conjugate vaccines for Hib and group C meningococci have reduced the incidence of these pathogens as a cause of bacterial meningitis. Vaccine against meningococcus serogroups A, C, W135 and Y confers protection for up to 3 years to healthcare workers and overseas travellers. There is currently no vaccine available for group B meningococcus. Throat swabs should be taken from close household and 'kissing' contacts, who should be offered prophylaxis with oral rifampicin for 2 days.

Table 3.5.1 CEREBROSPINAL FLUID FINDINGS IN MENINGITIS

	Normal (adults)	Bacterial	Viral	Tuberculous
Appearance	Clear	Turbid purulent	Clear/opalescent	Clear/opalescent
Cells ($\times 10^3$/l)	0–5	5–2000	5–500	5–1000
Main cell type	Lymphocytes	Neutrophils	Lymphocytes	Lymphocytes
Glucose (mmol/l)	2.2–3.3[a]	Very low	Normal[b]	Low
Protein (g/l)	0.1–0.4	Often > 1.0	0.5–0.9	Often > 1.0
Other tests		Gram stain; capsular antigen detection for meningococci, pneumococci, Hib	PCR for herpes simplex, herpes zoster, paramyxovirus (mumps)	PCR and culture for *M. tuberculosis*

PCR, polymerase chain reaction; Hib, *H. influenzae* type b. [a]Approximately 60% of blood level. [b]Occasionally low in mumps meningitis.

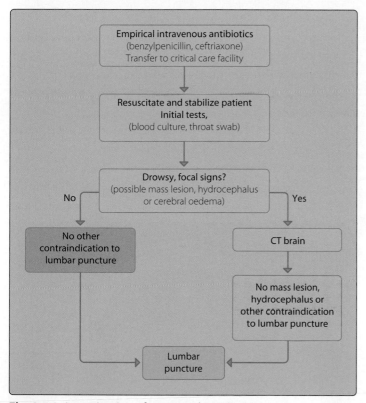

Fig. 3.5.2 Investigation of suspected meningitis.

Viral meningitis

Up to 90% of viral meningitis is caused by enteroviruses. Incidence is unknown but children are more commonly affected. Viral causes of meningitis include enterovirus (over 70 types, polio virus, coxsackievirus), echovirus (31 serotypes), herpes simplex virus, mumps virus, varicella-zoster virus and adenovirus.

Clinical features

Symptoms include acute onset of fever, headache and signs of meningeal irritation (i.e. photophobia, neck stiffness and jolt accentuation of headache). Non-specific symptoms include arthralgia, myalgia, sore throat, weakness and lethargy.

Most enteroviral infections are asymptomatic and up to 10% of the population has detectable enterovirus-specific IgM. Infection occurs in late summer and autumn, often in nurseries and daycare centres. A red macular papular rash may develop on the palms and soles and inside the mouth (as in hand, foot and mouth disease).

Primary genital herpes simplex infection may be associated with meningitis and occurs predominately in women (female: male ratio 6:1). Headache may be associated with genital recurrences. Reactivation of varicella–zoster virus usually presents as shingles but can also present as meningitis without a skin rash.

Mumps is becoming more common in young adults because of previous avoidance of MMR vaccine. Typically, mumps meningitis occurs 7–10 days after the onset of parotid swelling.

Investigations

In most mild infections, the diagnosis is clinical and investigation unnecessary. Enteroviruses can be cultured from throat swab and stool. Herpes simplex and varicella–zoster can be detected by serology and by PCR of CSF. Serology can also detect enterovirus IgM and mumps IgG. Lumbar puncture can exclude bacterial meningitis; in viral meningitis there is raised protein with predominance of lymphocytes.

Management

Treatment is supportive. Intravenous aciclovir should be given for herpes simplex or varicella–zoster infection.

6. Other CNS infections

Questions
- What investigations should be performed in suspected brain abscess?
- What are the causes of viral encephalitis?

Brain abscess

Epidemiology
Brain abscess may be secondary to focal infection in an adjacent site (e.g. otitis media or sinusitis), may follow penetrating trauma to the head or may arise from bacteraemia. However, in many patients there is no recognized source of infection.

Pathogenesis
An area of inflammation of the brain (**cerebritis**) develops, which may lead to an abscess associated with accumulation of pus and development of a capsule.

Clinical features
Clinical features are often non-specific and diagnosis may be delayed. Presenting symptoms are those of a space-occupying lesion and include headache, nausea, vomiting, lethargy, stupor and seizures. Focal neurological deficits are common and vary according to the size and location of the abscess. Surprisingly fever is not always present.

Investigations
Lumbar puncture should not be performed because of the risk of brainstem herniation. CT or magnetic resonance imaging (MRI) is essential for the diagnosis (Fig. 3.6.1). Inflammatory markers (e.g. white cell count and CRP) may be raised and blood culture should always be performed.

Management
Stereotactic needle aspiration to drain the abscess can be performed under CT or MRI guidance. Intravenous antibiotics are given for up to 6 weeks and should include cover for staphylococci. Patients with raised intracranial pressure may require additional treatment (e.g. mannitol, dexamethasone or hyperventilation).

Prognosis
Seizures occur in up to 50% of patients, and focal neurological deficits and learning difficulties are recognized complications. Outcome is poor in the newborn and elderly but mortality is now less than 30%.

Viral encephalitis

Epidemiology
Encephalitis is an uncommon outcome of many common viral infections. Across the world many cases of encephalitis are caused by arthropod-borne viruses.

Pathogenesis
Viruses reach the brain through the blood or neuronal route following a bite from a tick or mosquito. The neuronal route is typified by rabies and herpes simplex.

Clinical features
Onset is commonly acute with fever and headache. There is often disturbed higher mental function (e.g. behavioural change and confusion), which may progress to focal neurological signs and coma. These distinguish viral encephalitis from meningitis, in which there is no direct nervous tissue involvement.

Herpes simplex encephalitis
In developed countries herpes simplex is the most common cause of viral encephalitis although such cases are rare. One-third of

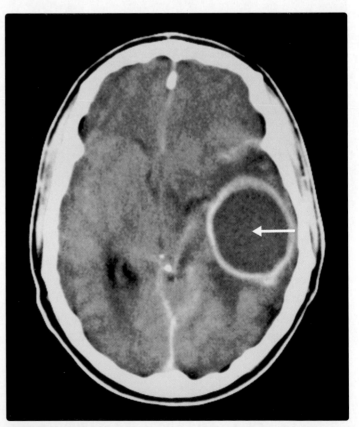

Fig. 3.6.1 Computed tomography of brain abscess (arrow) in the left cerebral hemisphere.

cases occur in those under 20 years and one-half in those over 50 years. The virus has a particular affinity for temporal lobes and may cause temporal lobe seizures, speech disorders, personality changes and altered behaviour.

Encephalitis in travellers

A history of recent travel should always be obtained from patients with suspected encephalitis. Herpes simplex virus, Epstein–Barr virus, cytomegalovirus, varicella–zoster virus, human herpes virus, non-polio enterovirus, mumps virus, rabies virus and West Nile virus have worldwide distribution. Others occur in specific geographical areas (Fig 3.6.2).

Rabies is only very rarely imported into the UK. It is universally fatal. The virus gains entry via a bite from a rabid animal (usually a dog). Preexposure vaccination is advisable in travellers spending longer periods in endemic areas. Postexposure active and passive vaccination is advisable after significant exposure.

Japanese encephalitis is commonly asymptomatic. However in symptomatic patients, mortality is up to 30%. The virus is transmitted by the mosquito *Culex tritaeniorhynnchus*, which acquires the virus from pig or bird reservoirs.

West Nile virus is spread by mosquitoes in Africa, Asia, parts of Europe and the USA.

Tick-borne encephalitis is present in forested and rural areas of Scandinavia, eastern Europe and Russia. It is common in forestry workers and shepherds and in travellers in late spring and summer. Mortality is < 2%.

Investigations

Before attempting lumbar puncture, head CT should be performed to exclude a space-occupying lesion. Typical CSF findings include mildly elevated protein and presence of lymphocytes. PCR analysis of CSF is available for various viruses including herpes simplex. Electroencephalography may be helpful.

Management

Herpes simplex encephalitis should be treated with high-dose i.v. aciclovir. Even with treatment, this form of encephalitis still has a 2 year mortality of up to 50% . In most other cases, treatment is supportive and includes adequate analgesia.

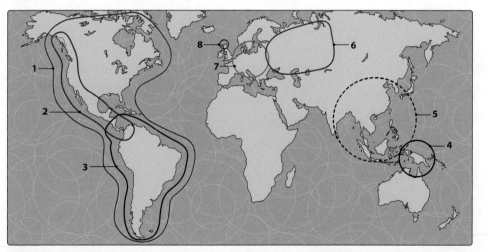

Fig. 3.6.2 Worldwide viral causes of encephalitis. 1, Eastern equine encephalitis; 2, western equine encephalitis; 3,Venezuelan equine encephalitis; 4, Murray Valley encephalitis; 5, Japanese encephalitis; 6, tick-borne encephalitis (eastern subtype); 7, tick-borne encephalitis (western subtype); 8, louping ill. Infections with a worldwide incidence are rabies (South and Southeast Asia, Central and South America) and dengue fever (South and Southeast Asia, Central and South America, southern USA, Africa).

7. Sexually transmitted infections

Questions
- What are the three stages of syphilis?
- What is the treatment of gonorrhoea?

Syphilis

Epidemiology

Syphilis is increasing in Europe and USA, mainly in homosexual men and commercial sex workers. In the UK, there are around 1600 new cases annually and in antenatal clinics the prevalence is 3–14%.

Pathogenesis

Syphilis is caused by the spirochaete *Treponema pallidum*, which is transmitted sexually. The treponemes enter through small abrasions during sexual intercourse, resulting in a primary chancre after 9–90 days. Circulating immune complexes lead to manifestations of secondary syphilis, which appear 6–8 weeks after exposure and may last for months (Fig. 3.7.1).

Clinical features

Primary syphilis presents as a painless anogenital ulcer with surrounding oedema (chancre). **Secondary syphilis** causes fever, headache, myalgia and malaise, sometimes preceded by a generalized rash affecting the palms and soles. There may be oral lesions with painless ulcerated patches (snail-tracked ulcers), flat warty anogenital mucosal lesions (condylomata lata) and generalized lymphadenopathy. Untreated primary and secondary syphilis resolve spontaneously and become latent.

After 5–15 years, approximately 40% of patients develop late complications, **tertiary syphilis**. This can include meningovascular syphilis, features of dementia (general paralysis of the insane) and tabes dorsalis involving the dorsal columns, leading to loss of proprioception and ataxic gait. Argyll Robertson pupils (small irregular pupils reactive to accommodation but not to light), Charcot's joints and aneurysm of the ascending aorta are all late features.

Infection in pregnancy can lead to premature birth or stillbirth, while **congenital syphilis** causes a generalized rash, cranial nerve palsies, acute keratitis, hepatosplenomegaly and Hutchinson's notched incisors.

Investigations

Treponemes can be seen on dark-field microscopy of swabs taken from a primary chancre, genital mucosal lesions or condylomata lata.

Treponeme-specific enzyme immunoassays are the test of choice for screening. Serological tests are shown in Fig. 3.7.2, including the changes detected in untreated syphilis. Tests identify

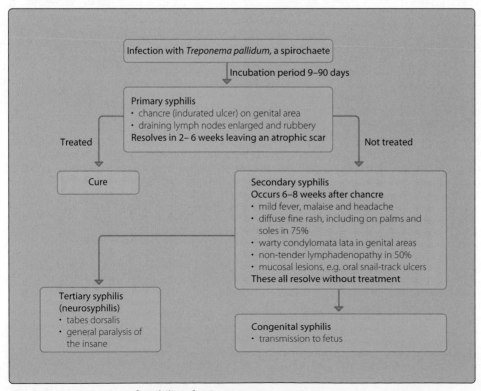

Fig. 3.7.1 Progression of syphilis infection.

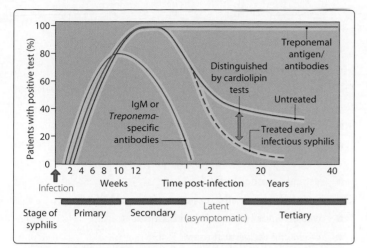

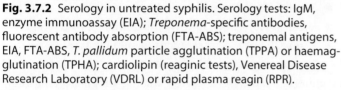

Fig. 3.7.2 Serology in untreated syphilis. Serology tests: IgM, enzyme immunoassay (EIA); *Treponema*-specific antibodies, fluorescent antibody absorption (FTA-ABS); treponemal antigens, EIA, FTA-ABS, *T. pallidum* particle agglutination (TPPA) or haemagglutination (TPHA); cardiolipin (reaginic tests), Venereal Disease Research Laboratory (VDRL) or rapid plasma reagin (RPR).

Treponema-specific antibodies, treponemal antigens, treponemal particle agglutination (TPPA) or haemagglutination (TPHA), and treponemal cardiolipin (reaginic tests: Venereal Disease Research Laboratory (VDRL) or rapid plasma reagin (RPR)).

Management

Early infectious syphilis should be treated immediately with a single dose of i.m. benzathine benzylpenicillin or with i.m. procaine benzylpenicillin daily for 10 days. For patients allergic to penicillin, oral doxycycline for 2 weeks or oral azithromycin for 1 week are effective. Later forms require more prolonged courses of i.v. benzylpenicillin. Treponemal enzyme immunoassay remains positive for life after treatment, but VDRL titre falls within 12 months.

Gonorrhoea

Epidemiology

Worldwide, approximately 62 million cases of gonorrhoea are diagnosed each year, with around 24 000 new cases in the UK. The incidence decreased in the late 1970s but rose 139% between 1995 and 2003.

Pathogenesis

The causative organism, *Neisseria gonorrhoeae*, is a Gram-negative diplococcus. It infects the mucosal surfaces of the genital tract and anal canal, oropharynx and eye. Transmission is always sexual and is more efficient from males to females. Approximately 30% of babies born to infected mothers develop eye infection, **ophthalmia neonatorum**.

Clinical features

Men with urethral infection usually develop discharge, often with dysuria, 3–10 days after exposure. Many men, however, remain asymptomatic. Cervical infection in women is asymptomatic in approximately 70%, but non-specific vaginal discharge or pelvic pain can occur. Rectal infection can cause pain or discharge but is more often asymptomatic. Pharyngeal infection is usually asymptomatic.

Investigations

Urethral or high vaginal swabs often confirm the diagnosis.

Management

Unfortunately, *N. gonorrhoeae* can be resistant to penicillin. Single doses of i.m. ceftriaxone, oral ciprofloxacin or high-dose amoxicillin with probenecid can been used.

Complications

In untreated infection, complications can occur in approximately 3% of women and 1% of men. These include salpingitis in females, with resulting infertility, and epididymitis in males. Less commonly, disseminated infection occurs, resulting in arthritis.

8. HIV infection

Questions
- What are the modes of transmission of HIV infection?
- What is the modern management of HIV infection?

Epidemiology

The acquired immunodeficiency syndrome (AIDS) caused by HIV (HIV-1 or HIV-2; Fig. 3.8.1) was first recognized in 1981. By 2004, there were 39.4 million people living with HIV/AIDS, 4.9 million new infections and 3.1 million deaths. The cumulative death toll is over 20 million, the vast majority of cases occurring in sub-Saharan Africa, where 25–40% of adults are infected. In industrialized nations, heterosexual transmission is now the dominant route. In the UK in 2003, 50% of infections were acquired heterosexually and 75% of these were acquired abroad in a country with a high prevalence of HIV.

Pathogenesis

Infection with HIV-1 eventually leads to AIDS; HIV-2 causes a less-aggressive illness and is restricted mainly to western Africa. HIV is a single-stranded RNA retrovirus from the lentivirus family. After mucosal exposure, HIV is transported to lymph nodes via CD4 lymphocytes. The virus replicates within cells (Fig. 3.8.1) and the viral genome can be incorporated into the host genome. It also lingers in sites less available to the body's natural defences or drugs (e.g. the brain). Continuous HIV replication leads to gradual attrition of the CD4 cell population, impairment of cell-mediated immunity and susceptibility to opportunist infections.

Modes of transmission

HIV is present in blood, semen and other body fluids such as breast milk and saliva. The modes of spread are:

- sexual (man to man, heterosexual and oral)
- parenteral (blood or blood product recipients, injection drug users and those experiencing needlestick injury)
- vertical (mother to fetus).

The transmission risk after exposure is thought to be:

- over 90% for blood or blood products
- 15–40% for the vertical route
- 0.5–1% for each injection drug use
- 0.2–0.5% for genital mucosal membrane spread
- < 0.1% for non-genital mucus membrane spread.

Worldwide, approximately 5–10% of new HIV infection is in children, mostly contracted during pregnancy, birth or breast-feeding. In developed countries, because of routine antibody screening, the likelihood of acquiring HIV from blood products is now less than 1 in 500 000. However, 5–10% of blood transfusions globally are with HIV-infected blood. There have been approximately 100 definite and 200 possible cases of HIV acquired in occupational and healthcare workers.

Clinical features

Primary infection causes sore throat, fever, fine rash, headache and myalgia in 70–80%. This coincides with a surge in plasma HIV RNA to $> 1 \times 10^6$ copies/ml. A period of asymptomatic infection follows, with sustained viraemia and declining CD4

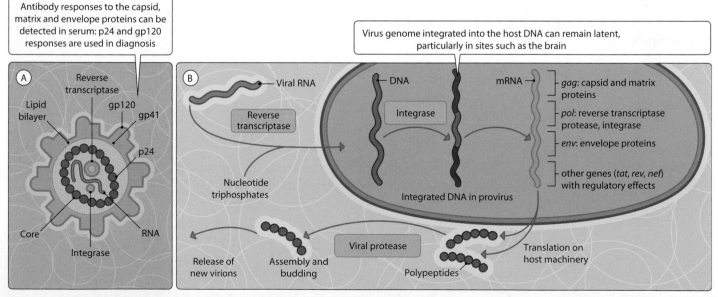

Fig. 3.8.1 HIV and its life cycle.

cell count. As the CD4 cell count falls below 500×10^6 cells/l (500 cells/μl), there is an increasing risk of opportunistic infection and specific malignancies (Fig. 3.8.2).

Most patients are unaware of their HIV infection and in the earlier stages general examination is unremarkable. As the immunodeficiency progresses, characteristic features arise such as weight loss, pharyngeal candidiasis, chronic diarrhoea, recurrent skin infections and herpes zoster infection.

Patients eventually present with AIDS-defining diseases, most commonly *Pneumocystis jirovecii* pneumonia (previously known as *P. carinii* pneumonia (PCP)), Kaposi's sarcoma (Fig. 3.8.3; purple non-tender papules over the skin and oral mucus membranes), oesophageal candidiasis, tuberculosis, cerebral toxoplasmosis, non-Hodgkin lymphoma or HIV-associated wasting and dementia.

Investigations

Specific IgG antibodies to HIV in serum (seroconversion) appear 3–12 weeks (median 8 weeks) after exposure. Prior to this, HIV RNA can be detected in the serum. Thereafter, measuring the CD4 lymphocyte count and HIV RNA viral load monitors progression.

Management

Management of HIV involves treatment of the virus and prevention of opportunistic infections. Aims include:

- reducing plasma viral load to an undetectable level (< 40 copies/ml)
- improving the CD4 lymphocyte count (to > 200×10^6 cells/l)
- improving quality of life without unacceptable drug-related side-effects.

Drugs for HIV

A combination of three drugs to which the virus is susceptible is required to produce lasting suppression of the viral load; this is known as combination antiretroviral therapy (CART). There are four major drug classes used in the treatment of HIV, with differing targets:

- HIV entry into T lymphocytes
- nucleoside inhibition of reverse transcription
- non-nucleoside inhibition of reverse transcription
- protease inhibition.

With appropriate choice of drugs, plasma HIV viral load falls to < 40 copies/ml at 24 weeks in over 80%. While this approach has greatly extended survival, the regimen is complex and unwelcome drug interactions and side-effects can reduce patient compliance. Lifelong commitment to take these medications is required.

Prevention of opportunistic infections

Patients should be immunized with hepatitis A and B vaccines and receive annual influenza vaccine. In patients with CD4 lymphocyte count < 200×10^6 cells/l, co-trimoxazole is used to prevent *P. jirovecii* infection and toxoplasmosis. Those with a positive tuberculin (Mantoux) skin test should be considered for rifampicin and isoniazid chemoprophylaxis. Azithromycin can be useful in preventing *Mycobacterium avium* infection.

Prevention of HIV infection

HIV infection is largely acquired sexually, and transmission can be greatly reduced by the use of condoms and safe sex practices. Vertical transmission of infection from mother to fetus can be reduced by giving zidovudine or nevirapine to mother and child over the birth period. Mothers should be advised not to breast-feed.

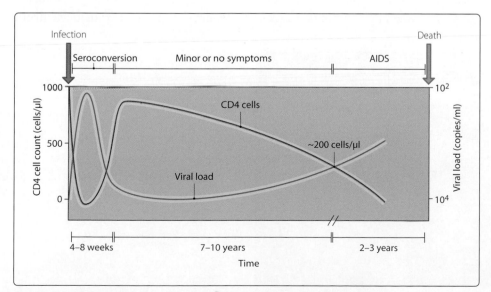

Fig. 3.8.2 Virological and immunological progression of HIV infection.

Fig. 3.8.3 Kaposi's sarcoma.

9. Malaria

Questions

- What is the life cycle of *Plasmodium falciparum*?
- How is malaria prevented and how is it treated?

Epidemiology

Malaria is one of the most important infections worldwide (Fig. 3.9.1). Approximately one-third of the world's population lives in malarial endemic areas (tropics and subtropics at altitudes below 1500 m) and each year there are approximately 250 million clinical cases worldwide. Falciparum malaria causes approximately 2 million deaths each year, predominately in young African children. Even in the UK, approximately 2000 cases are notified each year, with a mortality of 1–2%.

Pathogenesis

Malaria in humans is caused by four species of protozoan parasites: *Plasmodium falciparum*, *P. vivax*, *P. ovale* and *P. malariae*. Sporozoites are injected in the bite of a female *Anopheles* mosquito and multiply within the liver to produce thousands of merozoites, which invade red blood cells. In red blood cells, the parasites grow through the trophozoite stage to the schizont form, which ruptures and releases further merozoites (Fig. 3.9.2) The asexual forms of the parasite invade and destroy red blood cells, localize in tissues by binding to endothelial cells and induce the release of many cytokines (e.g. tumour necrosis factor alpha).

Clinical features

Malaria usually presents with a high fever after a visit to or residence in an endemic area. Symptoms occur within 6 weeks of leaving an endemic area in more than 90% of *P. falciparum* infections and within 1 year in *P. vivax* infection. There may be a short prodromal period of tiredness and aching that is followed by an abrupt fever, often with dramatic rigors during which the patient shakes visibly. Thereafter, the patient may be restless and excitable and may vomit or convulse. These features may last 6–10 h and are followed by a prolonged asymptomatic period. Headache, cough, myalgia, and mild diarrhoea are common, and jaundice can occur from haemolysis and liver dysfunction.

Malaria must be considered in all febrile patients living in or returning from an endemic country regardless of whether they have been taking antimalarial drugs. Examination is usually normal apart from fever, but in long-standing infection there may be enlargement of the liver and spleen (Fig. 3.9.3).

Investigations

Malaria is diagnosed by microscopic examination of thin blood films (Fig. 3.9.4). Initial blood films may be negative and daily films over 3 days off antimalarial drugs are required to exclude the diagnosis. Other laboratory tests include the antigen-capture test using a monoclonal antibody to *P. falciparum*, and rapid tests detecting parasite-specific lactate dehydrogenase for all four forms of malaria.

Management

Falciparum malaria

Chloroquine resistance is widespread across the world. Therefore, quinine is the drug of choice, with doxycycline or sulphadoxine and pyrimethamine (Fansidar) to eradicate asexual forms. Alternatives are artemisinin derivatives (e.g. artesunate) with amiodiaquine/mefloquine or artemether with lunefantrine.

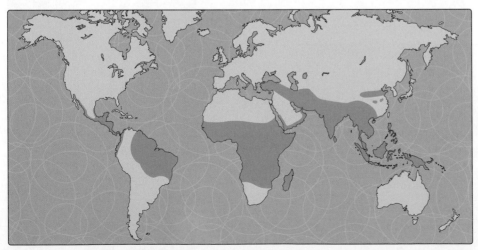

Fig. 3.9.1 Distribution of malaria.

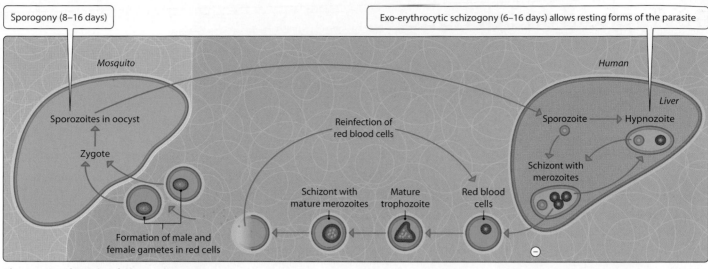

Sporogony (8–16 days)

Exo-erythrocytic schizogony (6–16 days) allows resting forms of the parasite

Mosquito

Human

Liver

Sporozoites in oocyst

Sporozoite → Hypnozoite

Zygote

Schizont with merozoites

Reinfection of red blood cells

Schizont with mature merozoites

Mature trophozoite

Red blood cells

Formation of male and female gametes in red cells

Fig. 3.9.2 Life cycle of *Plasmodium* sp.

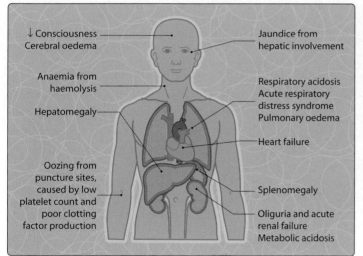

↓Consciousness Cerebral oedema

Jaundice from hepatic involvement

Anaemia from haemolysis

Respiratory acidosis Acute respiratory distress syndrome Pulmonary oedema

Hepatomegaly

Heart failure

Oozing from puncture sites, caused by low platelet count and poor clotting factor production

Splenomegaly

Oliguria and acute renal failure Metabolic acidosis

Fig. 3.9.3 Organ involvement in severe malaria.

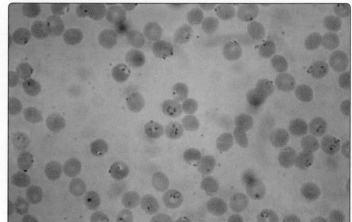

Fig. 3.9.4 Thin blood film.

Halofantrine should no longer be used as it can cause fatal cardiac arrhythmias.

Severe falciparum malaria is a medical emergency and requires i.v. quinine with electrocardiograph (ECG) monitoring. Intravenous fluids will be necessary and some patients will require treatment for hypoglycaemia, hyponatraemia and convulsions. Some patients lose consciousness with cerebral malaria, when the osmotic agent mannitol may be of value.

Non-falciparum malaria

Malaria caused by *P. vivax*, *P. ovale* or *P. malariae* is usually treated with chloroquine. Chloroquine has a half-life of over 7 days and is given in divided doses. When there is doubt about the infecting species, patients should be treated initially as for falciparum malaria. In *P. vivax* and *P. ovale* malaria, primaquine is given to eradicate the ex-erythrocytic forms present within the liver, which are responsible for relapses. Glucose-6-phosphate dehydrogenase (G6PD) should be measured before giving primaquine because of the danger of drug-induced haemolysis in individuals deficient in this enzyme. Chloroquine can aggravate psoriasis and often causes itching in individuals of African descent.

Prevention for travellers

Mosquitoes often bite in the evenings, when it is wise to cover arms and legs and use insect repellent creams. Sleeping in a mosquito net reduces the chances of contracting malaria.

P. falciparum resistance to chloroquine is common in many areas particularly sub-Saharan Africa, and in these regions mefloquine or Malarone (atovaquone + proguanil) is advised. Preventive drugs should be started before departure (e.g. 3 weeks for mefloquine, 1 week for chloroquine and 1 or 2 days for proguanil, doxycycline and Malarone) and taken throughout travel in a malarial area Chloroquine, proguanil, mefloquine and doxycycline should be taken for 4 weeks after returning home to cover the incubation period.

10. Typhoid and dengue

Question
■ What are the typical clinical features of typhoid and dengue fevers?

Typhoid

Epidemiology
There are 22 million cases of typhoid each year in sub-Saharan Africa, the Indian subcontinent and in central and southeast Asia, with 200 000 deaths. In Western countries, typhoid is found in returning travellers and in immigrants who return to visit their family.

Pathogenesis
Typhoid is caused by *Salmonella typhi* and is transmitted by contamination of food and water with faeces from infected individuals and carriers (Fig. 3.10.1). The incubation period is 10–14 days. The bacilli may live in the gallbladder of carriers for years after clinical recovery and pass intermittently in the stool and less commonly in the urine.

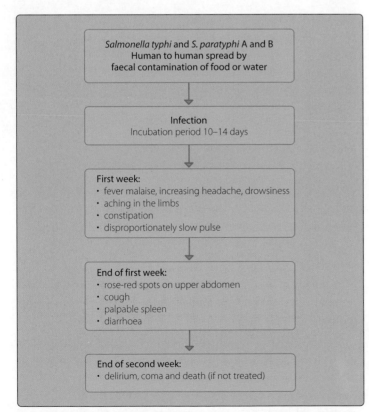

Fig. 3.10.1 Typhoid and paratyphoid fever (5% of those infected will become chronic carriers).

Clinical features
Classically, typhoid fever is of gradual onset in the first week, remittent in the second week and falling in the third week. Patients complain of headache, anorexia, vague abdominal pain, constipation or diarrhoea and a dry cough.

Early in the illness, patients appear well. At the end of the first week, sparse, slightly raised 'rose-red' spots that fade on pressure may appear on the upper abdomen. By day 10, the spleen may become palpable with abdominal distension. Untreated patients become profoundly ill from the second week onwards and may progress to coma.

Investigations
Typhoid should be considered in any febrile returned traveller when suspected malaria has not been confirmed.
■ blood culture is positive in up to 60% of those with typhoid fever
■ stool culture will contain the organism more frequently after the first week
■ Widal test (based on the detection of agglutinating antibodies to 'O' (somatic) and 'H' (flagellar) antigens) may give false-positive results, particularly in those previously vaccinated.

Management
Patterns of antibiotic resistance are changing. Fluoroquinolones (e.g. ciprofloxacin) are now the drugs of choice, although resistance is also emerging to these drugs, particularly in the Indian subcontinent. Alternatives are extended-spectrum cephalosporins and azithromycin. Treatment should continue for 14 days. Patients with confusion, shock and hypotension require intensive care and may benefit from parenteral steroids.

Chronic carriage
Patients still excreting *S. typhi* at 1 year are defined as chronic carriers. Up to 5% become chronic carriers, and in 25% of carriers, there is no history of acute typhoid. Eradication of carriage is difficult and requires prolonged high-dose antibiotics.

Prevention
Travellers to countries where enteric infections are endemic should be inoculated with one of three available typhoid vaccines (two inactivated injectable and one oral live attenuated).

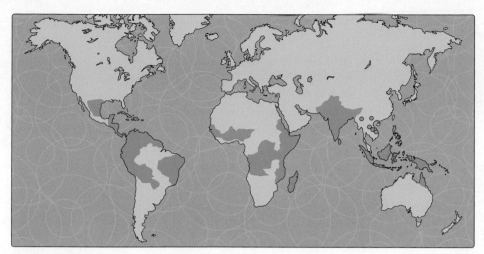

Fig. 3.10.2 Distribution of dengue.

Dengue

Epidemiology

Dengue is found throughout the tropics and subtropics, particularly southeast Asia and the Indian subcontinent (Fig. 3.10.2). It is estimated that 40–80 million are infected with dengue virus each year. Most cases imported into the UK are acquired in southeast Asia.

Pathogenesis

Dengue is a viral infection transmitted by *Aedes aegypti* mosquitoes, which live in urban areas, breeding in small collections of clean water in and around human habitats and bite during the day. Dengue viruses are flaviviruses, closely related to yellow fever and Japanese encephalitis viruses.

Clinical features

Dengue fever begins abruptly 3–15 days (usually 5–8) after a mosquito bite. Fever is often accompanied by severe headache, retro-orbital pain and intense myalgia with arthralgia (break-bone fever). A blanching rash may occur after a few days. Fever usually lasts 4–7 days and is followed by complete recovery. Dengue haemorrhagic fever is associated with coagulation disorders and encephalitis.

Investigations

Dengue viraemia is strongly correlated with temperature, and virus isolation (antigen detection or genome amplification) is usually successful in febrile patients. In later stages of the illness, IgM serology is more useful.

Management

There is no specific antiviral therapy for dengue virus. Aspirin should be avoided in dengue fever because of the increased bleeding tendency. Management is supportive with paracetamol and fluid replacement.

Patients with overt bleeding or a purpuric rash (dengue haemorrhagic fever) should be closely monitored. Steroids are widely used but there is little evidence of benefit.

Prevention and control

Vector control by elimination of urban mosquito breeding sites is often effective, but this needs to be constantly repeated. Effective vaccines are available for closely related mosquito-borne flaviviruses, yellow fever (live attentuated) and Japanese encephalitis (inactivated) but there is currently no vaccine for dengue virus.

11. Worm infestation

Question
■ What is the life cycle of *Schistosoma haematobium*?

Worm infections are common in developing countries, and coinfection with HIV is increasingly recognized. Worms are large, internal human parasites that reproduce sexually, generating millions of eggs (ova) or larvae.

Nematodes (roundworms)

Enterobius vermicularis *(threadworm)*
Threadworm is common in children throughout the world. Ova are swallowed and adult worms develop in the colon. Female worms lay ova around the anus, causing intense itching at night. Ova carried to the mouth cause reinfection (Fig. 3.11.1). A single dose of albendazole or piperazine is usually curative. If reinfection occurs, all family members should be treated.

Ancylostoma duodenale *(hookworm)*
The hookworm parasitizes the small intestine and can grow to 1 cm in length. Larvae cause allergic inflammation of the skin and blood eosinophilia if they reach the lung (Fig. 3.11.2A). **Ancylostomiasis** is a cause of anaemia in the tropics. Characteristic ova can be seen on stool microscopy. Single-dose albendazole or a 3 day course of mebendazole is usually effective.

Filariasis
Filarial worms are tissue-dwelling nematodes (Fig. 3.11.3A). Larvae are inoculated by biting insects. Microfilariae survive 2–3 years and adult worms 10–15 years. Lymphatic filariasis caused by *Wuchereria bancrofti* presents with fever, inflamed lymphatic vessels and epididymo-orchitis. Blood eosinophilia

and IgG antibodies are usually present. Diethylcarbamazine is usually effective.

Onchocerciasis (**river blindness**) is caused by the filarial worm *Onchocerca volvulus* transmitted by flies. The first symptom is itching and skin shavings can show wriggling microfilariae on microscopy. Blood eosinophilia is common. A single dose of ivermectin is usually effective.

Trematodes (flatworms)

Schistosomiasis
Worldwide, approximately 200 million people have schistosomiasis (Fig. 3.11.3B). Ova are passed in the urine or faeces and multiply in freshwater snails (Fig. 3.11.2B). Fork-tailed cercariae penetrate the skin or mucous membrane of humans. Itching occurs at the site of penetration (swimmer's itch); after 2–6 weeks, allergic manifestations (e.g. urticaria), muscle aches, abdominal pain and fever (Katayama fever) develop. Blood eosinophilia and IgG antibodies to schistosomae can be found.

Schistosoma haematobium causes painless haematuria and, later, urinary tract infection, a contracted calcified bladder and renal failure. *S. mansoni* causes abdominal pain, blood-stained diarrhoea and, later, hepatomegaly and portal hypertension. *S. japonicum* produces abdominal symptoms and in 5% CNS infection, causing epilepsy, blindness and stroke.

Praziquantel is the drug of choice for all forms of schistosomiasis, producing cure in 80%.

Cestodes (tapeworms)
Cestodes are ribbon-shaped worms with no alimentary system, absorbing nutrients through their surface. Humans acquire tapeworms by eating undercooked beef (*Taenia saginata*) or pork (*T. solium*). Adult worms may be several metres long and produce no intestinal upset. Patients may notice segments of worm or ova in their faeces. **Cysticercosis** is acquired by ingesting tapeworm ova, which penetrate intestinal mucosa and migrate to skeletal muscle or brain.

Niclosamide is useful for intestinal infection, while praziquantel or albendazole are used for cerebral cysticercosis.

Hydatid disease
Faecal–oral transmission of *Echinococcus granulosus*, a tiny tapeworm, occurs from an infected dog. Ova penetrate the small intestine, gaining access to the bloodstream and liver (Fig. 3.11.2C). The resulting cysts in the lung, bone or brain may calcify. IgG antibody tests are positive in 90%. Hydatid cysts can be excised and albendazole and praziquantel are effective.

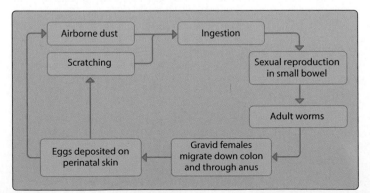

Fig. 3.11.1 Life cycle of threadworm.

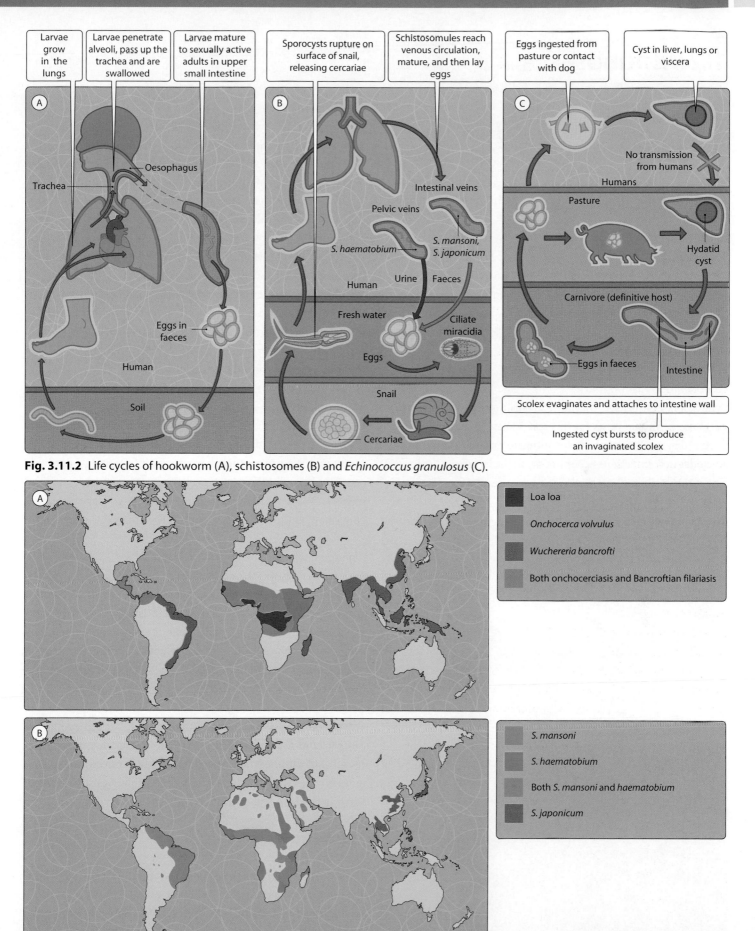

Fig. 3.11.2 Life cycles of hookworm (A), schistosomes (B) and *Echinococcus granulosus* (C).

Fig. 3.11.3 Worldwide distribution of filariasis (A) and schistosomiasis (B).

12. Zoonoses

Questions
- What are the clinical features of Lyme disease?
- What are the complications of toxoplasmosis?

Zoonoses are infections transmitted to humans from vertebrate animals.

Lyme disease

Epidemiology

Lyme disease is a common tick-borne infection particularly prevalent in southern Scandinavia, Germany, Austria and central Europe and also in the northeastern, mid-west and Pacific coast states of the USA. In the UK, approximately 500 cases are confirmed each year.

Pathogenesis

Lyme disease is caused by the tick-borne spirochaete *Borrelia burgdorferi*. Animal hosts for this spirochaete include deer, field mice and hares. Infection is transmitted to humans via the bite of an ixodes tick. Infections occur mainly in the late spring, summer and autumn when humans visit the countryside (Fig. 3.12.1).

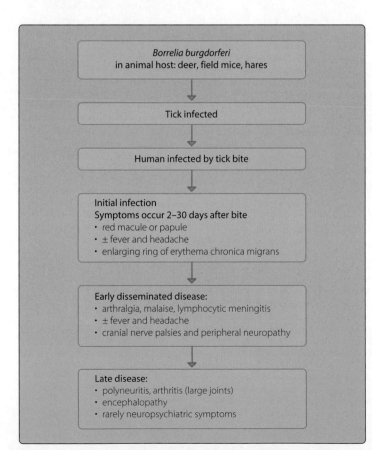

Fig. 3.12.1 The natural history of Lyme disease.

Clinical features

Infection can be asymptomatic. The most common manifestation is erythema chronica migrans, a localized rash appearing 2–30 days at the site of a tick bite. The rash may be faint, with a more pronounced margin that gradually migrates outwards.

Several months later, the organism affects other tissues producing a flu-like illness with myalgia and arthralgia, cranial nerve lesions, lymphocytic meningitis and small joint arthritis. In the USA, large joint arthritis is common. Acrodermatitis chronica atrophicans is a chronic skin manifestation found on the limbs and sometimes associated with peripheral neuropathy. Lyme disease may trigger a postinfection syndrome similar to chronic fatigue or fibromyalgia.

In the acute stages, examination may be normal but erythema chronica migrans should be sought.

Investigations

Diagnosis is largely clinical, particularly in the early stages. Borrelia IgG serology may be helpful, although a positive test may reflect past exposure rather than current infection. IgG antibody test may be negative in the early stages of erythema chronica migrans. Whole-cell antigens from different genospecies or recombinant antigens may give greater specificity.

Management

B. borgdorferi is slow to replicate and can disseminate widely to tissues that may be poorly penetrated by antibiotics. Prolonged courses of oral amoxicillin, doxycycline and cefuroxime have all been used. For severe infections, i.v. antibiotics including ceftriaxone, cefuroxime and benzylpenicillin are effective. A 14 day course is recommended for erythema chronica migrans, but more disseminated infection may require 2–4 weeks.

Prevention

Simple, common sense measures to avoid tick bites and prompt removal of attached ticks can greatly reduce infection. No vaccines are currently available and a vaccine previously manufactured in the USA was withdrawn in 2002.

Toxoplasmosis

Epidemiology

Worldwide toxoplasmosis is most common in warm, wet countries and increases with age. In France, 50–75% of the population is seropositive, while in UK approximately 20% of the population is seropositive.

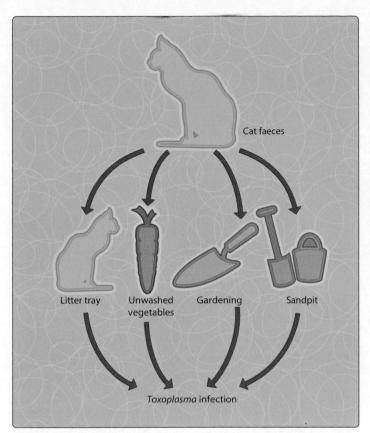

Fig. 3.12.2 Human toxoplasmal infection from cat faeces.

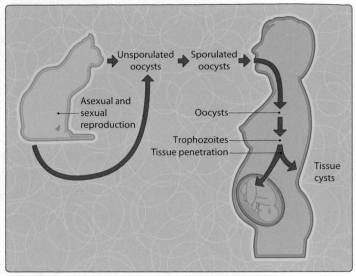

Fig. 3.12.3 Transmission of toxoplasmosis.

Pathogenesis

Toxoplasmosis is a zoonotic infection with a protozoan parasite, *Toxoplasma gondii*. The sexual phase of the life cycle of *T. gondii* occurs in cats, and oocysts are excreted in feline faeces (Figs 3.12.2 and 3.12.3). Infection can arise from other animals and birds, and unpasteurized milk, particularly goats' milk, has been identified as a source of infection.

Clinical features

Acute acquired infection has an incubation period of 3–21 days. Infection is asymptomatic in approximately 25% of those affected, and most patients have non-specific symptoms such as fever, malaise, myalgia and headache.

Lymphadenopathy, particularly in the neck, is common and can last for up to 6 months. The differential diagnosis includes infectious mononucleosis and lymphoma. Retinochoroiditis is usually regarded as caused by congenital infection.

Chronic infection can present with persistent tiredness. In the immunocompromised (e.g. HIV infection), toxoplasma cysts in the brain can reactivate, causing major neurological complications.

Investigations

Current infection is indicated by a fourfold increase in the dye test titre, an increase in toxoplasma-specific IgG or the presence of IgM:

- the gold standard is the **dye test**, which uses methylene blue to stain live toxoplasma not killed by specific antibody in the patient's serum
- in newborns, specific IgA denotes congenital infection
- during pregnancy, additional tests such as IgG Western blotting may be necessary
- CT and MRI of the head are useful in CNS toxoplasmosis, when serology is often non-diagnostic.

Management

Acute acquired infection does not usually require treatment except in pregnancy, when the aim is to prevent transmission of the infection to the fetus. Active eye disease should be treated, as should toxoplasmosis in the immunocompromised.

First-line treatment is pyrimethamine plus sulfadiazine and folinic acid for 6 weeks. Relapses are common and immunocompromised patients should receive lifelong treatment usually at 50% of the acute dose. In pregnancy and neonates, spiramycin may also be used. Drug toxicity is a frequent problem and alternative drugs include dapsone, azithromycin and atovaquone.

13. Healthcare-acquired infection

Questions
- Which situations can lead to healthcare-acquired infection?
- How can healthcare-acquired infections be prevented?

Although most infection found in primary and secondary care is acquired in the community, the transmission of infection during healthcare (healthcare-acquired infection or HAI) is becoming increasingly common. Previously known as hospital-acquired or nosocomial infection, HAIs now affect approximately 10% of all hospital admissions. The close proximity of ill patients, coupled with the concentrated use of antibiotics and ease of transmission by healthcare workers, has led to the selection of multidrug-resistant organisms, for example meticillin-resistant *Staphylococcus aureus* (MRSA), *Clostridium difficile* and extended-spectrum beta-lactamase-resistant Enterobacteriaceae (ESBL). There are a number of common situations where HAIs are a greater risk (Table 3.13.1).

Use of i.v. lines. One-third of cases of hospital-acquired bacteraemia are associated with an i.v. device. Almost 50% of isolates are staphylococci, the remainder being mainly Gram negative or the fungus *Candida*. Intravenous lines provide both a break in the skin allowing entry of organisms and a protected site for bacterial growth shielded from immune defences by a biofilm of platelets, fibrin and bacterial slime. Line infections are rarely eradicated by antibiotics and usually require line removal.

Respiratory infection. Pneumonia is responsible for approximately 25% of all hospital-acquired infections. After admission, the upper respiratory tract becomes colonized with organisms; this may progress to lower respiratory tract infection and pneumonia, particularly during endotracheal intubation. Gram-negative organisms are the usual cause, although MRSA is becoming increasingly common.

Surgical wounds. Despite antibiotic prophylaxis and aseptic surgical technique, surgical wound infection remains common. Infection usually arises from the patient's own skin flora, inoculating the wound during surgery. The lowest incidences (2–3.5%) are associated with orthopaedic procedures, while the highest (10–15%) are associated with amputations and abdominal surgery.

Urinary infection. Urinary catheters are routinely used in the care of acutely and chronically ill patients and can lead to bacteriuria. Greater age, debility and dehydration further increase the risk of urinary infection. As with line infections, it is usually impossible to eradicate the infection with antibiotics and catheter removal or replacement is usually necessary.

Antibiotic-associated diarrhoea. Use of broad-spectrum antibiotics can lead to overgrowth of the colonic bacterium *C. difficile*. This produces two cytotoxic and inflammatory exotoxins (A and B) that can cause an acute colitis and diarrhoea (see Part IV, Fig. 3.7.1). Around 5% of healthy adults and up to 20% of elderly patients in long-term care carry *C. difficile*. This overgrowth usually responds to withdrawal of the antibiotic but oral vancomycin or metronidazole can be used.

Prevention

The incidence of HAIs can be greatly reduced by good infection control (Fig. 3.13.1). This must always include good personal hygiene by healthcare staff, particularly effective hand washing, and wherever possible the avoidance of broad-spectrum antibiotics. Cultures of blood, urine, stool, etc. should always be taken before starting treatment and antibiotics should be targeted at the likely or confirmed pathogen.

Hand washing is the single most important method of reducing the spread of healthcare-acquired infection (Fig. 3.13.2).

Infections that can be transmitted on the hands of healthcare workers include:

- drug-resistant species: MRSA, *C. difficile*
- diarrhoeal infections: salmonella, shigella, *E.coli* O1571:H7, norovirus
- respiratory infections: influenza, common cold, respiratory syncytial virus
- others: hepatitis A.

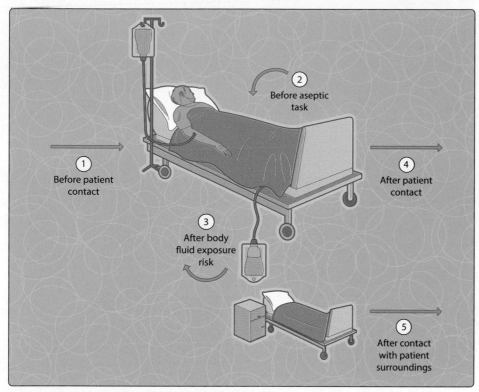

Fig. 3.13.1 Five moments for hand hygiene.

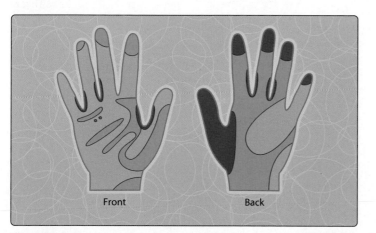

Fig. 3.13.2 Hand washing. Increasing shading indicates areas frequently missing effective cleansing.

Table 3.13.1 EXAMPLES OF HEALTHCARE-ACQUIRED INFECTING ORGANISMS

Organisms	Usual location	Risk factors	Typical infection
Meticillin-resistant *Staphylococcus aureus* (MRSA)	Nasal or skin	Antibiotic use, skin lesions, poor infection control	Skin/wound infection, orthopaedic or i.v. devices, bacteraemia, endocarditis, respiratory tract infection
Vancomycin-resistant enterococci (VRE)	Gut, hospital environment	Antibiotics, particularly i.v. broad-spectrum drugs	Low virulence, but causes bacteraemia in patients in intensive care
Multiresistant Gram-negative organisms	Gut, hospital environment, high-dependency units	Antibiotics, poor hygiene	Intra-abdominal, respiratory and blood-stream infections in vulnerable patients

PART II

Heart disorders

Andrew Gavin and Douglas Elder

The big picture

Heart disease includes not only coronary artery disease, the commonest cause of premature death in the UK, but also conditions affecting the pericardium, myocardium and valves. As vascular atherosclerosis is the major cause of heart disease in the developed world, we have included diseases affecting the major blood vessels in this part.

Mortality

Recent medical and surgical advances, together with a reduction in cigarette smoking and improvements in primary prevention, have led to a significant reduction in the incidence of cardiovascular disease. Despite this, cardiovascular disease remains the commonest cause of death in the developed world. In the UK, 38% of deaths occur as a result of cardiovascular disease (Fig. 1.1). Of these deaths, half result from coronary artery disease while 25% result from cerebrovascular disease. Coronary artery disease is the most common cause of premature death (under the age of 75 years) in the UK, accounting for 22% of premature deaths in males and 12% of females. Overall heart disease is responsible for over 20% of all premature deaths in the UK.

Morbidity

The incidence of myocardial infarction in the UK is estimated at over a quarter of a million per year. It is more common in males and the frequency increases with age. There are also estimated to be over 340 000 new cases of angina annually. Overall, 2.6 million individuals in the UK are estimated to have suffered from a myocardial infarction or angina. Over the age of 75 years, 1 in 4 males and 1 in 5 females are thought to be living with coronary artery disease. Improved survival rates following myocardial infarction has lead to increased numbers of patients requiring treatment for heart failure. As with ischaemic heart disease, the incidence of heart failure increases with age (Fig. 1.2). It is estimated that around 900 000 patients in the UK over the age of 45 years currently have varying degrees of heart failure.

Costs

Increased awareness of cardiovascular risk factors has led to improvements in both primary and secondary prevention. Since the mid-1990s, there has been a 17-fold increase in the number of prescriptions for lipid-lowering drugs. These drugs – mainly statins – now cost the NHS more than any other class of drug, with an annual cost of more than £759 million in 2004. The cost of effective blood pressure control has also significantly increased, accounting for £610 million of the NHS budget in 2004.

In 2003–4 there were approximately 415 000 inpatients treated for coronary artery disease in the UK: 5% of all male and 2% of all female inpatients. In addition, increased awareness of primary and secondary prevention has led to the introduction of rapid-access chest pain clinics, along with smoking cessation and cardiac rehabilitation services.

In 2003, cardiovascular disease was estimated to cost the NHS just under £15 billion – just under £250 per head of population. The majority of this money was taken up with inpatient care

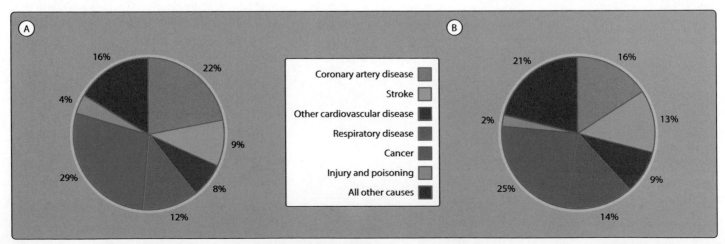

Fig. 1.1 Causes of death in the UK in 2003 of males (A) and females (B).

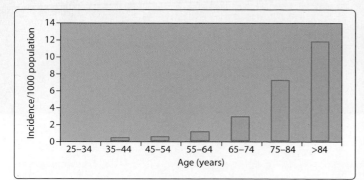

Fig. 1.2 Incidence of heart failure in the UK.

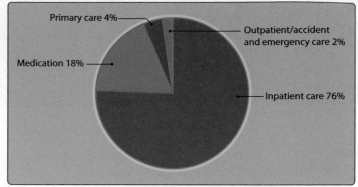

Fig. 1.3 Healthcare costs of cardiovascular disease in the UK.

(Fig. 1.3). When other costs such as loss of productivity are taken into account, this figure rises to £26 billion. With new drug and interventional developments and the need for a more specialist staff to meet the increasing burden of cardiovascular disease, this figure is likely to increase significantly over the next few years.

Risk factors

Hypertension

It is estimated that around a third of the adult population in the UK currently suffers from hypertension. Approximately 75% of these are not being treated, while more than 50% of the remainder are managed inadequately. The WHO has estimated that 11% of the disease burden in developed countries is a direct result of hypertension. A history of hypertension is thought to double the risk of myocardial infarction.

Hyperlipidaemia

A recent study has estimated that 45% of myocardial infarctions in western Europe are a consequence of abnormal blood lipids. Approximately two-thirds of adults currently have a total blood cholesterol of >5 mmol/l.

Smoking

Mortality from coronary artery disease is approximately 60% higher in smokers than non-smokers. Up to 30% of myocardial infarctions in western Europe are linked to smoking, with smokers having almost double the risk of non-smokers. Regular exposure to second-hand smoke increases the risk by 25%.

Diet

As well as being an independent risk factor for the development of cardiovascular disease, obesity increases an individual's likelihood of developing hypertension, hyperlipidaemia and type 2 diabetes mellitus. Western diets, which are typically high in salt, sugar and fat and low in complex carbohydrates, are thought to be a major factor in the high incidence of cardiovascular disease in the developed compared with the developing world. The WHO has estimated that just under 30% of coronary artery disease in developed countries is linked to low levels of fruit and vegetable consumption.

Physical activity

Physically active individuals have a significantly lower incidence of heart disease compared with those with a sedentary lifestyle. It is recommended that adults should undertake 30 min of moderate physical activity at least 5 days per week. Between two-thirds and three-quarters of adults in the UK currently fail to meet these guidelines.

Socioeconomic factors

There is a significant increase in the incidence of cardiovascular disease in manual workers compared with non-manual workers. This is partly a consequence of the increased incidence of smoking and poorer diet in low-income households.

High-return facts

1 **Ischaemic heart disease** is caused by deposition of fatty deposits or atheroma in the walls of coronary arteries. This reduces blood supply to heart muscle, which can result in chest pain on exertion (stable angina). Rupture of plaque or thrombus formation on the irregular surface of the plaque can result in chest pain at rest (unstable angina) or complete occlusion of the vessel (myocardial infarction). Risk factors for ischaemic heart disease include cigarette smoking, hypertension, diabetes mellitus, elevated cholesterol, family history and obesity. Management involves risk factor modification and drugs of different classes. More invasive treatment is based on restoring vessel patency.

2 **Acute coronary syndrome** is the collective term for ST elevation myocardial infarction, non-ST elevation myocardial infarction and unstable angina. ST elevation myocardial infarction is defined as necrosis of heart muscle (myocytes) caused by complete coronary artery occlusion. Patients usually present with central chest pain lasting >30 min radiating to the left arm, back, neck, teeth or gums. The ECG classically shows ST segment elevation in the area supplied by the occluded artery. Markers of cardiac muscle necrosis (creatinine kinase and troponin) are elevated. Management involves restoring vessel patency by thrombolysis or with a balloon and stent (angioplasty). Patients with non-ST elevation myocardial infarction (elevated biochemical markers with no ST elevation on ECG) are at high risk of developing a full-thickness infarct. Urgent angiography is required, and many undergo angioplasty and/or coronary artery bypass surgery. Thrombolysis is not indicated.

3 **Bradycardias** may be asymptomatic or present with dizziness or syncope. Underlying causes (e.g. rate-limiting drugs or ischaemic heart disease) should be identified and managed. Heart block (first-, second- and third-degree block) often results in bradycardia and may occur following a myocardial infarction. Some forms of heart block may require temporary or permanent pacemaker implantation.

4 **Tachycardias** (supraventricular or ventricular) often cause palpitation, chest pain, breathlessness and syncope. Treatment depends on the type of rhythm disorder and nature of any underlying heart disease. Significant tachycardia associated with haemodynamic compromise requires urgent electrical defibrillation to restore sinus rhythm and improve cardiac output. Patients with recurrent ventricular tachycardias are often considered for automated implantable defibrillator devices. **Atrial fibrillation** is the most commonly encountered rhythm disturbance and may be paroxysmal, persistent or permanent. Restoration of sinus rhythm either pharmacologically or by elective DC cardioversion is appropriate for some patients, while others, particularly those with significant comorbidity or significant structural heart disease, may require long-term pharmacological rate control. Anticoagulation prevents thromboembolism in atrial fibrillation.

5 **Cardiac arrest** is spontaneous loss of cardiac output with loss of consciousness. Irrespective of aetiology, basic life support should be initiated as soon as possible; without immediate intervention, irreversible hypoxic cerebral damage occurs after several minutes. Basic life support consists of maintenance and protection of the airway, assisted ventilation if required and chest compressions to maintain cardiac output. Advanced life support is necessary following basic life support and involves defibrillation, administration of drugs and treatment of reversible causes where indicated.

6 **Heart failure** occurs when cardiac output is insufficient for the demands of the body. Most individuals present with breathlessness due to pulmonary oedema. The main pathological features depend on the underlying cause but all result ultimately in increased sympathetic drive and activation of the renin–angiotensin–aldosterone system. Management includes removal of excess interstitial fluid with diuretics and the use of drugs to help to correct the neuroendocrine disturbances such as angiotensin-converting enzyme (ACE) inhibitors, beta-blockers and aldosterone antagonists. Underlying causes should be treated where appropriate.

7 **Pericarditis** is usually idiopathic but may be secondary to a variety of different conditions. Patients present with sharp central chest pain worse on inspiration and lying flat, and relieved by sitting forward. There is often widespread 'saddle-shaped' ST segment elevation on the ECG and there may be an associated pericardial effusion. Treatment is with non-steroidal anti-inflammatory drugs. **Constrictive pericarditis** occurs when there is thickening and fibrosis of the pericardium; impairment of diastolic filling results in impaired cardiac output and individuals usually present with breathlessness. Tuberculosis is the commonest cause worldwide. Diuretics improve symptoms and surgical removal of the fibrous pericardium is potentially curative. **Myocarditis** (myocardial inflammation) usually results from a self-limiting viral infection such as coxsackievirus B. Individuals are often asymptomatic or present with non-specific symptoms. Severe myocarditis may lead to heart failure. Treatment is supportive and most patients make a full recovery.

8 and 9 **Valvular heart disease** is characterized by narrowing of the valve outlet (stenosis) and/or leakage of blood back through a closed valve (regurgitation). The aortic and mitral valves are more commonly affected than the pulmonary and tricuspid valves. Clinical examination often reveals a characteristic heart murmur and the diagnosis is confirmed by echocardiography. Management involves dealing with any underlying cause, diuretics and, in severe disease, surgical repair or replacement.

10 **Hypertension** affects around 40% of the adult population. Although most individuals are asymptomatic, it is a major risk factor for coronary artery disease, stroke and heart failure. In the majority, there is no identifiable cause (essential hypertension) although in younger patients secondary causes (such as renal artery stenosis, Cushing's disease or phaeochromocytoma) should be considered. Management includes lifestyle advice and antihypertensive drugs. Several different classes of drug are often required to achieve satisfactory blood pressure control.

11 **Infective endocarditis** most commonly affects abnormal or prosthetic aortic and mitral valves, although the tricuspid valve is often affected in i.v. drug abusers. Patients present with lethargy, weight loss and night sweats, or acutely with heart failure from valvular insufficiency. A new murmur is often audible and there may be evidence of systemic embolization. Echocardiography, demonstrating a vegetation, and positive blood cultures confirm the diagnosis. Treatment is with prolonged i.v. antibiotics and valve replacement if significant destruction has occurred.

12 **Cardiomyopathy** describes dysfunction of the myocardium. The most common forms are dilated and hypertrophic cardiomyopathy. There is often no identifiable cause, although cardiomyopathy may be inherited or occur in association with systemic disorders such as haemochromatosis or alcoholism. Diagnosis is usually confirmed by echocardiography. Management includes treatment of underlying heart failure and prevention of significant arrhythmias.

13 **Atrial myxoma** is the most common primary cardiac tumour. The majority are benign and complete surgical excision is usually curative. **Aortic aneurysm** occurs when weakness of the aortic wall allows progressive dilatation and eventual rupture. The abdominal aorta is most commonly affected. **Aortic dissection** results from bleeding into the wall of the aorta. This can occur proximally in the ascending aorta or distal to the left subclavian artery. **Peripheral vascular disease** occurs when atheromatous plaques impair blood flow. This most commonly affects the lower limb, resulting in cramp-like calf pain on walking (intermittent claudication); severe disease can lead to rest pain and gangrene. Treatment includes risk factor modification, statins and antiplatelet agents. Revascularization, either surgically with bypass or by balloon and stenting (peripheral angioplasty), may be required.

14 **Congenital heart disease** usually means structural defects arising during fetal development, although the term also covers congenital arrhythmias and cardiomyopathies. Congenital heart disease occurs in approximately 1% of live births either in isolation or in conjunction with other abnormalities. Ventricular septal defect is the most common structural congenital heart defect, followed by atrial septal defect and patent ductus arteriosus. Many individuals with severe congenital heart disease now survive. Mild forms of congenital heart disease may not present until adulthood following discovery of a heart murmur or investigation of breathlessness or palpitation.

1. Ischaemic heart disease

Questions
- What lifestyle factors should be addressed in patients with ischaemic heart disease?
- What drugs are used in the management of ischaemic heart disease?
- What investigations are performed in suspected ischaemic heart disease?

Myocardial ischaemia is defined as inadequate oxygen delivery to heart muscle. **Angina pectoris** literally means 'strangling in the chest' and describes the discomfort experienced as a result of myocardial ischaemia. It is usually caused by increased myocardial oxygen demand distal to a stable atheromatous plaque. Figure 3.1.1 shows the arterial supply to the heart.

Epidemiology
Approximately one-quarter of deaths in males and one-fifth of deaths in females in the UK are attributable to ischaemic heart disease. This figure has not changed significantly despite many recent advances in management, and 20% of patients who suffer myocardial infarction still die before reaching hospital.

Pathogenesis
The development of **atheroma** is the key pathological process in ischaemic heart disease. Atheroma is characterized by the formation of atherosclerotic plaques, which consist of a cholesterol core surrounded by smooth muscle cells. Ulceration on the surface of the plaques can lead to intense platelet aggregation and subsequent thrombus formation. This leads to complete arterial occlusion. In the stable state, atheromatous plaques reduce the lumen diameter and blood flow. If atheroma occurs in the lumen of coronary arteries, cardiac muscle can become ischaemic. Myocardial infarction will occur if the blood supply is completely lost. Modifiable risk factors in the development of ischaemic heart disease include smoking, hyperlipidaemia, hypertension and good glycaemic control in diabetes mellitus. Non-modifiable risk factors include increasing age, family history of ischaemic heart disease in a first-degree relative aged < 60 years and male sex.

Clinical features
Myocardial ischaemia causes a tightness or heaviness in the chest. Important features to illicit from the history are:
- discomfort: character, site, radiation, severity
- duration of symptoms
- pattern: are the symptoms stable and predictable or are they increasing in frequency?
- activity: what activity brings on the symptoms?

Many forms of angina exist, which can often be identified from the history (Table 3.1.1).

Clinical examination can often be normal in patients with ischaemic heart disease. However, evidence of hyperlipidaemia (xanthalasma, xanthomata and corneal arcus) is sometimes found.

Investigations
The 12-lead ECG (Figs 3.1.2 and 3.1.3) is often normal although T wave inversion and ST segment depression can be found during an episode of angina. An exercise test (where individuals complete as much of a predetermined exercise programme as

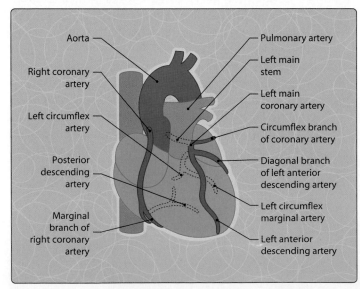

Fig. 3.1.1 The arterial supply to the heart.

Table 3.1.1 CLASSIFICATION OF ANGINA

Type of angina	Clinical feature
Stable angina	Develops on exercise and eases at rest
Crescendo angina (also unstable angina)	Develops with increasing frequency and decreasing exertion over a period of time
Unstable angina	Unpredictable and occurs at rest
Nocturnal angina	Occurs during sleep, often as a result of vivid dreams
Variant or Prinzmetal's angina	Develops at any time, unrelated to exertion, associated with normal coronary arteries, may be caused by coronary artery spasm

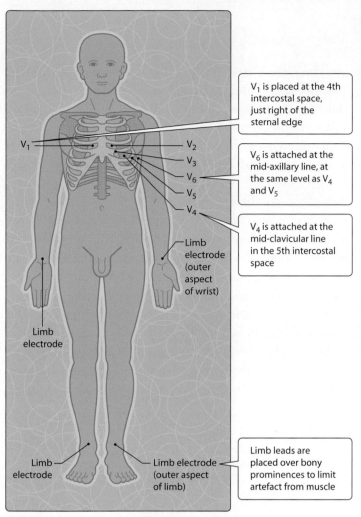

V₁ is placed at the 4th intercostal space, just right of the sternal edge

V₆ is attached at the mid-axillary line, at the same level as V₄ and V₅

V₄ is attached at the mid-clavicular line in the 5th intercostal space

Limb electrode (outer aspect of wrist)

Limb electrode

Limb electrode

Limb electrode (outer aspect of limb)

Limb leads are placed over bony prominences to limit artefact from muscle

Fig. 3.1.2 The position of ECG electrodes on the praecordium and limbs.

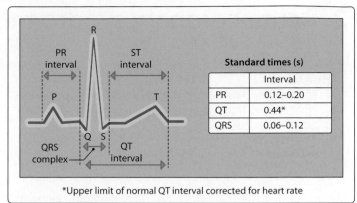

	Interval
PR	0.12–0.20
QT	0.44*
QRS	0.06–0.12

Standard times (s)

*Upper limit of normal QT interval corrected for heart rate

Fig. 3.1.3 The normal ECG complex.

Table 3.1.2 DRUGS USED IN THE MANAGEMENT OF STABLE ISCHAEMIC HEART DISEASE

Drug	Mode of action
Beta-blockers	Lower myocardial oxygen demand by decreasing heart rate, blood pressure and myocardial contractility
Calcium antagonists	Cause coronary artery dilatation; rate-limiting drugs (verapamil or diltiazem) act in a similar way to beta-blockers
Nitrates	Dilate the venous and arterial system
Potassium channel activator	Act in a similar fashion to nitrates
Aspirin	Prevents platelet aggregation
Clopidogrel	Acts in a similar way to aspirin; used if aspirin not tolerated
Statins	Inhibit an enzyme involved in cholesterol synthesis (HMG-CoA reductase)

possible with ECG monitoring) shows ST segment depression in ischaemic heart disease. This test has a sensitivity of 80% in identifying those with significant coronary artery disease. Exercise testing is also used for risk stratification after myocardial infarction.

Myocardial perfusion scintigraphy identifies areas of myocardium that do not receive adequate blood supply during cardiac stress.

Echocardiography may demonstrate a wall motion abnormality and can identify valvular pathology and estimate left ventricular function.

Coronary angiography involves the injection of contrast into the coronary arteries via a catheter in the femoral or radial artery. This may be helpful for those with:

- angina despite medical therapy
- unstable angina

- non-ST segment elevation myocardial infarction
- strongly positive exercise ECG
- ventricular arrhythmias.

Other tests include full blood count (FBC), U&Es and creatinine, glucose and lipids. The cardiac markers creatinine kinase and troponin are normal in stable angina but elevated following myocardial infarction.

Management

Risk factor modification is central to improving survival, and smoking cessation is essential. Drug therapy is well established in the management of angina (Table 3.1.2). Invasive treatment is based on restoring vessel patency by balloon and stent (angioplasty) or by coronary artery bypass surgery.

2. Acute coronary syndromes

Questions
- What are the different types of acute coronary syndrome?
- What is the management of an ST segment elevation myocardial infarction?
- What is the management of a non-ST elevation myocardial infarction?

There are three types of acute coronary syndrome associated with sudden rupture of plaque inside the coronary artery

Non-ST segment elevation myocardial infarction (NSTEMI). Patients have elevated serum troponin without ST segment elevation. ECG often shows T wave inversion or ST depression. Subtotal vessel occlusion occurs and ischaemic tissue subsequently infarcts.

ST segment elevation myocardial infarction (STEMI). Patients present with ST segment elevation (Fig. 3.2.1). Complete occlusion of the affected coronary artery by thrombus formation requires urgent attention.

Unstable angina. This is defined as chest discomfort provoked by minimal exercise or at rest. Plasma troponin and creatine kinase are normal. ECG is normal or shows ST segment depression and/or T wave inversion. Usually atheromatous plaque rupture causes platelet aggregation, lumen narrowing and tissue ischaemia.

Clinical features
The chest pain is similar to angina pectoris but often more severe, lasts longer and can be accompanied by autonomic symptoms (e.g. sweating, nausea and vomiting). In the elderly or in those with diabetes mellitus, these symptoms may be minimal or absent.

Examination is often unremarkable; however, it is important not to miss features of pulmonary oedema or the systolic murmurs of aortic stenosis or mitral regurgitation.

Investigations
ECG is essential (Fig. 3.2.2). Chest radiograph may be normal or show features of pulmonary oedema; a widened mediastinum suggests aortic dissection.

Echocardiography is useful to diagnose complications (e.g. ventricular septal defect), wall motion abnormalities and overall left ventricular function.

Management
Secondary prevention includes lifestyle advice, smoking cessation, and medication. Aspirin should be continued indefinitely. Clopidogrel is indicated in patients with raised troponin: 75 mg daily for 1 month in STEMI and for up to a year in other groups. Beta-blockade should be continued indefinitely in those without contraindications. Statins reduce future ischaemic events. Angiotensin-converting enzyme (ACE) inhibitors should be commenced irrespective of left ventricular systolic function in patients with STEMI or NSTEMI.

Acute coronary syndrome without ST segment elevation
In suspected acute coronary syndrome, patients should be admitted to hospital urgently and treated immediately with oxygen, aspirin 300 mg, clopidogrel 300 mg, low-molecular-weight heparin and beta-blockers. Ongoing chest pain may require i.v. opiates and oral, sublingual or i.v. nitrates. Coronary angiography should be considered in patients presenting with unstable angina or raised troponin in the absence of ST segment elevation (NSTEMI). Patients may continue with medical management, have coronary artery stenting or coronary artery bypass grafting (Fig. 3.2.3).

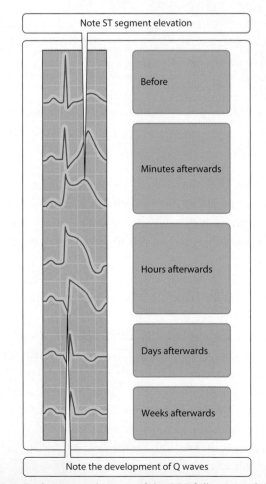

Note ST segment elevation

Before

Minutes afterwards

Hours afterwards

Days afterwards

Weeks afterwards

Note the development of Q waves

Fig. 3.2.1 Evolutionary changes of the ECG following a full-thickness myocardial infarction (STEMI).

Acute coronary syndrome with ST segment elevation
In STEMI, patients should be considered for either primary angioplasty (if available) or immediate thrombolysis.

Thrombolysis. Fibrinolytic drugs i.v. directly dissolve the thrombus but there is a 1–2% risk of life-threatening haemorrhage and not all patients will achieve adequate reperfusion.

Primary angioplasty. This is at least as efficient as thrombolysis but may carry less risk. The bleeding risk is not negligible as many procedures require the administration of powerful antiplatelet agents (e.g. glycoprotein IIb/IIIa inhibitors and heparin).

Patients who receive successful thrombolysis should be given secondary prevention and usually undergo exercise tolerance testing 6 weeks after the infarct. Those with a positive exercise test or anginal symptoms should undergo coronary angiography. Patients who undergo primary angioplasty at the time of their infarct may later require further angioplasty or coronary artery bypass grafting.

Complications following a myocardial infarction
Tachyarrhythmias. Most common is atrial fibrillation, although ventricular arrhythmias are a major cause of death.

Bradyarrhythmias. May complicate inferior myocardial infarction as the atrioventricular node derives its blood supply from the right coronary artery. No treatment is required in most, but atropine or a pacemaker may be necessary.

Continuing angina. This reflects ongoing ischaemia.

Mitral regurgitation. Often caused by rupture of a papillary muscle.

Ventricular septal defect. Ischaemia of the intraventricular septum can lead to rupture, blood shunting and circulatory collapse.

Ventricular aneurysm. Occurs in approximately 5–7% of patients following STEMI.

Cardiac tamponade. Rupture can lead to haemopericardium, cardiac tamponade and death.

Cardiogenic shock. If there is insufficient functional myocardium to maintain adequate cardiac output, pulmonary oedema can occur and mortality is high.

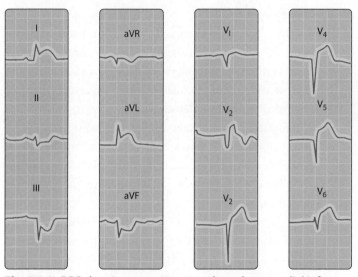

Fig. 3.2.2 ECG showing an acute anterolateral myocardial infarction. Note the ST segment elevation in leads V_2 through to V_6 and I and aVL; reciprocal ST segment depression is present in the inferior leads (II, III and aVF).

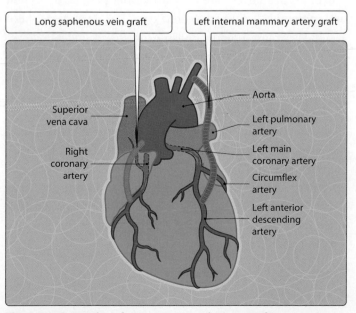

Fig. 3.2.3 Principles of coronary artery bypass grafting.

3. Rhythm disorders I: bradyarrythmias, heart block

Question

- What are the ECG features of first-, second- and third-degree heart block?

Heart rate and rhythm are usually controlled by the sinoatrial node in the right atrium (Fig. 3.3.1). The cells here are under the influence of sympathetic and parasympathetic stimulation, which increase and decrease the heart rate, respectively. All cardiac muscle cells are capable of automaticity. This means that if an area of the heart fails to keep the rate and rhythm, a lower centre will assume control. The atrioventricular (AV) node is the gateway from atria to the ventricles. In the normal heart, it is the only pathway between the atrium and the ventricle through which electrical signals can pass.

Rhythm disorders are divided into bradycardias (heart rate < 60 beats/min) and tachycardias (heart rate > 100 beats/min; Ch. 4). Narrow-complex (QRS width < 120 ms) tachycardias or bradycardias originate at or above the AV node. Broad-complex arrhythmias originate below the AV node, above the AV node with aberrant conduction down the bundle of His, or from the ventricle itself.

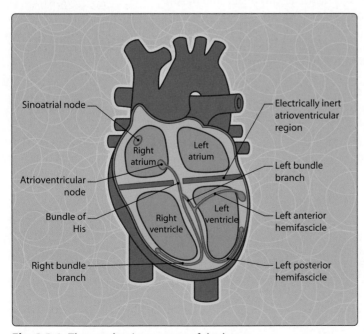

Fig. 3.3.1 The conducting system of the heart.

Bradyarrythmias

Sinus bradycardia is common in athletes and normal fit individuals, particularly during sleep. Intervention is rarely required.

Heart block

Heart block usually results from abnormal AV nodal conduction and can be divided into three main types (Fig. 3.3.2).

- first degree: prolonged PR interval > 200 ms; requires no treatment
- second degree
  - Mobitz type I or Wenckebach phenomenon: progressive PR prolongation followed by a non-conducted P wave; the Wenckebach phenomenon can be physiological (in athletes) or in those with high vagal tone and does not usually require intervention
  - Mobitz type II: constant PR interval with intermittent non-conducted P waves; this is always sinister and is usually caused by a conduction disturbance within the bundles of His. It usually requires permanent pacemaker insertion
- third degree: complete AV node dissociation, causing a ventricular escape rhythm, usually at 30 beats/min; the QRS wave may be narrow if it originates above the bundle of His or broad if it originates within the ventricle. It usually requires permanent pacemaker insertion.

Stokes–Adams attacks

Stokes–Adams attacks are caused by brief periods of asystole and commonly occur with Mobitz type II or third-degree heart block. They cause a sudden collapse for a few minutes, followed by central flushing and rapid recovery (but not always) of consciousness.

Sick sinus syndrome

Sick sinus syndrome or tachy/brady syndrome is thought to be secondary to disease of the sinoatrial node. It occurs with increasing frequency with increasing age. The sinoatrial node discharges irregularly and this can lead to sinus bradycardia or tachycardia, which is often associated with atrial fibrillation. Beta-blockade often improves symptoms but permanent pacemaker insertion may be required in symptomatic individuals.

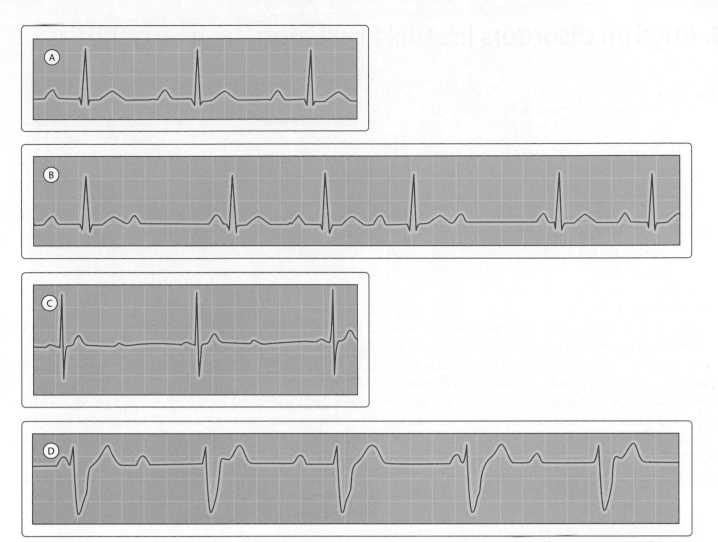

Fig. 3.3.2 ECG strips showing heart block. (A) First-degree heart block, note the prolonged PR interval; (B) second-degree heart block (Wenckebach phenomenon), note the progressive lengthening of the PR interval with eventual failure of the P wave to generate a QRS complex; (C) second-degree heart block (Mobitz type II), note the failure to produce a QRS complex on every second P wave; (D) third-degree (complete) heart block, note the lack of association between the P waves and the slow widened QRS complexes. P waves occur regularly but may be hidden by the QRS complex.

4. Rhythm disorders II: atrial fibrillation, tachyarrythmias

Questions
- What are the causes of atrial fibrillation?
- What drugs are used in the management of atrial fibrillation?
- What are the most common ventricular tachyarrythmias?

Tachycardias are defined as a heart rate >100 beats/min and are usually divided into narrow-complex and broad-complex. Narrow complex is defined as QRS duration of <120 ms (three small boxes on an ECG).

Atrial fibrillation

Atrial fibrillation is characterized by disorganized atrial electrical activity, which is transmitted through the atrioventricular (AV) node to the ventricles (Fig. 3.4.1). It is the most common arrhythmia and can be paroxysmal, persistent or permanent. Ventricular electrical activity shows a characteristic irregular rhythm (Fig. 3.4.2). There are many causes of atrial fibrillation, including ischaemic heart disease, hypertension, valvular disorders, electrolyte imbalance, sepsis, pericardial and myocardial disease, thyrotoxicosis and pulmonary embolism.

Management
In all cases of atrial fibrillation, an underlying cause should be actively sought and managed. If the patient is hypotensive with ventricular rate >150 beats/min, specialist help should be obtained as DC cardioversion under sedation may be necessary. If the patient is not compromised and the onset of atrial fibrillation can be confirmed within the last 24 h, then cardioversion is appropriate. This can be achieved pharmacologically (e.g. with i.v. amiodarone or flecanide), or electrically by DC cardioversion. Attempting DC cardioversion in patients who have established atrial fibrillation for more than 24 h increases the risk of embolic stroke caused by stasis of blood within the atria, in particular the left atrial appendage. In patients with significant comorbidity or significant structural heart disease, pharmacological rate control with digoxin and beta-blockers is more appropriate. Young patients with structurally normal hearts should be given low-dose aspirin while patients over the age of 65 years, those with significant risk factors for vascular disease, those with structurally abnormal hearts and those with a history of cerebrovascular disease should be considered for full anticoagulation with warfarin.

Long-standing atrial fibrillation requires a decision as to whether the goal is rhythm control (establishing and maintaining sinus rhythm) or rate control (controlling the ventricular rate to limit symptoms and maximize cardiac output) (Fig. 3.4.3).

The main risk to patients with persistent atrial fibrillation is ischaemic stroke, which occurs in approximately 5% per year. Many studies have investigated anti-platelet and anticoagulant strategies for reducing this risk.

Atrial flutter

Atrial flutter is similar to atrial fibrillation in aetiology, sequelae and management. However, in atrial flutter the atrial activity is organized but rapid. The atria support electrical activity at approximately 300 beats/min. The ECG shows a characteristic 'saw tooth' wave pattern with completely regular QRS complexes. In atrial flutter with 2:1 block, the ventricular will be 150 beats/min, whereas 4:1 block will produce a rate of 75 beats/min.

Supraventricular tachycardia

Supraventricular tachycardia affects approximately 1 in 1000 individuals. It is not usually a life-threatening arrhythmia but can cause significant morbidity. Patients usually present with rapid palpitation, often associated with shortness of breath or chest tightness. It involves a re-entry circuit either involving the AV node or an accessory pathway that permits electrical connection between atria and ventricles.

Supraventricular tachycardia can sometimes be terminated by using the Valsalva manoeuvre. If this is unsuccessful, i.v. adenosine should be considered. Adenosine acts by transiently

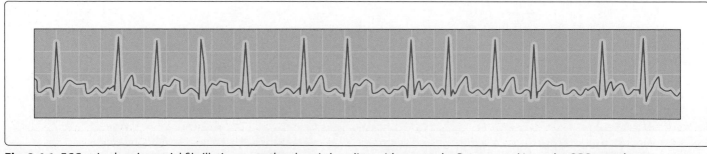

Fig. 3.4.1 ECG strip showing atrial fibrillation; note the chaotic baseline with no regular P waves and irregular QRS complexes.

blocking the AV node and breaking the circuit, leading to termination of the arrhythmia. It should not be administered to patients with severe asthma or those with atrial fibrillation who have an accessory pathway.

Broad-complex tachycardias

Broad-complex tachycardias may be life threatening and it is vital to identify and manage these appropriately.

Ventricular tachycardia

Ventricular tachycardia is defined as three or more broad-complex beats occurring at a rate >120 beats/min. Sustained ventricular tachycardia occurs when there are at least 30 beats in succession. Ventricular tachycardia is caused by coronary artery disease or conditions that cause structural damage to the ventricles, such as cardiomyopathy or valvular heart disease.

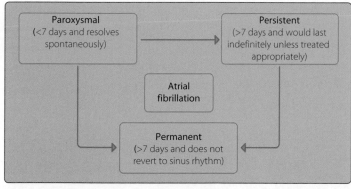

Fig. 3.4.2 Classification of atrial fibrillation.

Patients with haemodynamic collapse require immediate DC cardioversion after appropriate sedation. In more stable patients, initial management is with i.v. amiodarone. If this fails, DC cardioversion should be considered. Ventricular tachycardia occurring within 24 h of myocardial infarction does not usually confer risk of recurrence. Patients with spontaneous ventricular tachycardia where a reversible ischaemic focus is not demonstrated should be considered for an automated implantable cardiac defibrillator.

Torsades de pointes is a specific polymorphic form of ventricular tachycardia, usually the result of a prolonged QT interval. It may be congenital or caused by drugs (e.g. antipsychotic agents). In haemodynamic compromise, DC cardioversion is usually necessary, although overdrive pacing is occasionally required.

Supraventricular tachycardia with aberrancy describes any supraventricular rhythm that results in a broad-complex tachycardia. This can occur in the presence of left or right bundle branch block and often causes diagnostic uncertainty.

Ventricular fibrillation

Ventricular fibrillation is never associated with a cardiac output sufficient to preserve consciousness. The rhythm is easily recognized on the ECG as chaotic and irregular with no recognizable complexes. It is usually caused by ischaemic heart disease and should be cardioverted without delay. Individuals with spontaneous ventricular fibrillation in whom a reversible ischaemic focus is not demonstrated should be considered for automated cardiac defibrillator implantation.

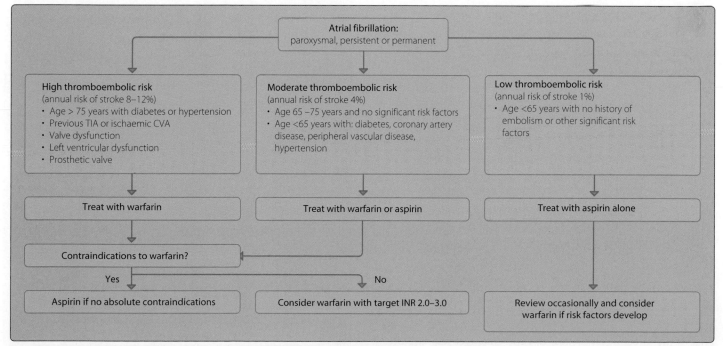

Fig. 3.4.3 Algorithm illustrating the use of anticoagulants in atrial fibrillation. TIA, transient ischaemic attack; CVA, cardiovascular accident (stroke); INR, international normalized ratio.

5. Cardiac arrest

Questions
- What is basic life support?
- What is advanced life support?
- What are the ECG features of ventricular fibrillation, ventricular tachycardia and asystole?

Cardiac arrest is defined as a sudden loss of cardiac output with loss of consciousness. The rhythm in cardiac arrest usually predicts survival. In individuals with ventricular fibrillation or ventricular tachycardia who receive prompt defibrillation, the likelihood of restoring a perfusing rhythm and subsequent survival is greater than in patients with asystole. In patients who suffer an unexpected cardiac arrhythmia after a myocardial infarction, early access to a trained resuscitation team is often associated with a successful outcome.

It is inadvisable to attempt cardiopulmonary resuscitation in all patients. For example, it is inappropriate in patients who have completed advanced life directives or who are nearing their natural end of life.

Pathogenesis

Cardiac arrest can be caused by a primary cardiac problem or be secondary to non-cardiac pathology. The common cardiac rhythm abnormalities (Fig. 3.5.1) include:

- **ventricular fibrillation**: irregular chaotic baseline with broad-complex QRS wave forms; patients are pulseless
- **ventricular tachycardia**: regular, broad-complex tachycardia; this rhythm may be associated with a pulse
- **asystole**: flat baseline with a low-grade fluctuation (always ensure that all ECG leads are connected appropriately); pulses will be absent

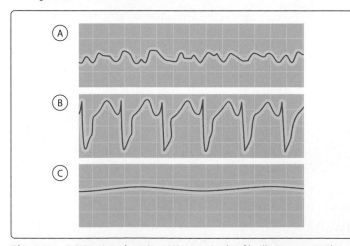

Fig. 3.5.1 ECG strips showing (A) ventricular fibrillation, note the chaotic rhythm and complexes; (B) ventricular tachycardia, note the regular broad complex tachycardia; (C) asystole, note the essentially flat baseline.

- **pulseless electrical activity**: a rhythm (e.g. sinus rhythm) that would usually be expected to accompany an adequate cardiac output is identified, but pulse is absent.

Clinical features

There is usually sudden collapse with loss of consciousness. Other features vary, although if cardiac arrest is secondary to a ventricular arrhythmia following a myocardial infarction, there may be recent chest pain or breathlessness. Cardiac arrest is diagnosed when there is no palpable proximal pulse (usually carotid pulse) in an unconscious patient with no respiratory effort.

Management

Once diagnosed, help must be summoned immediately. Basic Life Support (BLS; Fig. 3.5.2) underpins management in cardiac arrest. The main principles are to maintain a patent airway and provide adequate ventilation and circulation while awaiting expert help with equipment (usually drugs and a defibrillator) to perform Advanced Life Support (ALS; Fig. 3.5.3).

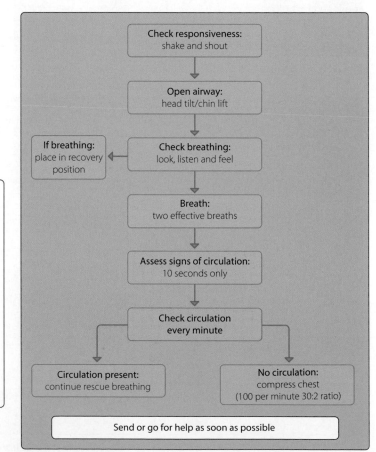

Fig. 3.5.2 Algorithm showing features of Basic Life Support.

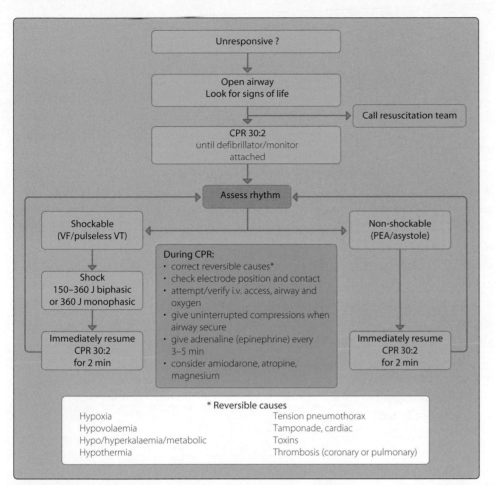

Fig. 3.5.3 Algorithm showing features of advanced life support. VF, ventricular fibrillation; VT, ventricular tachycardia; CPR, cardiopulmonary resuscitation; PEA, pulseless electrical activity.

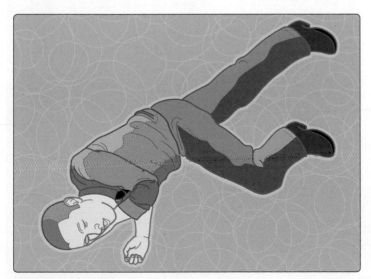

Fig. 3.5.4 The recovery position.

Once cardiorespiratory arrest has been confirmed, expired air ventilation followed by 30 chest compressions at a rate of approximately 100/min followed again by ventilation is required. This is continued until a cardiac defibrillator is available and ALS can begin. If the patient begins to breathe, they can be moved to the recovery position (Fig. 3.5.4).

Drugs routinely used in cardiac arrest

Few drugs influence outcome although several are advised by the European Resuscitation Council:

■ adrenaline (epinephrine): should be given to all patients in cardiac arrest every 3–5 min; it has both α- and β-adrenergic effects, resulting in vasoconstriction and increased venous return as well as increasing heart rate

■ atropine: blocks the parasympathetic action of the vagus nerve and may increase heart rate

■ amiodarone: may be of use in refractory ventricular arrhythmias.

Care after resuscitation

Care should be in a high-dependency or critical care setting. A full physical examination is required and investigations include blood electrolytes, lipids and glucose; cardiac enzymes or troponin; 12-lead ECG; chest radiograph; and arterial blood gases.

6. Heart failure

Questions
- What are the causes of heart failure?
- What is the management of acute congestive heart failure?
- What drugs are used in the management of heart failure?

Heart failure occurs when cardiac output is insufficient to keep up with demands. Although symptoms usually result from reduced cardiac output, high-output cardiac failure can occur. The underlying disease process may affect both ventricles, although commonly signs and symptoms are specific to left- or right-sided heart failure. Ischaemic heart disease is the most common cause but other common causes include hypertension and valvular dysfunction (e.g. mitral or aortic stenosis).

Epidemiology

Heart failure is a major public health problem with a prevalence of 1–2% and a 5-year mortality approaching 50%. Median age at presentation is 76 years and males are more commonly affected.

Pathogenesis

Different pathologies affect different aspects of heart function, all reducing cardiac output. Impaired cardiac filling can result from tamponade (infection, malignancy, direct trauma or myocardial infarction), constrictive pericarditis (tuberculosis, rheumatic heart disease or following haemopericardium) or restrictive cardiomyopathy (amyloidosis, sarcoidosis, haemochromatosis, scleroderma, Loeffler's endocarditis and endomyocardial fibrosis). Circulatory factors can increase preload (e.g. fluid overload in renal failure or use of anti-inflammatory drugs) or increase afterload. **High-output cardiac failure** occurs when the normally functioning heart cannot keep up with a dramatically increased demand for blood flow to one or more organs in the body. This can occur in severe anaemia, arteriovenous malformations, thyrotoxicosis, Paget's disease, beriberi and very occasionally in pregnancy.

Pathophysiology depends on the underlying cause, although all increase sympathetic drive and activate the renin–angiotensin–aldosterone system. Initially this is a physiological attempt to maintain cardiac output and tissue perfusion, although over-activation of these pathways contributes to disease progression.

Clinical features

Individuals may present acutely, with breathlessness, or more insidiously with a range of symptoms such as fatigue. Heart failure should be considered in individuals complaining of breathlessness, especially with a history of previous myocardial infarction or valvular heart disease. If left-sided heart failure is predominant, increased venous return when supine leads to orthopnoea (breathlessness lying flat that is relieved by sitting up), paroxysmal nocturnal dyspnoea (acute breathlessness wakening from sleep, forcing the patient to sit or stand up) and production of pink frothy sputum. If right heart failure predominates, fluid accumulates in the systemic veins, resulting in nausea and abdominal distension with ascites, hepatomegaly and peripheral oedema.

Physical examination can be normal in heart failure. Typical signs are shown in Fig. 3.6.1. A third heart sound or murmurs consistent with valve disease may also be present. The severity of heart failure can be classified according to the New York Heart Association (NYHA) scheme (Table 3.6.1).

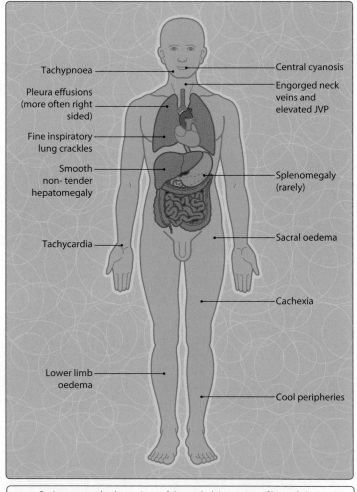

Tachypnoea	Central cyanosis
Pleura effusions (more often right sided)	Engorged neck veins and elevated JVP
Fine inspiratory lung crackles	
Smooth non-tender hepatomegaly	Splenomegaly (rarely)
Tachycardia	Sacral oedema
Lower limb oedema	Cachexia
	Cool peripheries

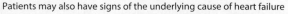
Patients may also have signs of the underlying cause of heart failure

Fig. 3.6.1 Clinical features of heart failure. JVP, jugular vein pressure.

Table 3.6.1 NEW YORK HEART ASSOCIATION CLASSIFICATION OF HEART FAILURE SEVERITY

Class	Symptoms
I (mild)	No limitation of physical activity
II (mild to moderate)	Slight limitation of physical activity, comfortable at rest but dyspnoea and fatigue on ordinary physical activity
III (moderate)	Marked limitation of physical activity; comfortable at rest but dyspnoea and fatigue on less than ordinary physical activity
IV (severe)	Symptoms at rest

Investigations

Chest radiograph features are shown in Fig. 3.6.2.

ECG may show evidence of ischaemia, previous myocardial infarction or left ventricular hypertrophy.

FBC excludes anaemia. Elevation of cardiac enzymes or troponin in serum indicate myocardial damage, usually as a result of myocardial infarction.

Echocardiography should be arranged in all patients with suspected heart failure. As well as confirming ventricular dysfunction this may reveal the cause (e.g. valvular disease or left ventricular hypertrophy secondary to long-standing hypertensive heart disease).

Management

Contributing features (e.g. anaemia, hypertension or thyroid disease) should be treated.

A number of drugs can be used:

- diuretics: promote fluid loss thereby reducing ventricular preload and relieving breathlessness and peripheral oedema
  - loop diuretics (e.g. furosemide) result in a brisk and short-lived diuresis with rapid relief of symptoms
  - spironolactone is a weak potassium-sparing diuretic aldosterone antagonist used in moderate-to-severe heart failure
  - metolazone, a powerful thiazide diuretic, is generally reserved for use in severe intractable heart failure
- ACE inhibitors: reduce levels of circulating catecholamines, vascular resistance and afterload; they can cause renal dysfunction and should be introduced in low doses with close biochemical monitoring and avoided in aortic stenosis
- angiotensin II receptor blockers: used either with ACE inhibitors or as an alternative in individuals who are intolerant of ACE inhibitors

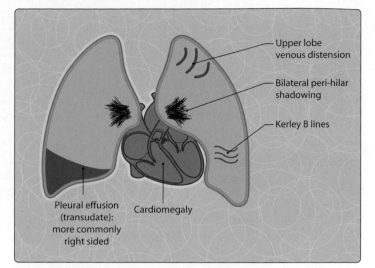

Fig. 3.6.2 Chest radiograph features of pulmonary oedema.

- beta-blockers: improve left ventricular ejection fraction and in the absence of contraindications (e.g. asthma) are recommended for all patients with stable heart failure caused by left ventricular systolic dysfunction
- hydralazine + isosorbide mononitrate: reduce afterload but are less effective than ACE inhibitors and are used only in individuals who are intolerant to both ACE inhibitors and angiotensin II receptor blockers
- inotropic drugs: are occasionally used in patients with low cardiac output (e.g. i.v. dobutamine).

Non-pharmacological approaches include advice regarding a low-salt diet and abstaining from smoking and alcohol. In the longer term, exercise may reduce morbidity and mortality.

Cardiac resynchronization therapy utilizing biventricular pacing reduces symptoms in individuals with ventricular dyssynchrony who remain symptomatic on medical therapy. In some cases, coronary revascularization, valve surgery or cardiac transplantation may also be considered.

Management of acute heart failure

Patients should sit upright and be given oxygen. Morphine relieves distress and also acts as a vasodilator, thereby reducing preload and afterload. Large i.v. doses of diuretics (e.g. furosemide 40–80 mg) should be given and repeated if necessary. Reduction of preload with i.v. nitrates should be considered in individuals without hypotension. If patients fail to respond, continuous positive airways pressure or non-invasive ventilation may improve oxygen delivery.

7. Pericarditis and myocarditis

Questions
- What are the clinical features of pericarditis?
- What are the clinical features of myocarditis?

Acute pericarditis

The heart is surrounded by two protective layers called the visceral (inner) and parietal (outer) pericardium (Fig. 3.7.1). Pericarditis is defined as inflammation of the pericardium. In the UK, acute pericarditis most commonly occurs in males between the ages of 20 and 50 years.

Pathogenesis

Pericarditis is caused by acute inflammation with leukocyte infiltration and fibrin deposition within the pericardium. Causes include:

- cardiovascular disorders: following myocardial infarction (Dressler's syndrome) or cardiac surgery
- viral infection: coxsackie B virus, adenovirus, echovirus, influenza, mumps, HIV
- bacterial infection: staphylococci, streptococci, *Escherichia coli*, pseudomonas, salmonella, shigella, tuberculosis
- fungal infection: histoplasma, aspergillus
- autoimmune disorders: rheumatoid arthritis, systemic lupus erthymatosus (SLE), scleroderma
- metabolic disorders: renal failure, hypothyroidism
- malignancy: usually metastatic
- drugs: procainamide, hydralazine, doxorubicin
- irradiation
- trauma.

Clinical features

Chest pain is worse on inspiration and lying flat, and relieved by sitting forward. There may be breathlessness, especially if a pericardial effusion is present. Patients are febrile, tachycardic and tachypnoeic. A pericardial friction rub, best heard at the lower left sternal edge, is often present. There may be signs of tamponade if a significant pericardial effusion is present.

Investigations

Cardiac enzymes, renal and thyroid function and autoantibodies may help identify a cause. FBC may show a leukocytosis and erythrocyte sedimentation rate (ESR) and CRP are often elevated.

Chest radiograph is often normal, although it may suggest a pericardial effusion. ECG shows generalized upwardly concave or 'saddle-shaped' ST elevation, which may be difficult to distinguish from acute myocardial infarction (Fig. 3.7.2). Echocardiography can distinguish pericarditis from myocardial infarction and may identify a pericardial effusion.

Management

Any underlying cause should be treated. Management includes bed-rest and non-steroidal anti-inflammatory drugs (NSAIDs), although these should be avoided immediately after myocardial infarction. In prolonged or recurrent pericarditis, other anti-inflammatory drugs (e.g. steroids or colchicine) may be useful.

Constrictive pericarditis

Constrictive pericarditis occurs when thickening and fibrosis of the pericardium causes cardiac compression, impaired diastolic filling, elevated diastolic pressures and reduced cardiac output. It can be infective (tuberculosis, pneumococci, staphylococci, coxsackie B, adenovirus), induced by radiation, postsurgical (following cardiac bypass surgery) autoimmune (SLE, rheumatoid arthritis, scleroderma), caused by uraemia (in patients on long-term dialysis) or drug related (procainamide, hydralazine). Most cases in the developed world are idiopathic; tuberculosis is the most common infectious cause worldwide.

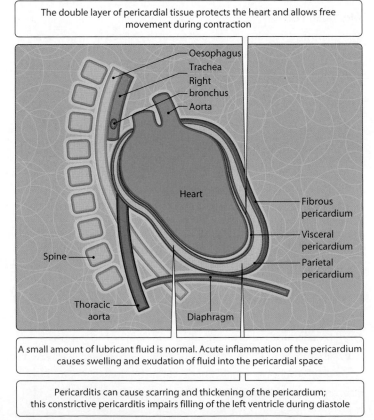

The double layer of pericardial tissue protects the heart and allows free movement during contraction

Oesophagus
Trachea
Right bronchus
Aorta
Heart
Fibrous pericardium
Visceral pericardium
Parietal pericardium
Spine
Thoracic aorta
Diaphragm

A small amount of lubricant fluid is normal. Acute inflammation of the pericardium causes swelling and exudation of fluid into the pericardial space

Pericarditis can cause scarring and thickening of the pericardium; this constrictive pericarditis impairs filling of the left ventricle during diastole

Fig. 3.7.1 Anatomy of the pericardium.

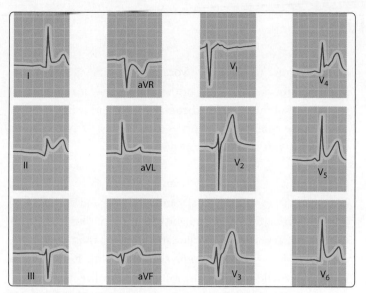

Fig. 3.7.2 Typical ECG changes in pericarditis; note the widespread concave ST segment elevation.

Clinical features

Breathlessness is the most common presenting feature and is accompanied by fatigue and orthopnoea. The jugular venous pressure is elevated, with prominent X and Y descents and a paradoxical rise on inspiration (Kussmaul's sign). The apex beat is soft or impalpable and heart sounds are difficult to hear, although a third heart sound in diastole may be audible. There may be pulsatile hepatomegaly, ascites and peripheral oedema.

Investigations

ECG changes are non-specific but chest radiograph may show a small heart and pericardial calcification. Pleural effusions are often present and the superior vena cava may be dilated. High-resolution CT or MRI shows the thickened pericardium directly as may echocardiography.

Cardiac catheterization may help in diagnosis and pericardial biopsy is occasionally required. Mantoux skin testing may suggest tuberculosis.

Management

Management consists of diuretics and treatment of any underlying condition. Surgical resection of the pericardium is definitive, although it has a high complication rate.

Myocarditis

Myocarditis is an acute and potentially reversible inflammatory process affecting the heart muscle (myocardium). Most recover although some have a persistent low-grade myocarditis and present with dilated cardiomyopathy 10–20 years later.

Pathogenesis

An infective organism (usually coxsackie B), toxin or autoimmune process results in inflammation of the myocardium:

- viral: coxsackie B, adenovirus, echovirus, influenza, rubella
- bacterial: diphtheria, chlamydia, coxiella, *Borrelia burgdorferi* (Lyme disease)
- protozoal: *Trypanosoma cruzi* (Chagas' disease)
- autoimmune: sarcoidosis, connective tissue disease
- miscellaneous: lead poisoning, chloroquine, radiation.

Clinical features

There may be a history of recent viral illness. Symptoms are variable and include fatigue, dyspnoea and chest pain. Focal inflammation can result in arrhythmias, which may present as palpitation or occasionally sudden death. Patients often have a resting tachycardia. The first heart sound is soft and a gallop rhythm may be present. There may also be murmurs of associated mitral and tricuspid regurgitation. If pericarditis is present, a pericardial rub may be heard. If the inflammatory process is widespread, features of congestive heart failure may be present.

Investigations

ECG may show non-specific changes, sinus tachycardia or heart block. Chest radiograph may be normal or show cardiac enlargement, venous congestion or pleural effusions. Echocardiography may show focal or generalized wall motion abnormalities.

Serum creatine kinase may be raised, indicating myocyte damage. Serial assays for coxsackie B titres may be helpful.

Endomyocardial biopsy is rarely performed but shows acute inflammatory changes and viral mRNA within myocardial cells.

Management

Management is mainly supportive and involves bed-rest and avoidance of exercise for several months. Diuretics, ACE inhibitors, beta-blockers and spironolactone are used if heart failure is present. Oral steroids are sometimes used in biopsy-proven acute myocarditis.

8. Valve disorders I: mitral valve

Questions
- What are the causes of mitral valve disease?
- How do mitral stenosis and mitral regurgitation differ clinically?

Disorders of the heart valves (Fig. 3.8.1) are common. Most are discovered during the investigation of breathlessness, chest pain, fatigue, heart murmurs, or ECG abnormalities (especially atrial fibrillation). The character of a murmur and where it occurs in the cardiac cycle (systole or diastole) depends on which valve is malfunctioning (Figs. 3.8.2 and 3.8.3).

ECG and chest radiograph features are usually non-specific and echocardiography is required to confirm the presence or absence of valvular disease/dysfunction. In the assessment of some disorders, cardiac catheterization provides additional information of the type and severity of valve abnormality.

Mitral valve
Malfunction of the mitral valve can alter blood flow into the left atrium and ventricle. Mitral stenosis results in reduced blood flow into the left ventricle in diastole and mitral regurgitation leads to reflux of blood into the left atrium during systole.

Mitral stenosis
Mitral stenosis is narrowing of the mitral valve; it is almost always the result of previous rheumatic fever and is two to three times more common in females than males. It is becoming increasingly rare in the developed world.

Pathogenesis

Rheumatic fever occurs usually in childhood and is caused by infection with group A haemolytic streptococci. This leads to inflammation and scarring of the cardiac valves, most commonly the mitral. The leaflets become thickened with fusion of the commissures and chordae, the mitral valve orifice narrows, the left atrium enlarges and pulmonary hypertension develops.

Clinical features

Mitral stenosis usually presents late with breathlessness, fatigue and palpitation. The enlarged left atrium is often associated with atrial fibrillation. It can also act as a source of systemic emboli and can compress surrounding structures, resulting in dysphagia and hoarseness (caused by left recurrent laryngeal nerve palsy). Patients may notice blood-streaked sputum. Pulmonary hypertension results in features of cor pulmonale. Patients with mitral stenosis classically have a malar flush over the cheeks.

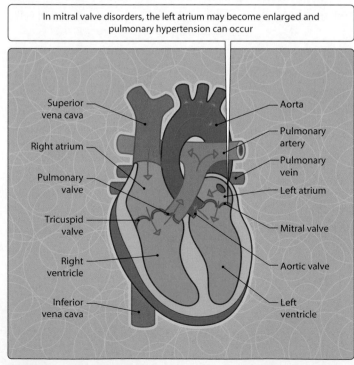

Fig. 3.8.1 The heart and its valves.

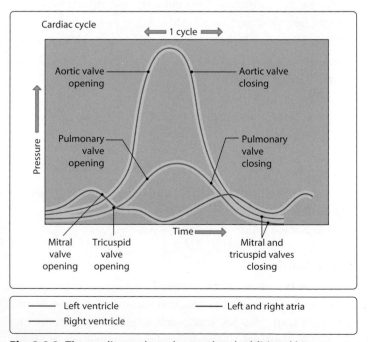

Fig. 3.8.2 The cardiac cycle and normal and additional heart sounds.

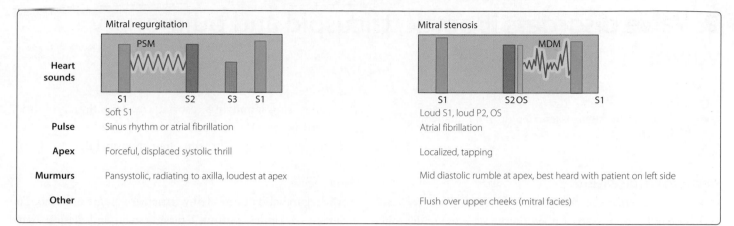

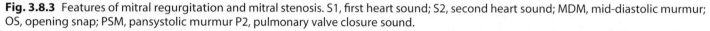

Fig. 3.8.3 Features of mitral regurgitation and mitral stenosis. S1, first heart sound; S2, second heart sound; MDM, mid-diastolic murmur; OS, opening snap; PSM, pansystolic murmur P2, pulmonary valve closure sound.

Investigations

ECG may show atrial fibrillation, P-mitrale (if in sinus rhythm) and right ventricular hypertrophy. Chest radiography may show a calcified mitral valve, enlarged left atrium, pulmonary oedema and cardiomegaly.

Management

Digoxin is used for rate control in atrial fibrillation together with warfarin anticoagulation to reduce the risk of systemic emboli and stroke. Diuretics are used to treat congestive heart failure. Antibiotic prophylaxis has previously been recommended before any invasive or dental procedure to reduce the risk of infective endocarditis. Definitive treatment in severe stenosis requires balloon valvuloplasty, open valvotomy or mitral valve replacement.

Mitral regurgitation

Trivial mitral regurgitation is common and is found in over 75% of the population.

Pathogenesis

Mitral regurgitation may be

- **structural**: as a result of abnormalities of the mitral valve leaflets (mitral valve prolapse, rheumatic fever, infective endocarditis, connective tissue disorders, e.g. Marfan's syndrome) or supporting structures (papillary muscle rupture, chordae tendinae rupture, annular calcification)
- **functional**: as a consequence of left ventricular dilatation (dilated cardiomyopathy, left ventricular wall motion abnormality post myocardial infarction).

It can also be congenital, either isolated or in conjunction with other cardiac abnormalities.

Resultant left ventricular volume overload leads to compensatory ventricular dilatation and impaired contractility. Increased backflow into the left atrium results in left atrial enlargement, atrial fibrillation and pulmonary hypertension.

Clinical features

Mitral regurgitation usually results in progressive breathlessness, fatigue and palpitation. Peripheral oedema indicates the development of pulmonary hypertension and cor pulmonale. Embolism from the dilated left atrium occurs less commonly than in mitral stenosis. Mitral regurgitation can occur acutely following myocardial infarction, as a result of papillary muscle necrosis, or in mitral valve endocarditis. This may result in a sudden rise in left atrial pressure and cardiogenic shock.

Investigations

ECG and chest radiograph changes are non-specific. An echocardiogram is required to confirm the diagnosis.

Management

Diuretics, ACE inhibitors and anticoagulation (if atrial fibrillation is present) are used in symptomatic disease. Mitral valve repair or replacement should be considered in advanced symptomatic disease or sudden mitral regurgitation following rupture of papillary muscle or infective endocarditis.

Mitral valve prolapse

In mitral valve prolapse, the anterior and posterior leaflets prolapse into the left atrium during systole. It occurs in 5% of the population and may be associated with mitral regurgitation. It is often asymptomatic but may present with atypical chest pain and palpitation. No treatment is usually required although beta-blockers are sometimes tried in symptomatic individuals.

9. Valve disorders II: aortic, tricuspid and pulmonary valves

Question
■ How do aortic stenosis and aortic regurgitation differ clinically?

Aortic valve disease

Conditions affecting the aortic valve result in either reduced excursion of the aortic valve leaflets (aortic stenosis) or diastolic reflux of blood through the valve into the left ventricle (aortic regurgitation). Many diseased aortic valves exhibit a degree of both stenosis and regurgitation (mixed aortic valve disease) but other conditions can also obstruct flow from the left ventricle (Fig. 3.9.1).

Aortic stenosis

Aortic stenosis is the most common valvular heart disease in the developed world and is usually caused by calcific degenerative disease. A congenital bicuspid aortic valve occurs in 2% of the population; these individuals present with symptomatic aortic stenosis at an earlier age.

Pathogenesis

Thickening and calcification of the valve leaflets (aortic sclerosis) increases with time. As the leaflets become increasingly immobile and obstruct blood flow, aortic stenosis and compensatory left ventricular hypertrophy can occur.

Clinical features

Patients with aortic stenosis commonly have a long asymptomatic period and present with moderately severe valve disease. The three typical symptoms are:
■ angina caused by reduced flow into the coronary arteries
■ breathlessness
■ syncope on exercise caused by inability to increase cardiac output during sudden exercise.

Aortic regurgitation

Aortic regurgitation can be acute or chronic and caused by a primary aortic valve problem or secondary to aortic root dilatation. Causes include:
■ valvular disease: infective endocarditis, rheumatic fever, autoimmune diseases (e.g. rheumatoid arthritis, systemic lupus erythrematosus), pseudoxanthoma elasticum
■ aortic root disease: hypertension, aortic dissection, Marfan's syndrome, trauma, seronegative spondyloarthropathies (e.g. ankylosing spondylitis, psoriatic arthropathy), syphilitic aortitis
■ congenital: isolated or with other abnormalities.

Pathogenesis

Aortic regurgitation causes left ventricular volume overload. To maintain net cardiac output, left ventricular end-diastolic size and total stroke volume are increased. The dilated left ventricle is less efficient and has greater oxygen demands.

Clinical features

Patients with aortic regurgitation complain of angina or breathlessness. Acute aortic regurgitation can lead to pulmonary oedema, hypotension and cardiogenic shock (Table 3.9.1).

Management

Aortic valve replacement with a prosthetic or tissue valve is the definitive treatment in severe aortic stenosis or regurgitation. Balloon valvuloplasty may be used as an alternative to surgery in elderly patients with aortic stenosis unfit for surgery.

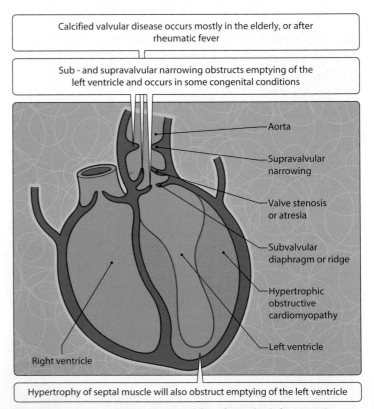

Calcified valvular disease occurs mostly in the elderly, or after rheumatic fever

Sub - and supravalvular narrowing obstructs emptying of the left ventricle and occurs in some congenital conditions

Aorta

Supravalvular narrowing

Valve stenosis or atresia

Subvalvular diaphragm or ridge

Hypertrophic obstructive cardiomyopathy

Left ventricle

Right ventricle

Hypertrophy of septal muscle will also obstruct emptying of the left ventricle

Fig. 3.9.1 Causes of obstruction of flow from the left ventricle.

Antibiotic prophylaxis against endocarditis is no longer routinely advised in all patients undergoing dental or invasive procedures. Medical treatment is of limited use in aortic valve disease. Vasodilators may exacerbate exertional syncope in aortic stenosis and should be avoided.

Tricuspid valve disease

Right-sided valve abnormalities are much less common than left-sided lesions.

Epidemiology

Mild tricuspid regurgitation is very common. Significant tricuspid regurgitation is often secondary to other pathology. Tricuspid stenosis is increasingly rare but is found in up to 30% of individuals with rheumatic mitral stenosis.

Pathogenesis

The competence of the tricuspid valve depends on the valve leaflets, papillary muscles and chordae as well as right ventricular size and function. Tricuspid regurgitation is usually secondary to conditions producing pulmonary hypertension and right ventricular dilatation. Tricuspid valve endocarditis is common in i.v. drug abusers and often requires surgical excision. Tricuspid stenosis is almost always caused by rheumatic fever but it can also occur in carcinoid syndrome.

Clinical features

Patients with tricuspid valve disease usually present with fatigue, ascites and peripheral oedema (Table 3.9.2).

Management

Primary tricuspid regurgitation in the absence of pulmonary hypertension is well tolerated without treatment. In the presence of pulmonary hypertension, replacement of the tricuspid valve may be required. In secondary tricuspid regurgitation caused by right ventricular overload, treatment is that of the underlying condition plus diuretics and ACE inhibitors. Diuretics form the mainstay of treatment in tricuspid stenosis. Balloon valvuloplasty or surgical repair/replacement should also be considered.

Pulmonary valve disease

Mild pulmonary regurgitation of no clinical significance is a common finding on echocardiography. Significant pulmonary regurgitation is usually secondary to pulmonary hypertension. Pulmonary stenosis is almost always congenital. It may rarely be acquired in carcinoid syndrome or rheumatic fever.

Clinical features

Patients with pulmonary valve disease usually present with fatigue, ascites and peripheral oedema.

Management

Management of pulmonary regurgitation involves treating the underlying cause. Mild-to-moderate pulmonary stenosis is well tolerated and usually requires no treatment but severe stenosis may require balloon valvuloplasty or surgical valvotomy.

Table 3.9.1 ECG AND CHEST RADIOGRAPH FEATURES OF AORTIC VALVE DISEASE

	Stenosis	**Regurgitation**
ECG	Left ventricular hypertrophy with strain pattern	Left ventricular hypertrophy
Chest radiograph	Left ventricle normal size; calcified aortic valve may be visible	Cardiomegaly, dilated ascending aorta

Table 3.9.2 CLINICAL SIGNS, ECG AND CHEST RADIOGRAPH FEATURES OF RIGHT-SIDED VALVULAR HEART DISEASE

	Tricuspid regurgitation	**Tricuspid stenosis**	**Pulmonary regurgitation**	**Pulmonary stenosis**
Jugular venous pressure	Elevated; large V wave and prominent Y descent	Elevated; large A wave and slow 'y' descent	Elevated	Elevated; large A wave
Right ventricular heave	Yes	No	Yes	Yes
Auscultation	Pansystolic murmur lower sternal edge, louder on inspiration	Opening snap; rumbling diastolic murmur lower left sternal edge, louder on inspiration	Crescendo diastolic murmur, louder on inspiration	Ejection systolic murmur left upper sternal edge, louder on inspiration
Chest radiograph	Enlarged right atrium and ventricle	Enlarged right atrium	Dilated right atrium, ventricle and pulmonary artery	Poststenotic pulmonary artery dilatation
ECG	Non-specific; may show incomplete right bundle branch block	Tall right atrial P waves (leads II and V_1)	May show right ventricular hypertrophy	Right atrial and ventricular hypertrophy

10. Hypertension

Questions
- What is the management of essential hypertension?
- What are the causes of secondary hypertension?

Hypertension is defined as a systolic blood pressure (BP) of >140 mmHg and/or diastolic BP of >90 mmHg (>140/90 mmHg). Although morbidity and mortality (risk factors for coronary artery disease, stroke and heart failure) increase with increasing BP, most individuals with hypertension are asymptomatic. More than 95% have essential hypertension with no single identifiable cause. Secondary hypertension, usually as a result of underlying renal or endocrine disease, is less common. A number of mechanisms are involved in controlling arterial BP and all can be modulated to cause hypertension; many are sites where antihypertensive drug therapy can target

(Fig. 3.10.1). Factors predisposing to the development of hypertension include:

- sympathetic nervous system stimulation
- activation of the renin–angiotensin system
- endothelial dysfunction (reduced production of nitric oxide, a potent vasodilator)
- genetic factors
- intrauterine factors (low birth weight)
- lifestyle factors (smoking, alcohol, obesity).

Essential hypertension

Epidemiology
Essential hypertension is a major cardiovascular risk factor, affecting approximately 40% of the adult population. Incidence increases with age and it is more common in black Americans and Japanese. Lowering BP reduces mortality and morbidity caused by stroke and coronary artery disease.

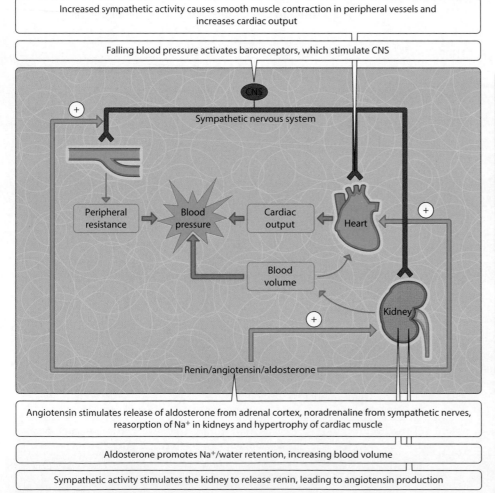

Fig. 3.10.1 Control of blood pressure.

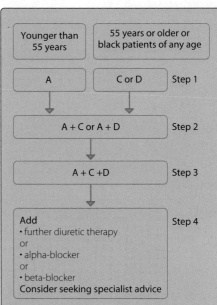

Fig. 3.10.2 Algorithm for the treatment of newly diagnosed hypertension. Black patients are those of African or Carribean descent, and not mixed race, Asian or Chinese. ACE, angiotensin-converting enzyme; A, ACE inhibitor (consider angiotensin II receptor antagonist if ACE intolerant); C, calcium-channel blocker; D, thiazide-type diuretic.

Pathogenesis

In 70% of individuals with hypertension, there is a family history and it is likely that multiple genes contribute. Activation of the autonomic nervous system and the renin–angiotensin system leads to the production of angiotensin II (a potent vasoconstrictor) and aldosterone (causing salt and water retention). Other vasoactive substances and dysfunction of the vascular endothelium also contribute. Ultimately the internal elastic lamina thickens and there is hypertrophy of smooth muscle of blood vessels thus increasing peripheral resistance and hypertension.

Clinical features

Individuals with hypertension are usually asymptomatic and raised BP is usually detected during a routine examination or when complications arise.

BP should be checked in both arms while sitting and lying down. Anxiety alters BP so repeated measurements are needed. Simply measuring BP can cause it to rise ('white coat' hypertension) and ambulatory monitoring avoids this problem.

If hypertensive heart disease is present there may be a loud aortic second heart sound and fourth heart sound. The eye is often affected (hypertensive retinopathy). This can be graded as follows:

1. Increased vessel tortuosity and silver wiring
2. As grade 1 with arteriovenous nipping where thickened retinal arteries cross over veins
3. As grade 2 with soft (cotton wool) exudates and flame-shaped haemorrhages
4. As grade 3 with papilloedema.

Investigations

Urinalysis may show proteinuria or haematuria. Urea and creatinine may demonstrate renal failure. There may be hyperlipidaemia. Chest radiograph may show cardiomegaly. ECG and echocardiograph may show left ventricular hypertrophy.

Management

Treatment is aimed at maintaining a systolic BP <140 mmHg and diastolic BP <90 mmHg. In patients with diabetes, renal impairment or established cardiovascular disease, the target is a systolic BP <130 mmHg and diastolic <85 mmHg. All individuals with hypertension should be given lifestyle advice regarding smoking cessation, reducing alcohol consumption, weight loss, limited dietary salt intake and greater exercise where necessary and appropriate.

Drug choice depends on the age, ethnicity and comorbidity of the patient. Most require at least two agents to achieve adequate (BP) control (Fig. 3.10.2). Other drug classes may be needed in persistent hypertension.

Malignant hypertension

Diastolic BP >130 mmHg increases risk of acute vascular damage and encephalopathy. Malignant hypertension is rare but potentially serious, requiring inpatient care.

Secondary hypertension

Epidemiology

Secondary hypertension accounts for <5% of those presenting with newly diagnosed hypertension. Of these, underlying renal disease is the cause in 80%. Females who develop hypertension in pregnancy usually become normotensive after delivery but are at increased risk of developing hypertension in later life. Causes of secondary hypertension include:

- renal disease: renal artery stenosis, chronic glomerulonephritis, chronic pyelonephritis, polycystic kidney disease
- endocrine disorders: phaeochromocytoma, Conn's disease, Cushing's disease or acromegaly
- cardiovascular disease: coarctation of the aorta
- physiological change: pregnancy
- drugs: oral contraceptive pill, steroids and ciclosporin.

Clinical features

Secondary hypertension should be considered in all hypertensive patients aged <40 years. Individuals may have features suggestive of an underlying cause.

Investigations

U&Es and urinalysis may be abnormal in renal disease. In those with suspected endocrine or metabolic disorders, measurement of cortisol (Cushing's syndrome), growth hormone (acromegaly) or urinary catecholamines (phaeochromocytoma) are required.

Chest radiograph may show rib notching in coarctation of the aorta. Renal ultrasound may show abnormalities. MRI is used to confirm renal artery stenosis and coarctation of the aorta.

Management

Any underlying disease should be managed but otherwise treatment is similar to that of essential hypertension.

11. Infective endocarditis

Questions
- What factors predispose to the development of infective endocarditis?
- What are the clinical features of infective endocarditis?

Infective endocarditis is an infection of the endocardial surface of the heart, which consists of the cardiac valves and lining of the cardiac chambers. Infection may follow an acute or subacute clinical course.

Pathogenesis

Infective endocarditis occurs as a result of bacteraemia, with bacteria lodging on damaged endocardium (Fig. 3.11.1), most commonly an abnormal valve (e.g. congenital bicuspid aortic valve). Bacteraemia can result from dental procedures or invasive investigations (e.g. colonoscopy or pacing wire insertion). The valve becomes inflamed and eroded and a vegetation develops. The most common organism associated with endocarditis is the mouth commensal *Streptococcus viridans*, but many other bacteria can be involved including *Staphylococcus aureus*, coagulase-negative staphylococci, enterococci, other Gram-negative bacilli and chlamydia.

Clinical features

Figures 3.11.2 and 3.11.3 show the main clinical features.

Acute endocarditis

Patients present with an acute febrile illness. This is characterized by prominent, changing cardiac murmurs, and embolic events often occur early in the course of the disease (e.g. ischaemic fingers or toes). Symptoms and signs of severe valvular incompetence are often present.

Subacute endocarditis

Subacute endocarditis is a more insidious form of endocarditis characterized by a longer illness, often over months, with intermittent fever, sweats, general malaise and weight loss. Patients often have structural cardiac abnormalities (e.g. valvular heart disease, atrial or ventricular septal defects). Clinical signs include a changing cardiac murmur, splinter haemorrhages (Fig. 3.11.3)

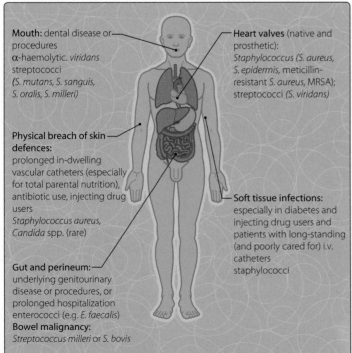

Fig. 3.11.1 Causes and sources of valve infection in infective endocarditis.

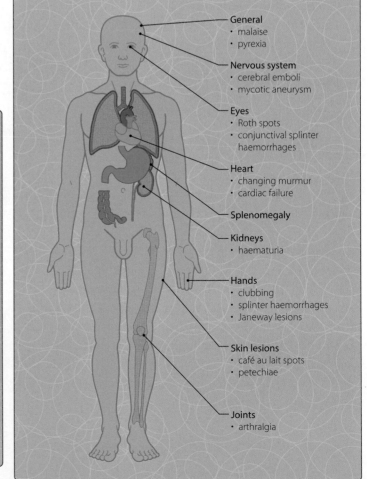

Fig. 3.11.2 Clinical features of infective endocarditis.

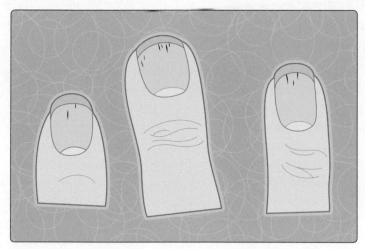

Fig. 3.11.3 Splinter haemorrhages in a patient with infective endocarditis.

caused by circulating immune complexes, finger clubbing, Roth spots on the retina, Janeway lesions on the palms and café au lait spots.

The Duke criteria for diagnosis require the presence of two major criteria, one major and three minor, or five minor criteria:

- **major criteria**:
  - positive blood culture with an organism known to cause infective endocarditis
  - evidence of vegetation, abscess or prosthetic valve dehiscence or new valvular regurgitation on echocardiography
- **minor criteria**:
  - predisposing heart condition or i.v. drug abuse
  - persisting fever >38°C
  - vascular phenomenon, e.g. emboli, splinter haemorrhages
  - immunological phenomenon, e.g. Roth spots
  - positive blood cultures not meeting major criteria
  - echocardiography features consistent with infective endocarditis but not meeting the major criteria above.

Investigations

Multiple blood cultures are required at different times and from different sites. FBC often shows an elevated white cell count and low haemoglobin. CRP and ESR are elevated.

Transthoracic echocardiography can identify vegetations as small as 3 mm in diameter. Transoesophageal echocardiography may provide a greater sensitivity and identify vegetations as small as 1 mm. Serial ECGs are important, especially with aortic valve involvement, as atrioventricular block can suggest aortic root abscess formation.

Management

Patients who are haemodynamically unstable should be managed in a high-dependency setting with early cardiothoracic involvement. Isolation of the organism is key to management and, therefore, multiple blood cultures are essential. Appropriate i.v. antibiotic therapy should be tailored to this, although empirical 'best guess' antibiotics with benzyl penicillin and gentamicin may be started early. Antibiotics are usually given for 6 weeks, of which at least 3 weeks are by the i.v. route. Valve replacement is usually required for prosthetic valve endocarditis or if significant valve damage has occurred.

12. Cardiomyopathy

Questions
- What are the different types of cardiomyopathy?
- What tests are used in the investigation of suspected cardiomyopathy?

Cardiomyopathy is a disorder of cardiac muscle (myocardium, the muscle between the endocardium and the pericardium; Fig. 3.12.1) that leads to cardiac dysfunction. The four main types (Fig. 3.12.2) are:

- hypertrophic cardiomyopathy (HCM)
- dilated cardiomyopathy (DCM)
- restrictive cardiomyopathy (RCM)
- arrhythmogenic right ventricular cardiomyopathy (ARVC).

Hypertrophic cardiomyopathy

The prevalence of HCM may be as high as 1 in 500 of the population. It is characterized by asymmetrical or symmetrical left ventricular wall thickening. This results in obstruction to left ventricular outflow, with an increased risk of sudden death. HCM is usually familial, with autosomal dominant transmission of mutations in the genes coding for myofibrillary proteins. It is often asymptomatic although patients may complain of exertional breathlessness, chest pain or syncope and there may be a family history of sudden death.

Left ventricular outflow obstruction in HCM causes a steep-rising jerky pulse and systolic murmur of mitral regurgitation. Beta-blockers and calcium channel blockers are used to treat symptoms. ACE inhibitors and digoxin worsen the outflow

obstruction and should be avoided. Atrial fibrillation is often poorly tolerated and amiodarone may help to maintain sinus rhythm. Surgical myomectomy or septal ablation may be required if a significant gradient across the outflow tract persists despite drug treatment. Individuals considered at high risk of sudden cardiac death should be considered for an implantable defibrillator.

Dilated cardiomyopathy

DCM accounts for up to 4% of heart failure. In DCM, individual myocytes increase in length and lose intracellular myofibrils, resulting in ventricular dilatation and impaired contractility. Coronary artery disease and hypertension must be excluded to make the diagnosis. There is a familial pattern in 25%. It may be idiopathic, although it can be associated with:

- alcohol abuse
- postpartum
- infection (influenza, coxsackievirus, toxoplasma, diphtheria)
- haemochromatosis
- thiamine deficiency (beri-beri)
- muscular dystrophies
- hyper- and hypothyroidism
- connective tissues disorders
- drugs such as the cytotoxic antibiotics (anthracyclines e.g. daunorubicin).

DCM usually presents with breathlessness and features of heart failure. Management includes diuretics, ACE inhibitors and beta-blockers. If atrial fibrillation develops, digoxin and anticoagulation may be required.

Restrictive cardiomyopathy

RCM occurs when the myocardium fails to relax in diastole with reduced filling of one or both ventricles. This can be caused by endomyocardial fibrosis in infiltrative diseases (amyloidosis), storage diseases (haemochromatosis) or malignancy (metastases or following radiotherapy). RCM presents with breathlessness and features of heart failure. Diuretics are often used but the prognosis is poor.

Arrythmogenic right ventricular cardiomyopathy

ARVC is familial in >30% of those affected and more common in males. It is characterized by fibrofatty replacement of the right ventricular myocardium and may lead to sudden death, often in the young and athletes. Examination may be normal. Treatment options include beta-blockers, catheter ablation and an implantable defibrillator.

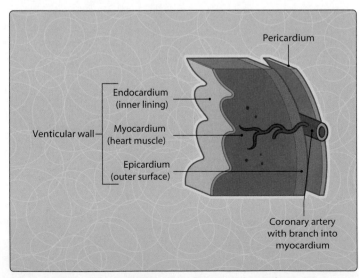

Pericardium

Endocardium (inner lining)

Venticular wall

Myocardium (heart muscle)

Epicardium (outer surface)

Coronary artery with branch into myocardium

Fig. 3.12.1 Cardiomyopathy arises from a variety of conditions that affects the myocardium.

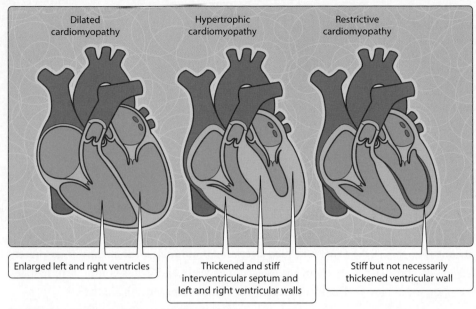

Dilated cardiomyopathy   Hypertrophic cardiomyopathy   Restrictive cardiomyopathy

Enlarged left and right ventricles

Thickened and stiff interventricular septum and left and right ventricular walls

Stiff but not necessarily thickened ventricular wall

Fig. 3.12.2 The main types of cardiomyopathy.

Investigations in cardiomyopathy

Since ECG changes in cardiomyopathy are non-specific, echocardiography is required to confirm the diagnosis. Coronary angiography is sometimes performed to exclude ischaemic heart disease in all types of cardiomyopathy. Other investigations include:

- 24h Holter monitoring for risk stratification in HCM and ARVC
- viral, autoimmune and biochemical screening may be useful in DCM
- endomyocardial biopsy is sometimes required to confirm the diagnosis of ARVC and RCM.

13. Miscellaneous cardiovascular disorders

Questions
- What is an atrial myxoma?
- What are the symptoms of a dissecting aortic aneurysm?
- What are the symptoms of peripheral vascular disease?

Atrial myxoma

Most tumours affecting the heart tend to be metastatic and primary cardiac tumours are rare. Atrial myxoma accounts for >50% of primary cardiac tumours of which most are benign; 90% are solitary and 75% occur in the left atrium (Fig. 3.13.1). Atrial myxoma is uncommon, with a prevalence of approximately 0.01% at postmortem. They are more common in females and can occur in any age group.

Myxomas are often polypoid with a smooth surface. The most common site of attachment is at the border of the fossa ovalis of the left atrium.

Clinical features and management

Symptoms are non-specific although patients may complain of breathlessness caused by obstruction of flow through the mitral valve. Embolization of part of the tumour may result in stroke or peripheral arterial embolus. The first heart sound is often loud and an early diastolic tumour 'plop' may be heard in diastole. Fever and finger clubbing may be present.

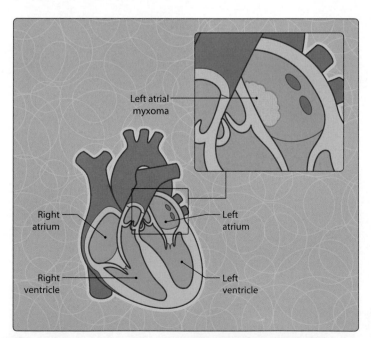

Left atrial myxoma

Right atrium

Left atrium

Right ventricle

Left ventricle

Fig. 3.13.1 Atrial myxomas are usually (75%) found in the left atrium. They arise from the intraventricular septum and grow into the atria.

Echocardiography and MRI allow identification of atrial myxoma, its size and site of attachment

Surgical resection is usually curative. Recurrence is only 2% and usually is a result of incomplete excision.

Diseases of the aorta

Aortic aneurysm

Aortic aneurysm is a progressive weakness of the media layer of the aortic wall resulting in dilatation and eventual rupture. It most commonly occurs in the abdominal aorta between the renal and iliac arteries. Abdominal aortic aneurysm is present in 5% of males aged >65 years and is less common in females. Rupture accounts for 2% of all male deaths in the UK.

The main risk factor predisposing to aortic aneurysm is atherosclerotic disease, leading to aortic wall weakening. It is also associated with hypertension, diabetes mellitus and smoking.

Clinical features and management

Small aneurysms are often asymptomatic, while larger aneurysms may present as acute or chronic back or abdominal pain. Aneurysmal rupture presents acutely with abdominal pain and hypovolaemic shock. An abdominal aortic aneurysm can be felt as a pulsatile mass in the epigastrium. A pulsatile mass below the umbilicus suggests an aneurysm of an iliac artery. There may be evidence of peripheral embolization.

Ultrasound or CT scans usually confirms the diagnosis.

Small aneurysms (<4 cm diameter) are at low risk of rupture and should be observed. Those with larger aneurysms should be considered for elective surgical repair. Ruptured abdominal aortic aneurysm is an emergency and requires immediate resuscitation and surgical intervention.

Aortic dissection

Type A dissection begins in the ascending aorta and may extend into the descending aorta and type B dissection is confined to the descending aorta distal to the origin of the left subclavian artery (Fig. 3.13.2). Aortic dissection is uncommon, with an incidence of <1% in the population and most common in males >40 years. Type A dissection is twice as common as type B.

Damage to the media layer of the aortic wall allows blood to enter below the intima, which separates to create a flap. This produces a false lumen that can expand and rupture externally or cause ischaemia to major organs. Conditions predisposing to aortic dissection include atherosclerosis, hypertension, trauma, Marfan's syndrome, Ehlers–Danlos syndrome, aortic coarctation, bicuspid aortic valve and syphilis.

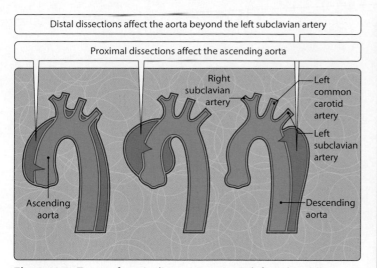

Fig. 3.13.2 Types of aortic dissection: type A, left and middle; type B, right.

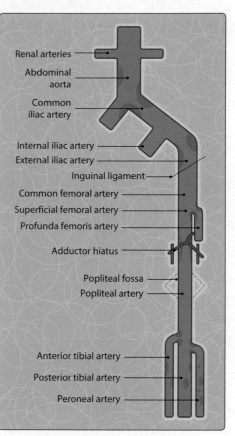

Fig. 3.13.3 Anatomy of the lower limb arterial tree and areas prone to atherosclerosis.

Clinical features and management

Patients present acutely and complain of 'tearing' chest and back pain, most commonly between the shoulder blades. Individuals are often hypertensive with a large discrepancy in blood pressure between the arms. In type A dissection, features of aortic regurgitation may be present.

Chest radiograph shows mediastinal widening and sometimes a small left pleural effusion. Transoesophageal echocardiogram, CT scan of thorax or MRI confirms the site of the dissection.

Blood pressure should be controlled, usually with i.v. beta-blockers. Type A dissection requires surgical repair. Type B can be managed medically with bed-rest and careful blood pressure control unless there is evidence of leakage or ischaemia to major organs.

Peripheral arterial disease

Peripheral arterial disease is caused by atherosclerotic narrowing of peripheral arteries, which reduces blood flow to the extremities (usually the legs; Fig. 3.13.3). Peripheral vascular disease is thought to occur in 15–20% of individuals >65 years of age, although only 10% of these suffer from classic intermittent claudication. The major risk factors are diabetes mellitus and smoking.

Atherosclerosis is caused by an accumulation of fatty deposits (plaques) in arterial walls. This ultimately results in narrowing of the arterial lumen and impaired blood supply.

Clinical features and management

Patients commonly complain of intermittent claudication (cramp-like pain, usually in the calves, brought on by exertion and relieved by rest). It is often bilateral although one leg is usually more affected than the other. Individuals may also present with leg ulcers that fail to heal or gangrene. The limb is usually cool to touch, with skin atrophy and hair loss. Dorsalis pedis and posterior tibial pulses are absent and bruits may be audible over more proximal arteries.

The ankle–brachial index compares the blood pressure in the arm with that in the ankle. Peripheral angiography allows direct visualization of the peripheral arteries.

Management involves smoking cessation, control of hypertension and diabetes, statins and anti-platelet agents. Surgical management depends on the site and severity of the disease. Where focal narrowing or stenosis is identified, angioplasty (bypass or balloon and stenting) may be useful. Bypass surgery may be appropriate for severe proximal disease. In severe ischaemia and gangrene, amputation may be required.

Acute lower limb ischaemia is usually caused by thrombosis at the site of an atheromatous plaque or embolization from the heart or an atheromatous central vessel. Patients present with an acutely painful, pale and pulseless limb. Treatment involves surgical removal of the clot or amputation if this is not possible.

14. Congenital heart disease

Questions
- What are the causes of congenital heart disease?
- What are the most common types of congenital heart disease?
- What is a ventricular septal defect?

Congenital heart disease occurs in approximately 1% of live births. The most common types are ventricular septal defect (VSD), atrial septal defect (ASD), patent ductus arteriosus, pulmonary stenosis, coarctation of the aorta, aortic stenosis and tetralogy of Fallot.

Many congenital heart defects occur spontaneously, although recognized associations include:
- fetal infections (e.g. rubella)
- prenatal hypoxia and birth at high altitude (patent ductus arteriosus)
- maternal alcohol abuse
- teratogens (e.g. thalidomide)
- ASD and VSD syndromes and chromosomal abnormalities (Down's syndrome is associated with ASD and VSD and Turner's syndrome with coarctation of the aorta).

Ventricular septal defects

VSD causes an abnormal communication between the left and right ventricles (Fig. 3.14.1). It may occur in isolation or be a component of more complex congenital heart disease such as tetralogy of Fallot (Fig. 3.14.2) and transposition of the great vessels. VSDs are the most common congenital malformation and occur in approximately 1 in 500 live births. The main implication is related to intracardiac shunting. Since the left side of the heart is at greater pressure than the right, blood from the left heart is circulated through to the right and repeats its transit through the pulmonary circulation. This increases left ventricular workload, increases pulmonary artery pressures and decreases cardiac output. Each of these haemodynamic consequences is progressive and can result in significant left ventricular failure.

Clinical features

Small VSDs are asymptomatic. Larger ones can cause breathlessness, fatigue and frequent chest infections. VSD usually results in a loud pansystolic murmur; signs of pulmonary hypertension may be present in those with progressive lesions.

Investigations

Chest radiograph may show enlarged pulmonary arteries and cardiomegaly. ECG may show left or right ventricular hypertrophy. Two-dimensional or Doppler echocardiography usually identifies the VSD.

Management

VSDs usually need surgical closure.

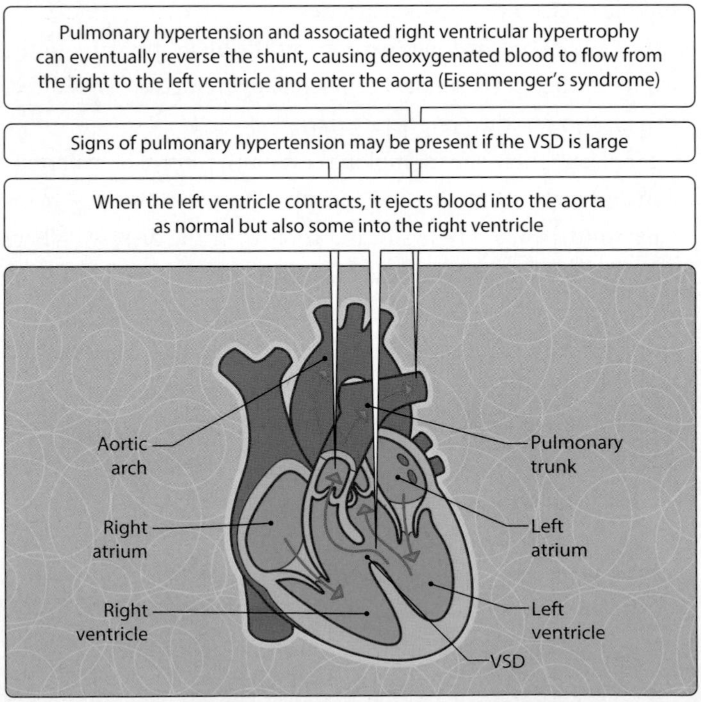

Atrial septal defect

The atria are separated by a fibromuscular sheet known as the atrial septum. Defects here allow communications between the atria. ASDs account for roughly a third of congenital heart

Pulmonary hypertension and associated right ventricular hypertrophy can eventually reverse the shunt, causing deoxygenated blood to flow from the right to the left ventricle and enter the aorta (Eisenmenger's syndrome)

Signs of pulmonary hypertension may be present if the VSD is large

When the left ventricle contracts, it ejects blood into the aorta as normal but also some into the right ventricle

Right ventricular overflow obstruction occurs at, above or just below the pulmonary valve

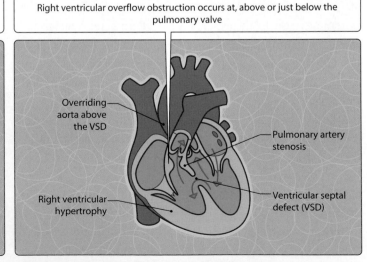

Aortic arch
Right atrium
Right ventricle
Pulmonary trunk
Left atrium
Left ventricle
VSD

Overriding aorta above the VSD
Right ventricular hypertrophy
Pulmonary artery stenosis
Ventricular septal defect (VSD)

Fig. 3.14.1 Features of a ventricular septal defect (VSD).

Fig. 3.14.2 Features of tetralogy of Fallot.

disorders and tend to be more common in females. The two main types are:

- ostium primum defects: anterior, inferior aspect of the septum
- ostium secundum defects (the most common): midseptum around the foramen ovale.

ASDs can result in left-to-right shunting of blood, which can lead to right ventricular hypertrophy and pulmonary hypertension (Fig. 3.14.3).

Clinical features
Many individuals are asymptomatic, although others complain of breathlessness, frequent chest infections, palpitation (from supraventricular arrhythmias) and may ultimately develop right heart failure. The classical auscultatory finding is fixed wide splitting of the second heart sound.

Investigations
Chest radiography shows enlarged pulmonary arteries and right ventricular hypertrophy. ECG may show right bundle branch block or right or left axis deviation. Echocardiography is usually diagnostic and may show the defect, abnormal blood flow, right ventricular hypertrophy and pulmonary hypertension

Management
Individuals with large defects usually require surgical closure. It is uncertain whether small asymptomatic defects need definitive intervention or not.

Patent foramen ovale
The foramen ovale allows oxygenated blood to bypass the lungs in the fetal circulation. It usually closes spontaneously and over 80% close by the age of 20 years. In the remainder, the foramen ovale remains patent and may allow shunting of blood from the right to the left heart, with increased risk of thrombotic stroke. In these individuals and also in deep-sea divers (who may develop cerebral artery air embolism), surgical closure should be considered.

Patent ductus arteriosus
The ductus arteriosus is an essential part of the fetal circulation and connects the aorta and pulmonary artery. If this fails to close after birth, the patent vessel allows blood to flow directly from the aorta into the pulmonary artery (Fig. 3.14.4).

Coarctation of the aorta
Coarctation of the aorta is caused by a narrowing of the aorta at the ductus arteriosus. It is more common in males. In females it can be associated with Turner's syndrome.

Clinical features include secondary systemic hypertension, weak leg pulses and radio-femoral delay. Auscultation of the heart reveals a mid to late systolic murmur audible over the upper praecordium or back. Chest radiograph typically shows rib notching caused by bone erosion by collateral intercostal arteries; it may also show the narrowed area of aorta. ECG shows left ventricular hypertrophy. Imaging such as aortography, CT and MRI can show the coarctation. Surgery or balloon dilatation is sometimes required in severe stenosis.

Blood can pass from left to right through the defect between the atria

The murmur is produced by increased flow across the pulmonary valve and an increased stroke volume

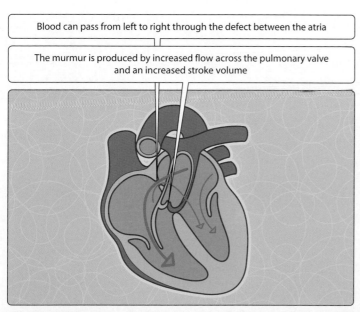

Fig. 3.14.3 Features of an atrial septal defect.

Blood from the aorta crosses into the pulmonary artery, creating a left-to-right shunt; its turbulent flow causes the murmur

If pulmonary hypertension develops, shunting may reverse, causing central cyanosis (Eisenmenger's syndrome)

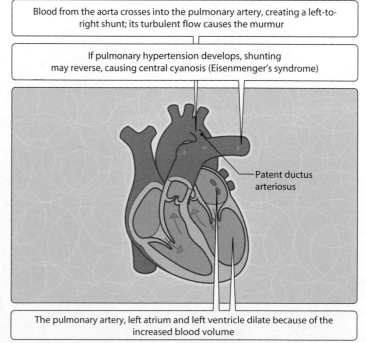

Patent ductus arteriosus

The pulmonary artery, left atrium and left ventricle dilate because of the increased blood volume

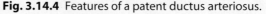

Fig. 3.14.4 Features of a patent ductus arteriosus.

PART III

Lung disorders

Graeme Currie and Graham Douglas

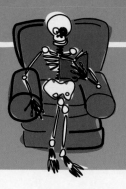

The big picture

Respiratory medicine covers a broad spectrum of disorders involving the airways, lung parenchyma, pulmonary vasculature, pleura and mediastinum, along with neuromuscular abnormalities affecting the diaphragm and chest wall. Patients, therefore, present not only with problems primarily affecting the respiratory system but also with many disorders secondarily affecting the airway, lung parenchyma and vessels, or that are part of a multisystem syndrome.

Mortality

Respiratory disease is extremely common throughout the world. According to the WHO, of all 50.5 million deaths in 1990, 9.4 million (18.7%) were from respiratory disease (4.3 million lower respiratory tract infections/pneumonia, 2.2 million chronic obstructive pulmonary disease (COPD), 2.0 million tuberculosis and 0.95 million lung cancer). In Europe, respiratory disease ranks second (after cardiovascular disease) in terms of mortality, incidence, prevalence and cost. However, as death from ischaemic heart disease declines across the Western world, the relative mortality from respiratory disease rises. In the UK, respiratory disease is now the overall leading cause of death, having taken over from heart disease.

Morbidity

Respiratory disease causes considerable morbidity and in the UK is currently the third most commonly reported long-term illness, involving over 7% of adults in 1998. Surveys in general practice show that almost a third (31%) of the population consults primary care for respiratory conditions at least once each year; this compares with 15% for musculoskeletal problems and 9% for cardiovascular problems. Around two-thirds of children under 5 years visit their GP with a respiratory condition at least once a year. The prevalence of respiratory disease also varies with social class. In 1998, manual workers reported rates 96% higher than non-manual workers in males and 43% higher in females. Rates of respiratory disease appear to be lower in the Indian and Chinese communities.

Respiratory disease causes considerable morbidity (Fig. 1.1) and can lead to respiratory failure. Classification into type 1 or type 2 relates to the absence or presence of hypercapnia (rise in arterial CO_2, $Paco_2$) (Table 1.1). Type 1 respiratory failure is typically caused by a mismatch of ventilation and perfusion, resulting in low Pao_2 (hypoxaemia) but $Paco_2$ is normal. It is caused by conditions that affect oxygenation (e.g. pneumonia and interstitial lung disease). In type 2 respiratory failure, Pao_2 is low and $Paco_2$ is high owing to hypoventilation (in advanced COPD, neuromuscular disorders or kyphoscoliosis).

Table 1.1 ARTERIAL BLOOD GAS FEATURES OF TYPES 1 AND 2 RESPIRATORY FAILURE

	Type 1	Type 2
Pao_2	↓	↓
$Paco_2$	No change or ↓	↑
HCO_3^-	No change	No change or ↑
pH	No change or ↑	No change or ↓

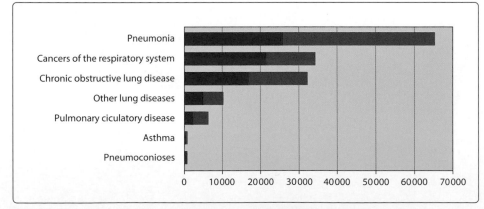

Fig. 1.1 Respiratory disease deaths by cause, 1999, UK. Red, men; orange, women.

Costs

The total financial burden of lung disease in Europe amounts to nearly £70 billion (102 billion euros). COPD contributes almost one half of this figure followed by asthma, pneumonia, lung cancer and tuberculosis. This includes direct as well as indirect costs of these diseases: inpatient care (17.5%), ambulatory care (8.9%), drugs (6.6%), mortality and rehabilitation (19.6%) and lost working days (47.4%).

In the UK, the total cost of respiratory disease to the NHS is around £2600 million per year. Within primary care, this amounts to around £650 million. In 2000, there were approximately 78 000 inpatient admissions to hospital, with an associated cost of over £1000 million. There were also over half a million outpatient attendances, costing around £41 million.

Drugs, particularly inhalers for asthma and COPD, are among the most common prescriptions in the UK and account for about 7% of the total NHS drug budget. The total cost associated with inhalers and other preparations for respiratory disease amounted to approximately £800 million in 2000. Chemotherapy for patients with lung cancer adds around £6 million yearly.

Prevalence and incidence

Asthma is arguably the most common chronic disease at all ages in the UK. Around 33% of adults and 28% of children aged 2–15 years have a history of wheezing. Studies in children suggest that the prevalences of both wheeze and asthma have increased considerably since the mid-1980s, and the prevalence of wheeze in adults appears to have increased from 16% in 1991 to 21% in 1996.

COPD has been diagnosed in around 1 million patients in the UK, but it is thought that as many as three times this number are undiagnosed. It is the only common chronic disease with a rising mortality and in the UK is currently the sixth commonest cause of death and is likely to rise to fourth within the next 10 years.

Lung cancer is the most common fatal cancer in males, representing 20% of all male cancers. Men in the UK have a 1 in 13 risk of lung cancer at some time during their lives.

The UK is one of the first countries to report that the incidence of lung cancer is higher than that of breast cancer in women, representing 12% of all female cancers. The incidence of lung cancer varies across the UK and is highest in Scotland. Survival rates for lung cancer are low, with a 1-year survival rate of 20% and 5-year survival rate of 5%. The only common cancer with a lower survival rate is pancreatic cancer.

Tuberculosis is very common in underdeveloped countries, but the incidence is again increasing in the UK, particularly in the London area.

Occupational lung disease

Occupational lung disease is becoming increasingly recognized. Occupational asthma is common in the community, with over 400 causative agents reported. In the UK, there are over 2000 deaths each year from occupational lung disease, over three-quarters of these from mesothelioma, a cancer of the lining of the lung (pleura) caused by inhalation of asbestos dust.

Smoking

Smoking is the greatest preventable cause of death in the developed world and is the usual causative factor in lung cancer and COPD. The decline in smoking in developed countries has been greater in males than in females, such that in many countries the prevalence in females is now close to that of males. In contrast, the prevalence of smoking continues to rise in many less-developed countries.

The main health hazards of cigarette smoke are tars (cancer), carbon monoxide and nicotine (cardiovascular disease), with both gas and particulates implicated in the decline in lung function seen in COPD. Environmental tobacco smoke (passive smoking) is associated with childhood respiratory infections, sudden infant death and asthma, and in adults with lung cancer and cardiovascular disease. Prevention of starting smoking is more effective than attempts at giving up, but smoking cessation at any age will bring health benefits.

High-return facts

2

1 The upper and lower airways share the same epithelial lining and release similar inflammatory mediators. Allergic rhinitis commonly coexists with asthma, and typical symptoms include intermittent runny and blocked nose, loss of sense of smell and conjunctivitis. Other conditions affecting the upper airway include the common cold, nasal polyps, tonsillitis, epiglottitis, sinusitis, foreign body inhalation and tumours.

2 **Asthma** affects around 10% of children and 6% of adults. Endobronchial inflammation leads to airway hyper-responsiveness and episodic airflow obstruction. There are five steps in management although inhaled steroids are fundamental in all but the mildest of disease. Acute severe asthma is a medical emergency and treated with O_2, steroids and nebulized bronchodilators. Occupational asthma accounts for around 10% of adult-onset asthma and should be considered in all adults presenting with asthma.

3 **Chronic obstructive pulmonary disease** (COPD) is largely caused by cigarette smoking. There is irreversible airflow obstruction that fails to change significantly over time. Treatment is with long-acting bronchodilators to prevent symptoms and short-acting bronchodilators for relief of symptoms. High-dose inhaled steroids can reduce exacerbations in those with forced expiratory volume in 1 s < 50% of predicted. Acute exacerbations of COPD are treated with O_2 (24% or 28%), nebulized bronchodilators, systemic steroids and usually antibiotics.

4 **Pneumonia** is an infection of the lung parenchyma that causes chest radiograph changes. It can be community-acquired, hospital-acquired (nosocomial) or occur in the immunocompromised. *Streptococcus pneumoniae* (pneumococcus) is the commonest cause of community-acquired pneumonia. Severity of pneumonia is assessed with the CURB-65 score, measuring parameters associated with poor outcome. Treatment is with high-flow O_2 and antibiotics, particularly against pneumococci.

5 **Tuberculosis** is a notifiable disease caused by *Mycobacterium tuberculosis*. Immigration, global poverty and HIV infection have caused an increase. If sputum is smear positive on Ziehl–Neelsen staining, the patient is infectious and should be isolated. Treatment is initially with a combination of four first-line drugs: rifampicin, isoniazid, pyrazinamide and ethambutol. Multidrug-resistant tuberculosis requires a different combination.

6 **Bronchiectasis** is a permanent dilatation of distal airways, predisposing to chronic infection. Symptoms include chronic cough, copious purulent sputum production and, occasionally, haemoptysis. Treatment is with daily physiotherapy and antibiotics when required. **Cystic fibrosis** is the most common serious autosomal recessive condition in Western populations. Malfunction of a chloride channel protein causes an increase in mucous viscosity in all systems. Management includes physiotherapy, nutritional and pancreatic supplements and antibiotics.

7 **Lung cancer** is the most common fatal malignancy in both men and women in the UK. Cigarette smoking is responsible for up to 90%. Histologically, it can be divided into small cell and non-small cell (squamous cell, adenocarcinoma, large cell) cancer. The latter is staged using a system based on tumour size, lymph node involvement and metastatic involvement (TNM). Small cell lung cancer is staged as limited or extensive disease. Fewer than 10% of patients are living 5 years after diagnosis.

8 **Pneumothorax** is accumulation of air in the pleural space. It can be primary, secondary, traumatic or iatrogenic. A large secondary pneumothorax causing chest pain or breathlessness usually requires an intercostal drain. A tension pneumothorax is a medical emergency. A **pleural effusion** caused by changes in hydrostatic or oncotic pressure (e.g. in heart failure) has a low protein content (transudate), while that from inflammatory, obstructive or malignant conditions has a high protein concentration (exudate). Large exudates should be drained and transudates require treatment of the underlying cause.

9 **Idiopathic pulmonary fibrosis** affects the interstitium of the lung (between the alveolar epithelium and capillary endothelium). The cause is unknown. There is no effective treatment but steroids and immunosuppressive drugs are tried. Lung transplantation is considered in advanced disease. **Extrinsic allergic alveolitis** is an inflammatory response (typically type III or type IV hypersensitivity reaction). Common causes are inhaled avian proteins (bird fancier's lung) or fungal spores on mouldy hay (farmer's lung). Breathlessness shortly after exposure can persist with chronic exposure. Removal of the allergen is usually effective, although oral steroids may be required.

10 **Sarcoidosis** is a multisystem granulomatous disorder that most commonly affects the lungs. Patients may be asymptomatic or have fever, weight loss and malaise. Acute sarcoidosis consists of bilateral hilar lymphadenopathy, erythema nodosum and joint pains. Symptoms often resolve with non-steroidal anti-inflammatory drugs. Patients with progressive pulmonary disease, hypercalcaemia, uveitis, disfiguring skin lesions, and cardiac, neurological or eye involvement may require oral steroids.

11 **Pneumoconiosis** is caused by inhalation of inorganic dusts such as coal or silica dust. There is no specific treatment and the most important issue is prevention and identification. **Asbestos** was widely used and many workers have previously been exposed to it. Asbestos exposure can cause several different types of benign (pleural plaques, thickening, effusions) or malignant (mesothelioma, lung cancer) lung disease that present at least 20 years following exposure. **Asbestosis** is a type of interstitial lung disease caused by inhalation of large amounts of asbestos fibres. There is no effective treatment for asbestosis but chemotherapy is becoming available for mesothelioma.

12 Factors predisposing to **deep venous thrombosis** (and subsequent **pulmonary embolism**) include venous stasis, injury to the vein wall and enhanced coagulability of the blood (Virchow's triad). Management of pulmonary embolism consists of O_2, low-molecular-weight heparin followed by warfarin for at least 3–6 months. Thrombolysis may be considered in acute massive pulmonary embolism with haemodynamic collapse. Prevention of pulmonary thromboembolism with low-molecular-weight heparin and early mobilization is important in patients admitted to hospital.

13 **Sleep apnoea syndrome** is associated with obesity, snoring, excessive daytime sleepiness and overnight apnoeic episodes. Diagnosis requires a high Epworth Sleepiness Score and positive overnight sleep studies. Management includes weight loss, avoidance of sedative drugs and alcohol and overnight continuous positive airways pressure (CPAP). **Narcolepsy** is less common and results in irresistible daytime sleepiness, cataplexy (sudden onset of muscle weakness when awake), hypnagogic hallucinations (vivid dreams at the onset of sleep) and sleep paralysis.

14 **Pulmonary hypertension** is present when the mean pulmonary artery pressure is >25 mmHg at rest or >30 mmHg on exercise. Secondary pulmonary hypertension is more common and can be caused by advanced chronic obstructive pulmonary disease, pulmonary embolism, left-to-right cardiac shunts, vasculitis, sarcoidosis and HIV infection. Treatment depends on the underlying cause and includes O_2, warfarin, vasodilator drugs and in some cases lung transplantation.

15 **Acute respiratory distress syndrome** (ARDS) is characterized by bilateral pulmonary infiltrates, hypoxaemia, lung fibrosis and normal pulmonary artery wedge pressure. Management includes treatment of the underlying condition (e.g. antibiotics, removal of infected tissue, etc), respiratory support (often with intubation and mechanical ventilation) and nutrition.

16 The lung can be damaged by inhaled or oral **drugs**, producing reactions including bronchoconstriction (beta-blockers, aspirin), cough (ACE inhibitors), alveolitis (amiodarone, methotrexate) and pulmonary embolism (contraceptives). **Connective tissue disorders** such as rheumatoid arthritis, systemic lupus erythematosus, systemic sclerosis, ankylosing spondylitis, Sjögren's syndrome and Behçet's syndrome all affect the lung in different ways.

17 The presence of **eosinophils** in lung tissue indicates a cellular response to an exogenous or endogenous agent; blood eosinophilia may also be present. Causes include idiopathic pulmonary eosinophilia (Löffler's syndrome) and tropical eosinophilic pneumonia (worms), an allergic reaction to drugs (e.g. penicillin, sulphonamides, chlorpropamide and carbamazepine) or environmental triggers (e.g. allergic bronchopulmonary aspergillosis), or an autoimmune disorder (Churg–Strauss syndrome, a small vessel multisystem vasculitis).

1. Upper airway disorders

Questions
- What conditions cause upper airway symptoms?
- What are the clinical features of quinsy and how is it managed?

The common cold

The common cold (coryza) is a self-limiting highly infectious illness characterized by mild systemic upset (fever, malaise, anorexia), sore throat, sneezing and a runny or blocked nose. It is most commonly caused by rhinovirus, but also by adenovirus or parainfluenza virus.

Sinusitis

Acute sinusitis affects the paranasal sinuses (Fig. 3.1.1). It sometimes occurs following a viral upper respiratory tract infection, although it can also be caused by bacteria such as *Streptococcus pneumoniae* or *Haemophilus influenzae*. Symptoms include frontal headache or facial pain, nasal stuffiness and discharge. It is usually self-limiting but broad-spectrum antibiotics are sometimes required. Chronic sinusitis causes facial fullness rather than actual pain. An uncommon complication of sinusitis is cerebral abscess.

Nasal polyps

Nasal polyps are smooth pale shiny polypoid structures that arise from the nasal or sinus mucosa (usually the ethmoid sinuses). They are often found bilaterally, although they can cause symptoms predominantly on one side. Aspirin sensitivity, asthma and nasal polyps often coexist. Symptoms from nasal polyps include

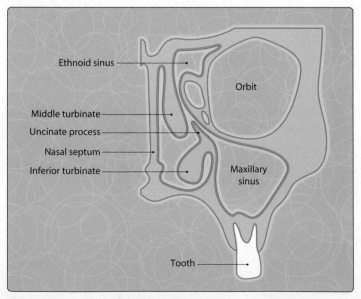

Ethnoid sinus

Orbit

Middle turbinate

Uncinate process

Nasal septum

Inferior turbinate

Maxillary sinus

Tooth

Fig. 3.1.1 Location of the sinuses.

anosmia, postnasal drip and blocked nose, which causes the individual to mouth breathe. Treatment is with decongestants and nasal steroids and, occasionally, endoscopic sinus surgery. Unfortunately, nasal polyps frequently recur following surgery.

Rhinitis

Rhinitis is an inflammatory condition affecting the nose, resulting in excess mucous production; typical symptoms include an intermittently blocked and runny nose, itchy nose, sniffing, sneezing and impaired sense of smell. It is frequently caused by allergens (e.g. house dust mite, grass and tree pollens, animal danders) and can be associated with conjunctivitis and wheezing. Many individuals with rhinitis have asthma and vice versa. Serum radioallergoabsorbant testing (RAST) can detect specific IgE levels to different allergens.

Not all rhinitis is allergic in nature; it can be non-allergic (vasomotor rhinitis) or occur as a consequence of exercise, cold weather or food intolerance. In patients with more severe disease, it can also cause systemic upset and difficulty in sleeping. Rhinitis has been classified as being either intermittent or persistent, and can also be considered mild, moderate or severe. Treatment includes allergen avoidance, topical steroids and antihistamines.

Postnasal drip syndrome

Postnasal drip syndrome is caused by nasal secretions, frequently from allergic rhinitis or sinusitis, tracking down the posterior pharyngeal wall. Symptoms include frequent throat clearing, and chronic cough. In non-smoking patients not using an ACE inhibitor who have a normal chest radiograph, the most common causes of chronic cough (in isolation or in combination) are postnasal drip, asthma or gastro-oesophageal reflux disease. Reasons for specialist referral in patients with a chronic (lasting >8 weeks) cough include:

- weight loss
- haemoptysis
- purulent sputum
- night sweats
- risk factors of immunosuppression
- difficult symptom control.

Tonsillitis

Tonsillitis can be caused by viruses or bacteria, and results in fever, malaise, sore throat and pain on swallowing (odynophagia) (Fig. 3.1.2). In young adults with suspected tonsillitis, especially when mild cervical lymphadenopathy is present, consider **infectious mononucleosis** (glandular fever). In these cases, a monospot test to detect heterophile antibody is useful.

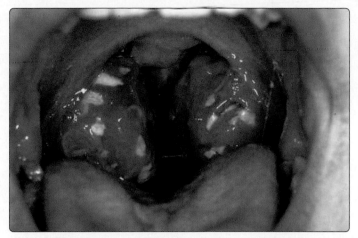

Fig. 3.1.2 Exudative tonsillitis.

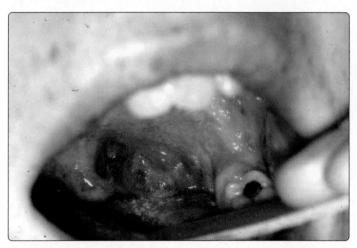

Fig. 3.1.3 A left-sided quinsy from which pus was aspirated.

Tonsillitis can be complicated by the development of a peritonsillar abscess (quinsy; Fig. 3.1.3). Features that suggest quinsy include unilateral sore throat, difficulty swallowing, difficulty opening the mouth owing to masseteric muscle spasm (trismus) and a nasal quality to the voice. Examination reveals a

BOX 3.1.1 THE HEIMLICH MANOEUVRE FOR DISLODGING INHALED FOREIGN BODIES

1. Stand behind the patient
2. Encircle your arms around the upper part of the abdomen just below the patient's rib cage
3. Give a sharp forceful squeeze, forcing the diaphragm sharply into the thorax.

This should expel sufficient air from the lungs to force the foreign body out of the trachea.

unilateral swollen tonsil. Treatment of uncomplicated tonsillitis is with oral phenoxymethylpenicillin (penicillin V). Aspiration of pus is required if a quinsy is present.

Epiglottitis

Epiglottitis is a potentially life-threatening disorder caused by *H. influenzae* type B, which can produce airway obstruction. It is less common in those over 5 years of age. Symptoms include fever, drooling and difficulty swallowing and breathing; affected individuals are usually systemically unwell. The epiglottis is swollen and reddened but should not be visualized unless immediate airway assistance is available. Treatment is with broad-spectrum antibiotics such as a third-generation cephalosporin.

Foreign body inhalation

Foreign body inhalation occurs more commonly in children, although adults can sometimes inhale foreign bodies such as a tooth or peanut. Foreign bodies usually become lodged in the right bronchial tree because the angle leading to the right main bronchus is less acute. In an emergency situation, the Heimlich manoeuvre (Box 3.1.1) should be performed, although some patients require removal of the foreign body through a rigid bronchoscope. Complications of foreign body inhalation include pneumonia, abscess formation or post-obstructive bronchiectasis.

2. Asthma

Questions
- What are the main steps in the pharmacological management of chronic asthma?
- What is the management of severe acute asthma?

Epidemiology

Approximately 7.2% of the world's population (100 million) has asthma, including 6% of adults and 10% of children. In the UK, approximately 5.2 million (1.1 million children and 4.1 million adults) are currently receiving treatment for asthma and 8 million have been diagnosed at some stage in their lives. Asthma affects people in one in five UK households and is more common in urban than rural areas. Although most patients control their asthma with inhaled therapy, it causes at least 40 000 deaths per year worldwide and a death every 7 h in the UK.

Pathogenesis

Both bronchial smooth muscle dysfunction and inflammation of the airways lead to symptoms of asthma (Fig. 3.2.1). Inflammatory cells release cytokines, resulting in oedema and epithelial cell damage with excess mucus production. Asthma is often triggered by IgE-mediated reactions to specific allergens (e.g. house dust mite, animal danders or pollens; Fig. 3.2.2). **Atopy** is an inherited predisposition to develop allergic disease (e.g. asthma, eczema or rhinitis) that is confirmed by positive skin prick tests or specific IgE antibodies to common allergens.

Clinical features

Classic symptoms include wheeze, chest tightness, breathlessness and cough. These symptoms are variable and intermittent, often nocturnal and cause night-time disturbance, and provoked by particular triggers or allergens. Chest examination may be normal, although expiratory wheeze is often present during an exacerbation.

Investigations

All patients with suspected asthma should have spirometry. If symptoms are typical and spirometry normal or obstructive, empirical treatment should be started. If spirometry has a restrictive pattern or the symptoms are not entirely typical of asthma, a challenge test (methacholine, mannitol or exercise) should be considered. Peak expiratory flow monitoring (PEF) (Fig. 3.2.3) can assess longer-term control.

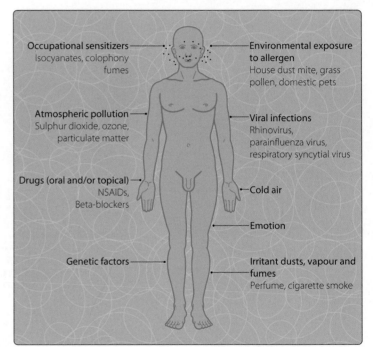

Fig. 3.2.2 Some of the causes and triggers of asthma.

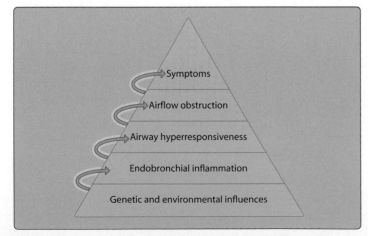

Fig. 3.2.1 The pathophysiological hallmarks of asthma.

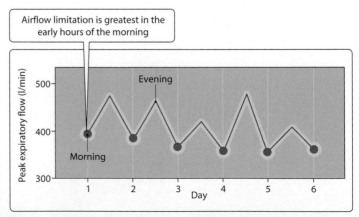

Fig. 3.2.3 Typical diurnal variation of poorly controlled asthma.

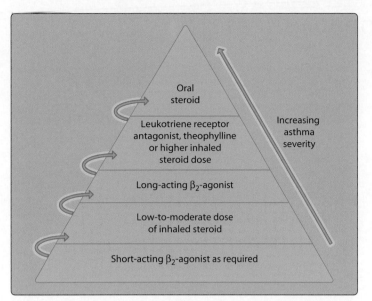

Fig. 3.2.4 The stepwise pharmacological management of chronic asthma.

Management

The most common delivery device is a pressurized metered dose inhaler (pMDI) but up to 50% of patients are unable to use this correctly and only 10% of the drug dose reaches the airways. Addition of a spacer reduces the problem of coordinating the activation of the device and inhalation.

Management (Fig. 3.2.4) aims to control symptoms, prevent of exacerbations and achieve best possible lung function. Good patient education is essential. Modern evidence-based guidelines advise a stepwise approach to drug therapy.

Step 1: mild intermittent asthma.   All patients should receive an inhaled short-acting β_2-agonist (e.g. salbutamol) for symptomatic relief. The use of two or more inhalers per month or greater than 10–12 puffs per day suggests poor control.

Step 2: introduction of regular preventative therapy.   Inhaled steroids are the drug of choice for prevention of asthma. In most adults, the starting dose is 400 µg beclometasone dipropionate per day in two divided doses or the equivalent dose of an alternative inhaled steroid. They should be considered for patients with any of the following: exacerbation of asthma requiring oral steroid in the last 2 years, using inhaled short-acting β_2-agonist three times a week or more or waking one night a week or more with respiratory symptoms.

Step 3: add-on therapy.   Adherence to treatment and inhaler technique should first be rechecked. The most effective add-on therapy in adults and children over 5 years is an inhaled long-acting β_2-agonist (LABA). These are available in combination inhalers with steroids. If there is no improvement, the LABA should be discontinued and inhaled steroid increased to 800 µg beclometasone dipropionate or equivalent.

Step 4: addition of a fourth drug.   For those with more severe asthma, a leukotriene receptor antagonist, higher dose of inhaled steroid or oral theophylline may be of benefit.

Step 5: continuous steroid tablets.   In a few patients with severe and brittle asthma, daily low-dose steroid tablets should be considered.

Prognosis

Many children will 'grow out of' asthma but most adults experience lifelong symptoms requiring treatment. However, if an allergic trigger or occupational cause can be found and removed, symptoms may resolve completely.

Acute asthma

Severe acute asthma is a common and life-threatening condition. Most deaths occur in those receiving inadequate inhaled or oral steroid or in those not followed up. Patients with severe acute asthma have any of the following:

- PEF < 50% best
- heart rate > 110/min
- respiratory rate > 25/min
- unable to complete sentences in one breath.

Treatment involves hospital admission for O_2, high-dose nebulized short-acting β_2-agonists and prednisolone 40 mg daily (or i.v. hydrocortisone). Magnesium i.v. or aminophylline may be necessary. Antibiotics are only necessary when there is purulent sputum, fever or consolidation on chest radiograph.

Occupational asthma

Occupational asthma is the commonest industrial lung disease and accounts for 10% of adult-onset asthma. Particularly helpful questions include whether symptoms improve on days away from work or on holiday. PEF recordings throughout the working week and during weekends and holidays can be diagnostic. Specific challenge tests and measurement of specific IgE may be helpful.

3. Chronic obstructive pulmonary disease

Questions
- What are the main clinical differences between asthma and chronic obstructive pulmonary disease?
- How do you manage an acute exacerbation of chronic obstructive pulmonary disease?

Chronic obstructive pulmonary disease (COPD) is characterized by progressive airflow obstruction that is not fully reversible and does not change markedly over several months. Around a million individuals in the UK have been diagnosed with COPD and it accounts for 5% of all deaths in the UK each year. Exacerbations of COPD are responsible for approximately 10% of all admissions to hospitals in the UK.

Pathogenesis
COPD is largely caused by prolonged cigarette smoking, although other factors (e.g. previous coal mining) have been implicated. An uncommon inherited form of progressive airflow obstruction is α_1-antitrypsin deficiency, which is characterized by development of symptoms at an early age. The main pathological features of COPD are mucous hypersecretion, tissue destruction and disruption of normal repair and defence mechanisms, causing small airway inflammation and fibrosis. These result in increased resistance to airflow in the small conducting airways, decreased compliance, air trapping and progressive airflow obstruction.

Clinical features
COPD should be considered in any current or previous smoker over 35 years of age who has any combination of breathlessness, chest tightness, wheeze, sputum production, cough, frequent chest infections and impaired exercise tolerance. Asthma is the main differential diagnosis (Table 3.3.1).

Physical examination can be normal in COPD but, signs include central cyanosis, hyperinflated chest, accessory muscle use, wheeze, diminished breath sounds and paradoxical movement of the lower ribs. **Cor pulmonale** is defined as right ventricular dilatation with consequent fluid retention caused by any chronic lung disorder with pulmonary hypertension (increasing afterload). Some patients with advanced COPD may have signs consistent with cor pulmonale (raised jugular venous pressure, loud P2 owing to pulmonary hypertension, tricuspid regurgitation, pitting peripheral oedema and hepatomegaly). Skeletal muscle wasting and weight loss are common in advanced COPD.

Table 3.3.1 CLINICAL DIFFERENTIATION OF ASTHMA AND CHRONIC OBSTRUCTIVE PULMONARY DISEASE (COPD)

	COPD	Asthma
Age	> 35 years	Any age
Cough	Persistent and productive	Intermittent and non-productive
Smoking	Almost invariable	Possible
Breathlessness	Progressive and persistent	Intermittent and variable
Nocturnal symptoms	Uncommon unless severe disease	Common
Family history	Uncommon unless family members also smoke	Common
Concomitant eczema or allergic rhinitis	Possible	Common

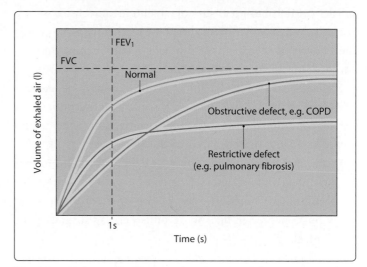

Fig. 3.3.1 Volume–time curves showing normal, restrictive and obstructive patterns with spirometry. In obstructive disease, the forced expiratory volume in 1s (FEV_1) is reduced and its ratio to the forced vital capacity (FCV) is < 0.7. In restrictive disorders, both the FEV_1 and the FVC are reduced and the FEV_1/FVC ratio is ≥ 0.7.

Investigations
Spirometry is essential in the diagnosis of COPD (Fig. 3.3.1). It measures the forced expiratory volume in 1 second (FEV_1) and forced vital capacity (FVC). In COPD, the FEV_1 is always reduced to < 80% predicted for a given patient's height, age and sex, and the FEV_1/FVC ratio is < 0.7.

Arterial blood gas measurement assesses pH, bicarbonate and the partial pressures of CO_2 and O_2 (Po_2 and Pco_2, respectively).

Type 1 or type 2 respiratory failure can occur in COPD (see The big picture).

Chest radiograph is useful in excluding other conditions and may show hyperinflation.

FBC may show polycythaemia secondary to hypoxia, with haematocrit > 0.55.

Echocardiogram may show right heart dilatation and elevated indirect pulmonary artery pressures confirms cor pulmonale.

Management

Management should be staged to meet the level of impairment (Fig. 3.3.2). Lifestyle advice includes smoking cessation, maintenance of optimal weight and pulmonary rehabilitation. Patients should be offered annual influenza immunization and a single pneumococcal vaccination.

A short-acting inhaled bronchodilator (β_2-agonist) is used as required. In persistent symptoms and exacerbations, a regular long-acting bronchodilator (β_2-agonist or anticholinergic drug) should be added. Regular high-dose inhaled steroid should also be prescribed for $FEV_1 < 50\%$ predicted and frequent exacerbations (over two per year).

Theophylline is an oral non-selective phosphodiesterase inhibitor with weak bronchodilator effects. It should be reserved for patients with advanced disease who have persistent symptoms or are intolerant of inhaled treatments. Oral steroids have a limited role in chronic management.

Long-term O_2 therapy for over 15 h/day improves survival and quality of life in patients who are sufficiently hypoxic ($Po_2 < 7.3$ kPa when clinically stable on two separate occasions 3 weeks apart) or who have cor pulmonale, secondary polycythaemia or pulmonary hypertension. Oxygen can be provided by an O_2 concentrator, which extracts nitrogen from room air. Long-term O_2 therapy is contraindicated in smokers because of the fire risk.

Exacerbations of disease

Exacerbations are mainly caused by viruses, bacteria or environmental pollutants, although the precise cause usually remains unknown. Typical features include increased breathlessness, cough, sputum volume or purulence, wheeze and chest tightness.

Management

Management involves controlled O_2 (24 or 28%), high-dose nebulized or inhaled bronchodilators and oral steroids. Aminophylline, the i.v. formulation of theophylline, is sometimes used in more severe exacerbations. Antibiotics are useful if bacterial infection is likely.

In exacerbations with mild-to-moderate respiratory acidosis (pH 7.26–7.35), a close-fitting face or nose mask connected to a cycled ventilator facilitates non-invasive respiratory support. This is useful in off-loading tiring respiratory muscles, reducing the work of breathing, improving alveolar ventilation and oxygenation and increasing CO_2 elimination.

Severity	At risk	Mild	Moderate	Severe
Spirometry	$FEV_1 > 80\%$	FEV_1 50–80% of predicted	FEV_1 30–50% of predicted	$FEV_1 < 30\%$ of predicted
Symptoms	With or without chronic cough and sputum production	Progression of symptoms + breathlessness	>2 exacerbations per year	Impaired quality of life, exacerbations life threatening
Treatment				Consider assessment for long-term oxygen therapy if non-smoker
			Consider specialist referral Add high-dose inhaled steroid to reduce exacerbations (this will usually be prescribed in combination with long-acting β_2-agonist) Add a further long-acting bronchodilator	
		Consider pulmonary rehabilitation Add a long-acting bronchodilator (anticholinergic or β_2-agonist)		
	If symptomatic: use short-acting β_2-agonist and or anticholinergic as necessary **Avoid risk factors:** influenza and pneumoccal vaccinations **Assess for anxiety and depression:** screen in all with COPD and treat conventionally			
	Offer help for smoking cessation at every opportunity			

Fig. 3.3.2 Overview of the management of chronic obstructive pulmonary disease.

4. Pneumonia

Questions
- What are the main clinical signs of pneumonia?
- How do you assess the severity of pneumonia?

Infections of the lower respiratory tract are very common, particularly during the winter months. They can involve the trachea or bronchi (tracheitis or bronchitis) or the parenchyma of the lung (pneumonia). Pneumonia can be classified into community-acquired, hospital-acquired (nosocomial) or those occurring in the immunocompromised.

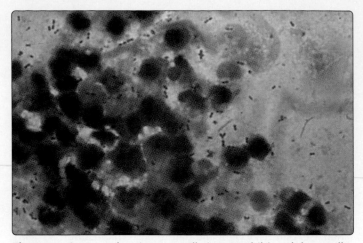

Fig. 3.4.1 Sputum showing pus cells (neutrophils) and the small Gram-positive diplococci of *S. pneumoniae*.

Epidemiology
Community-acquired pneumonia occurs in 5–11 per 1000 adult population per year and each GP in the UK deals with approximately 10 adults and 12 children with pneumonia annually. Between 22 and 42% of adults with community-acquired pneumonia are admitted to hospital and 5–10% of these require intensive therapy. Mortality in the community is <1%. In hospital, mortality rises to 6–12% and may be as high as 50% for those requiring intensive care. Despite modern antibiotics, pneumonia remains the second commonest cause of death in the Western world.

Pathogenesis
Streptococcus pneumoniae (pneumococcus) remains the commonest cause of community-acquired pneumonia. *Mycoplasma pneumoniae* is probably the next most common pathogen and has a cyclical pattern with clusters of cases every 4 years. *Legionella* spp. infection is associated with water systems in modern buildings. Pneumonia caused by *Staphylococcus aureus* occurs during influenza epidemics and has a high mortality. Occasionally there are chemical causes such as aspiration pneumonia.

Clinical features
Community-acquired pneumonia is usually an acute illness, sometimes preceded by symptoms of upper respiratory tract infection. Most patients are breathless, with cough and sputum production (classically rusty coloured in pneumococcal pneumonia; Fig. 3.4.1), sometimes associated with pleuritic chest pain. Pneumonia caused by mycoplasma and chlamydia presents with more general symptoms such as malaise, sweating, myalgia, arthralgia and headache. Haemoptysis does not generally occur in pneumonia, and its presence should raise the possibility of malignancy.

High fever and rigors are common in younger patients and in those with pneumococcal and legionella infection. Herpes labialis (cold sore) is seen in approximately one-third of those with pneumococcal pneumonia. Classical signs of lung consolidation are often found and include dullness to percussion, bronchial breathing and localized inspiratory crackles. Patients with severe pneumonia may also have signs of septicaemia, confusion, hypotension and rapid respiratory rate.

Investigations
The following investigations are used:
- sputum: Gram stain can give rapid indication of the pathogen involved, and subsequent culture should be arranged
- blood cultures should always be performed in hospital before giving antibiotics
- chest radiograph shows consolidation or in some cases a pleural effusion (parapneumonic effusion; Fig. 3.4.2).
- pleural fluid should be aspirated, cultured and examined for cytology; most effusions are straw coloured (parapneumonic) but if pH <7.2 a complicated parapneumonic effusion or empyema (pus in the pleural space) is present
- urinary antigen tests for pneumococci and legionella are increasingly useful
- serology for IgG antibodies and cold agglutinins (IgM) are needed for *M. pneumoniae*.

Assessment of severity
Severity assessment is important to guide management. A widely used score is CURB-65, which identifies five simple parameters that are associated with increased risk of death (Table 3.4.1):
- confusion
- urea >7 mmol/l: indicating multiorgan failure and septicaemia
- respiratory rate ≥30/min: strongly associated with hypoxia and increased mortality
- blood pressure: diastolic ≤60 mmHg or systolic <90 mmHg
- aged 65 years or over.

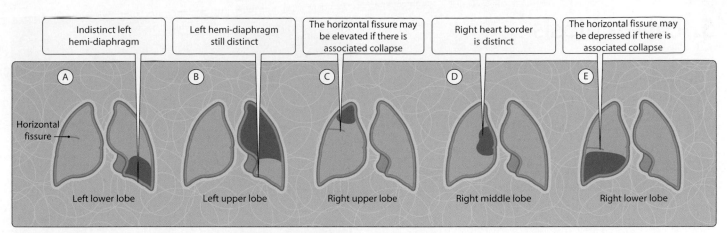

Fig. 3.4.2 Typical areas of consolidation in lobar pneumonia on a chest radiograph.

Table 3.4.1 USE OF THE CURB-65 SCORE TO ASSESS SEVERITY IN PNEUMONIA

Score	Management	Mortality
0–1	Likely to be suitable for home treatment	Low (2%)
2	Consider hospital admission	Intermediate (9%)
≥3	Manage as 'severe pneumonia'; assess for admission to intensive care, particularly if score is 4 or 5	High (22%)

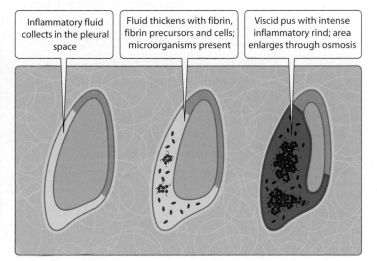

Fig. 3.4.3 Features of a developing empyema.

Other poor prognostic signs are multilobe involvement and hypoxia (pulse oximetry (S_pO_2) < 92%).

Management

Patients should be advised to rest, take plenty of fluids and be encouraged not to smoke. Paracetamol may be helpful for relief of fever or pleuritic pain. Continuous O_2 may be required if O_2 saturation < 94% or Po_2 < 8 kPa. Antibiotics should cover the likely organism including *S. pneumoniae*.

Non-severe pneumonia treated at home or in hospital. Oral antibiotics, amoxicillin, for 7 days or a macrolide (clarithromycin) or quinolone (e.g. levofloxacin) for those with penicillin allergy.

Hospital-treated severe pneumonia. Intravenous antibiotics, coamoxiclav and clarithromycin, and assess the patient rapidly for the need for high-dependency or intensive care.

Complications

Patients with pneumonia who fail to improve should be reviewed for an alternative or additional diagnosis such as lung cancer or pulmonary oedema. While uncomplicated parapneumonic effusions (pH > 7.2) do not usually require drainage, a complicated pleural effusion (pleural fluid pH < 7.2) or empyema (Fig. 3.4.3) should be drained. Lung abscess is rare and often caused by anaerobic bacteria.

Prevention

Annual influenza vaccination is recommended for those at 'high risk' of death from influenza or pneumonia: chronic lung, heart, renal and liver diseases, diabetes mellitus, immunosuppression or those aged over 65 years. Pneumococcal polysaccharide vaccine is also recommended for those aged 2 years or older, in whom pneumococcal infection is likely to be more common, particularly high-risk groups and those aged over 65 years. Pneumococcal vaccination should not be repeated within 3 years.

5. Tuberculosis

Questions
- What factors are causing a rise in tuberculosis?
- What is the treatment of pulmonary tuberculosis?

Tuberculosis (TB) is at least as old as mankind and remains one of the major infectious diseases across the world. Global poverty and HIV are largely responsible for its persistence into the 21st century.

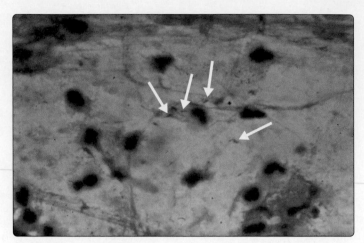

Fig. 3.5.1 Gram stain showing acid– and alcohol-fast bacilli (red rods, arrowed).

Epidemiology

Of the current 6 billion world population, approximately 2 billion are infected with *Mycobacterium tuberculosis* and 8–9 million of these present as new cases of TB each year; 10% of infections occur as coinfection with HIV. Additionally, 3–4 million are sputum smear positive and, therefore, highly infectious. Half the new cases of TB occur in India, China, Indonesia, Pakistan and Bangladesh. Across the world, there are 3 million deaths from TB each year.

Notifications for TB have declined across western and central Europe and the Middle East since 1980, have remained relatively static in southeast Asia and Latin America, and have increased in Africa and eastern Europe. Factors contributing to the rise in TB include the HIV pandemic, displacement and migration, poverty, disruptions to healthcare infrastructure, poorly managed TB programmes and drug resistance. In the UK, the progressive fall in TB notifications during the 20th century has now stopped and there is a notable rise in London, largely in those born abroad. TB in individuals born in the UK remains commonest in the elderly, while TB in those born abroad peaks in those aged 20–40 years.

Pathogenesis

TB is caused by *M. tuberculosis*. Patients with pulmonary TB should be considered infectious if they have a cough productive of sputum that is smear positive on Ziehl–Neelsen staining for acid- and alcohol-fast bacilli (Fig. 3.5.1). Individuals with pulmonary cavitation tend to be more infectious, while children under the age of 12 years with primary pulmonary tuberculosis are rarely infectious.

Clinical features

Nearly all primary infections are asymptomatic, even in close household contacts of sputum smear-positive cases. Occasionally in children, local hilar lymphadenopathy can cause bronchial narrowing and pleural effusion (Fig. 3.5.2).

Weight loss, fever and night sweats are common. Chest auscultation is often normal, despite gross abnormalities on the chest radiograph.

Miliary tuberculosis results from tubercle bacilli spreading through the bloodstream and producing widespread miliary lesions, most notably in the lungs. Symptoms are usually insidious and include fever, weight loss, malaise and anorexia.

Symptoms of post-primary pulmonary TB include malaise together with a cough, which may become productive of purulent sputum, and haemoptysis. Post-primary non-pulmonary TB can occur in a wide variety of sites including the kidneys, bone and joints, abdomen (causing ascites), female genital tract and the CNS (causing TB meningitis).

Investigations

Sputum examination by auramine (screening) and Ziehl–Neelsen staining with eventual culture are essential to the diagnosis of pulmonary TB. PCR techniques can confirm M. tuberculosis infection before full sputum culture is available. In patients with non-pulmonary TB, samples for culture should be obtained before starting treatment, for example ascitic fluid, pleural effusion, early morning urine in renal TB and CSF in suspected TB meningitis. The sensitivity of PCR in these situations is low. Occasionally, biopsy with culture (e.g. of liver or bone) may be necessary.

Chest radiograph may show areas of consolidation and cavitation (Fig. 3.5.3), particularly in the lung apices. Cavitation is less likely in immunosuppressed patients coinfected with HIV. Other chest radiograph changes include widespread nodules or pleural effusion.

Bronchoscopy with culture of bronchial washings is necessary in some cases of suspected but unproven TB.

Management

Tuberculosis is a notifiable disease. Patients infectious with smear-positive pulmonary tuberculosis should be isolated for 2 weeks while those with non-pulmonary TB are not infectious.

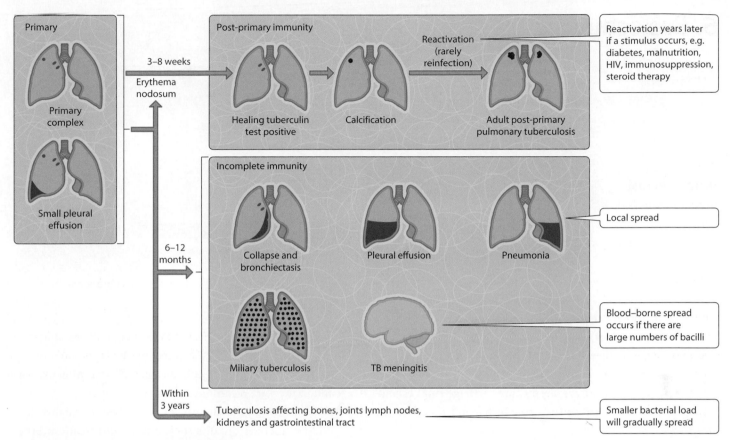

Fig. 3.5.2 Features of primary and post-primary tuberculosis.

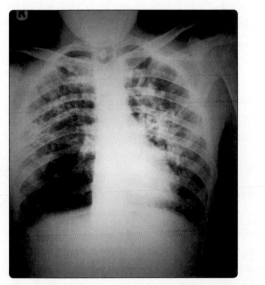

Fig. 3.5.3 Chest radiograph showing bilateral cavitation and consolidation in the upper zone caused by untreated pulmonary tuberculosis.

Treatment of tuberculosis should start with four first-line drugs: rifampicin, isoniazid, pyrazinamide and ethambutol. These drugs are all taken once daily before breakfast, with the first three usually in the form of a combination tablet. This regimen is continued for 2 months, while waiting confirmation of the diagnosis and full drug sensitivities. Thereafter, the regimen is simplified into two drugs to which the organism is sensitive (usually rifampicin and isoniazid). This continuation phase is completed after 4 months, a total of 6 months of treatment, except for CNS infection and meningitis, when a continuation phase of 10 months is recommended.

Multidrug-resistant tuberculosis
In the UK, approximately 10% of TB isolates have single drug resistance, most commonly to isoniazid. Unfortunately, multidrug-resistant *M. tuberculosis* (MDRTB), resistant to both rifampicin and isoniazid, is becoming increasingly common. This has occurred because of the use of rifampicin or isoniazid as single agents. MDRTB is no more infectious than 'ordinary' TB. Management of MDRTB is complex, relies on second-line drugs with significant side-effects and should be carried out in specialist units.

Prevention
BCG vaccine is made with an attenuated strain of *Mycobacterium bovis*. The efficacy of BCG varies across the world and seems least effective in those countries bordering the equator. Because the prevalence of TB is relatively low in the UK, the school BCG vaccination programme was disbanded in 2005, but BCG should still be offered to high-risk populations such as children born into immigrant populations.

6. Bronchiectasis and cystic fibrosis

Questions
- What are the underlying causes of bronchiectasis?
- What are the main features of cystic fibrosis in an adult?

Bronchiectasis

Bronchiectasis is defined as an irreversible dilatation of the distal airways (bronchi) which predisposes to chronic infection. Its prevalence is not known but it is less common where antibiotics are available.

Pathogenesis

Although the precise aetiology can remain unknown, in many individuals, a cause of bronchiectasis can be identified (Table 3.6.1). Damage to the bronchial wall leads to pooling of secretions, permanent airway dilatation and chronic infection (Fig. 3.6.1). Where there are supporting cartilage rings dilatation is prevented and it is the bronchi beyond this that are affected.

Clinical features

Typical features include cough, breathlessness, excessive sputum production, haemoptysis, weight loss and malaise. During an exacerbation, patients typically report worsening cough and breathlessness in conjunction with a greater volume and purulence of sputum. Clinical signs include coarse lung crackles, typically heard in inspiration and expiration, and wheeze over the affected areas of lung. In long-standing disease, finger clubbing can develop. Complications of bronchiectasis include:

- bronchopneumonia, lung abscess, empyema
- infective metastatic spread, e.g. cerebral abscess
- massive and life-threatening haemoptysis
- secondary amyloidosis
- progressive respiratory failure
- cor pulmonale.

Investigations

Chest radiograph may show dilated bronchi with thickened walls (so-called tramlines). High-resolution CT typically shows large-calibre bronchioles that fail to taper and have a greater diameter than the associated pulmonary artery (Fig. 3.6.2). Sputum culture helps to tailor antibiotic therapy and exclude active tuberculosis. Spirometry can be normal in bronchiectasis but airflow obstruction may occur.

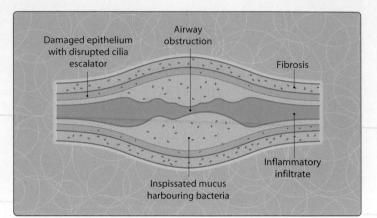

Fig. 3.6.1 Pathological features of the airway in bronchiectasis.

Management

Autogenic drainage. Patients should be taught the technique to enable them to clear airway secretions daily.

Immunization. Pneumococcal vaccination and influenza immunization are recommended for most patients.

Antibiotics. Antibiotics are usually prescribed in a higher dose and for a longer duration (e.g. 2 weeks) to treat exacerbations of bronchiectasis. In those with repeated infections and deteriorating lung function, long-term oral or nebulized antibiotics are sometimes used. In advanced disease, *Pseudomonas aeruginosa* can colonize the airways.

Inhaled treatment. Inhaled long-acting bronchodilators are used if airflow obstruction is present, while inhaled steroids may slow disease progression.

Surgery. Occasionally patients with very localized disease can have the affected lobe removed.

Cystic fibrosis

Cystic fibrosis is a multisystem disease characterized by increased mucous viscosity and resulting in frequent respiratory tract infections and pancreatic insufficiency (Fig. 3.6.3). It commonly presents in neonates and infants and is the most common serious autosomal recessive condition affecting young people in Western populations. In the UK, the incidence is approximately 1 in 2500 live births, with a carrier rate of the responsible gene of 1 in 25.

Pathogenesis

The gene responsible for cystic fibrosis is found on chromosome 7 and encodes a protein known as the cystic fibrosis transmembrane conductance regulator (CFTR). This is found in many parts of the body (e.g. pancreas, reproductive tract, liver and sweat glands) and is part of a chloride channel. Mutated *CFTR* results in defective sodium and chloride transport across epithelial

Table 3.6.1 CAUSES OF BRONCHIECTASIS AND RELEVANT INVESTIGATIONS

Cause	Investigation
Post-infection	
Childhood measles, whooping cough or pneumonia	History
Chronic aspiration	History
Tuberculosis	Chest radiograph, sputum culture, microscopy and sensitivity
Hypersensitivity	
Allergic bronchopulmonary aspergillosis	*Aspergillus* precipitins, blood eosinophilia
Obstruction	
Inhalation of foreign body	Bronchoscopy
Tumour	Bronchoscopy, CT
Extrinsic compression from a lymph node	Bronchoscopy, CT
Systemic disease	
Rheumatoid arthritis	History, examination, rheumatoid factor
Coeliac disease	Endomysial antibodies
Inflammatory bowel disease	History
Abnormal host defence	
Immunoglobulin deficiency	Immunoglobulin levels
α_1-Antitrypsin deficiency	α_1-Antitrypsin levels
Ciliary dyskinesia/Kartagener's syndrome	Ciliary kinetic studies, electron microscopy of cells from nasal brushings

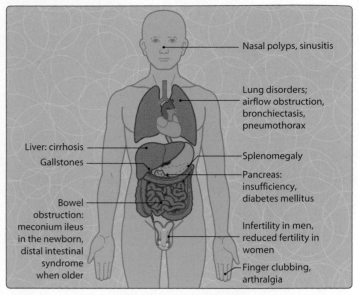

Fig. 3.6.3 The clinical features of cystic fibrosis.

cells. The most common mutation (ΔF508) is associated with severe respiratory disease and pancreatic insufficiency.

Clinical features

Newborn infants can present with meconium ileus, while young children present with failure to thrive, short stature, steatorrhoea and frequent chest infections.

Investigations

Immunoreactive trypsinogen is increased in newborns with cystic fibrosis (checked by a heel prick several days after birth). The sweat test uses pilocarpine iontophoresis (applying an electric current across a small portion of skin) to measure sodium and chloride in sweat, which is increased (especially chloride) in cystic fibrosis. Chest radiograph typically shows shadows and exaggerated bronchial markings consistent with chronic infection and eventually bronchiectasis. Lung function tests usually become obstructive as the disease progresses.

Management

Treatment is centred around a multidisciplinary approach.

Respiratory care. Infections are treated promptly with oral or i.v. antibiotics. Physiotherapy and autogenic drainage are also vital.

Nutrition. Adequate dietary intake must be ensured and fat-soluble vitamins are also required by most individuals. Pancreatic enzyme supplementation is necessary to aid absorption. Nasogastric or gastrostomy feeding may be required.

Liver disease. Ursodeoxycholic acid may reduce progression.

Transplantation. Lung transplantation in end-stage respiratory disease and liver transplantation in serious liver disease may be necessary.

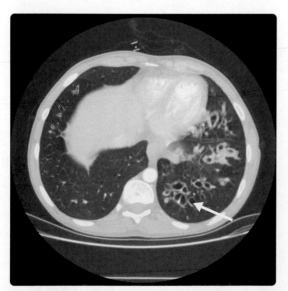

Fig. 3.6.2 High-resolution CT of bronchiectasis in a patient with cystic fibrosis showing dilated bronchi (arrow).

7. Lung cancer

Questions
- What investigations should be carried out in suspected lung cancer?
- What treatment options are available?

Lung cancer is a global health problem, particularly in developing countries, where cigarette smoking is increasing. Lung cancer is the most frequent cause of cancer death in both males and females in the UK. There are approximately 50 000 new cases and 45 000 deaths in the UK each year; 85% of cases occur in patients over 60 years and the incidence is higher, and survival poorer, in people of low socioeconomic status.

Pathogenesis
Lung cancer usually arises from the bronchial epithelial mucosa but can also originate in the lung parenchyma; it is divided histologically into small cell and non-small cell (squamous, adenocarcinoma and large cell). Current or previous cigarette smoking is responsible for up to 90% of cases. Risk is dependent and related to the tar content. Other risk factors implicated include passive smoking, asbestos, nickel, chromium, arsenic, radon and idiopathic pulmonary fibrosis.

Clinical features
Features suggesting lung cancer include haemoptysis, weight loss, poor appetite, increasing breathlessness and cough, especially in those aged over 50 years. Lung cancer may also present with diffuse chest pain caused by displacement of mediastinal structures, or more localized pain caused by pleural or bony metastasis (Fig. 3.7.1). **Pulmonary signs** include pleural effusion, monophonic wheeze, lobar collapse, stridor, hoarseness (recurrent laryngeal nerve involvement causing vocal cord paralysis). **Extrapulmonary signs** include finger clubbing, hypertrophic pulmonary osteoarthropathy, cervical lymphadenopathy and superior vena cava obstruction (facial and upper limb swelling and plethora, dilated superficial chest wall veins, engorged jugular veins). Ipsilateral partial ptosis, enophthalmos, miosis (small pupil) and periorbital loss of sweating can follow involvement of the cervical sympathetic nerve (Horner's syndrome). Wasting of the small muscles of the hand (Pancoast's syndrome) may occur with an apical lung cancer invading the brachial plexus.

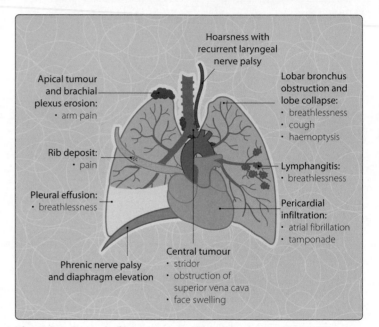

Fig. 3.7.1 Spread of lung cancer within the chest and associated symptoms.

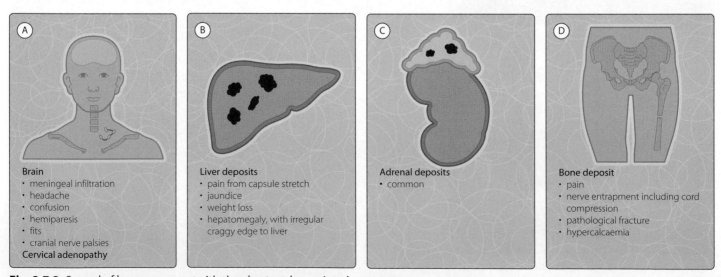

Fig. 3.7.2 Spread of lung cancer outwith the chest and associated symptoms.

Paraneoplastic syndromes (syndrome of inappropriate anti-diuretic hormone production and parathyroid-related peptide production causing hypercalcaemia) may occur in association with lung cancer.

Investigations

Chest radiograph may show a pulmonary mass, hilar lymph-adenopathy, pleural effusion, lobar collapse or rib metastasis.

Direct visualization and biopsy during bronchoscopy is usually needed. Cells for cytology can also be obtained from pleural fluid and from enlarged lymph nodes or metastases.

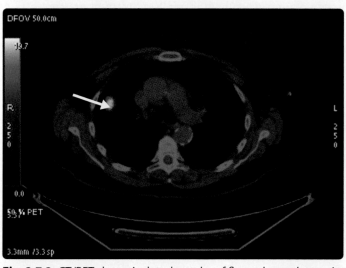

Fig. 3.7.3 CT/PET shows isolated uptake of fluorodeoxyglucose in a right upper lobe tumour (arrow).

Mediastinoscopy may be required to assess mediastinal lymph node involvement. In potentially operable early-stage cancer, positron emission tomography (PET) may be helpful to exclude distant metastases. Isotope bone scan is required in bony pain. CT head scan should be arranged if signs and symptoms suggestive of brain metastases are present.

Management

Management should be multidisciplinary. Non-small cell lung cancer is staged for prognosis and management using the TNM staging system (Table 3.7.1).

Small cell lung cancer is staged as being either limited (confined to the hemithorax of origin) or extensive. Those with limited disease should be treated with chemotherapy and radiotherapy if they are fit. As small cell lung cancer is very sensitive to chemotherapy, a complete response can be expected in up to 60% of patients. In patients with extensive disease, the prognosis is poor. Palliative chemotherapy for patients fit enough can assist symptom control, particularly haemoptysis, chest pain, dyspnoea and cough, but does not prolong life.

The 5-year survival in non-small cell lung cancer depends on stage and surgery with adjuvant chemotherapy offers the best chance of cure in early disease. Regardless of stage, the prognosis of small cell lung cancer is poor. Fewer than 10% of patients with lung cancer are alive 5 years after diagnosis.

Table 3.7.1 TNM CLASSIFICATION, STAGING, MANAGEMENT AND PROGNOSIS OF NON-SMALL CELL LUNG CANCER

Stage	Classification	Management options	5-year survival (%)
I	T1–2, N0	Surgery if fit; radical radiotherapy if not fit	60–80
II	T1–2, N1 or T3, N0	Surgery if fit; radical radiotherapy if not fit	25–40
IIIa	T1–2, N2 or T3, N1–2	Surgery in selected cases; chemo-radiotherapy	10–30
IIIb	T4, any N, M0 or any T, N3, M0	Chemo-radiotherapy	<5
IV	Any M1	Chemotherapy if fit or best supportive care	<5

T, tumour size, N, lymph node involvement; M, metastatic involvement.

8. Pleural disorders

Questions
- How do you manage a tension pneumothorax?
- What are the main causes of a pleural effusion?

Pneumothorax

A pneumothorax is a collection of air in the pleural space and can be divided into primary, secondary, iatrogenic or traumatic according to aetiology. **Tension pneumothorax** occurs when the intrapleural pressure exceeds atmospheric pressure, resulting in reduced venous return to the heart, falling cardiac output and eventual cardiac arrest. In patients with preexisting lung disease, even a small pneumothorax can cause tension. In the UK, the annual frequency of a primary pneumothorax is approximately 18–28/100 000 for males and 1.2–6/100 000 for females. It is more common in current cigarette smokers.

Pathogenesis
Primary pneumothorax tends to occur in young, tall, thin males with no underlying lung disease. Rupture of an underlying small subpleural bleb or bulla is usually responsible. Secondary pneumothorax occurs when there is an underlying lung abnormality such as chronic obstructive pulmonary disease, asthma or rare conditions (e.g. lymphangioleiomymatosis or histiocystosis X). Iatrogenic pneumothorax is most commonly encountered during central vein cannulation or during a pleural procedure. Intubated patients being mechanically ventilated can develop a pneumothorax when high inspiratory inflation pressures cause pulmonary barotrauma. Traumatic pneumothorax can follow injury to the thorax.

Clinical features
Typical symptoms include an abrupt onset of pleuritic pain and breathlessness. Examination findings include reduced breath sounds, reduced chest expansion, hyper-resonant percussion note, tachycardia, tachypnoea, hypotension and (in tension) mediastinal shift to the contralateral side. Most individuals have reduced O_2 saturation with type 1 respiratory failure.

Investigations
Chest radiograph shows absent lung markings extending from the edge of visceral pleura (Fig. 3.8.1A). CT is performed when diagnostic uncertainty exists, prior to a surgical procedure or to exclude rare lung disorders.

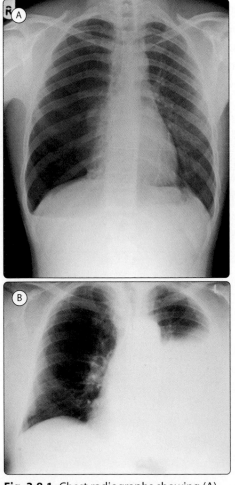

Fig. 3.8.1 Chest radiographs showing (A) a right-sided pneumothorax and (B) a left-sided pleural effusion.

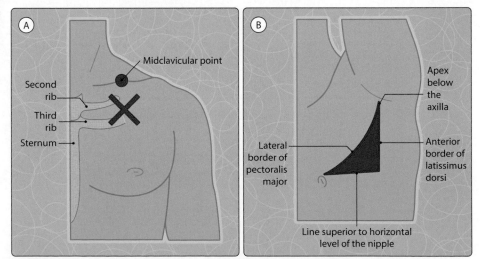

Fig. 3.8.2 Insertion of drains. (A) A venflon should be inserted into the second intercostal space in the mid-clavicular line in tension pneumothorax. (B) A chest drain should usually be inserted into the 'safe triangle' of the chest.

Management

Management depends on the severity of symptoms, size and presence of any underlying lung disease; 'small' size being < 2 cm between the lung edge and chest wall and 'large' when the rim is > 2 cm.

Primary spontaneous pneumothorax. If small and with few symptoms, no active intervention is required. Symptomatic or larger pneumothorax should undergo needle aspiration; if the pneumothorax fails to resolve, an underwater intercostal drain is required.

Secondary pneumothorax. If small with few symptoms, overnight observation is required but a symptomatic or larger pneumothorax usually requires chest drain insertion as needle aspiration tends to be less successful (Fig 3.8.2B).

Tension pneumothorax. This is a medical emergency and treatment will be necessary immediately (Fig. 3.8.2A).

Recurrent pneumothorax. The recurrence rate for primary pneumothorax is at least 20% after the first episode, 40% after the second. Patients with a first spontaneous pneumothorax who have a second ipsilateral pneumothorax, bilateral pneumothorax or first contralateral pneumothorax should be referred for surgical pleurodesis to ablate the pleural space.

Pleural effusion

A pleural effusion is an accumulation of an abnormal amount of fluid in the pleural space. It should be distinguished from a haemothorax, chylothorax and empyema, which are collections of blood, chyle and pus, respectively, in the pleural space.

Pathogenesis

The pleural surfaces (visceral and parietal pleura) are normally lubricated by a small amount of fluid. Changes in the hydrostatic or oncotic pressure can result in the accumulation of pleural fluid with low protein content (**transudate**, protein < 30 g/l); while inflammatory, obstructive or neoplastic conditions produce an **exudate** of higher protein concentration (> 30 g/l). Causes of a transudate include heart, liver or renal failure, hypothyroidism, peritoneal dialysis, or constrictive pericarditis. Causes of an exudate include infection, pulmonary embolism, cancer, connective tissue disease, subphrenic abscess, pancreatitis, drugs (e.g. amiodarone), Meig's syndrome (benign ovarian fibroma with pleural effusion) and Dressler's syndrome (after myocardial infarction or cardiac surgery).

Clinical features

Progressive breathlessness is the most common symptom of a pleural effusion. Features which can help to determine its cause include:

- haemoptysis, weight loss and previous or current smoking (malignant effusion)
- purulent sputum and fever (parapneumonic effusion)
- previous asbestos exposure (mesothelioma or benign asbestos effusion)
- pleuritic chest pain (pulmonary embolism)
- orthopnoea and ankle swelling (heart failure).

Typical findings include stony dull percussion note, reduced breath sounds, reduced chest expansion, bronchial breathing on top of the effusion and mediastinal shift in massive effusions.

Investigations

Chest radiograph shows an obliterated costophrenic angle with dense opacification and a curved upper border (Fig 3.8.1B). Chest wall ultrasound can localize the area most suited to aspirate pleural fluid. Fluid should be sent for sugar and protein measurement, microscopy, culture and cytology. Other tests include amylase (high in pancreatitis), pH (<7.2 in empyema) and lactate dehydrogenase (LDH, high in exudates). A blood-stained effusion suggests pulmonary embolism or malignancy; straw colour is consistent with any cause, and blood, pus and milky fluid suggest a haemothorax, empyema and chylothorax, respectively. Pleural biopsy is useful in diagnosing tuberculosis, mesothelioma or other malignancies. CT and bronchoscopy may be needed.

Some patients with an undiagnosed pleural effusion require inspection and biopsy of the pleural cavity using a video-assisted thoracoscopic (VATS) surgery.

Management

Management depends on the underlying cause. A transudate and a clinical picture in keeping with heart failure is treated with diuretics. In many exudates, the pleural fluid should be drained by an intercostal tube (Fig 3.8.2B), although care should be taken not to drain > 1.5 l/day. If cancer is identified, following complete drainage of fluid, a reaccumulation of fluid can be prevented by instillation of an irritant (such as talc) through the intercostal tube.

9. Interstitial lung disorders I

Questions
- What investigations should be carried out in suspected interstitial lung disease?
- What are the clinical features of extrinsic allergic alveolitis?

Idiopathic pulmonary fibrosis

Idiopathic pulmonary fibrosis (IPF) is a disease affecting the interstitium of the lung (Fig. 3.9.1). This is the microscopic space forming part of the blood–gas barrier. IPF is associated with the light microscopy appearance of 'usual interstitial pneumonia', in which 'pneumonia' is used to indicate inflammation (rather than infection).

Epidemiology

IPF is relatively uncommon, with prevalence estimated at 7–20/100 000 population. It is a disease predominately of the elderly, with a mean age of onset of 67 years. It is also slightly more common in males and in those with a history of smoking (Fig. 3.9.2). Familial IPF is rare, although clustering within families is recognized.

Pathogenesis

The exact cause of IPF is unknown. Various environmental stimuli have been suggested as risk factors for developing IPF, such as cigarette smoking, antidepressants, chronic aspiration, metal and wood dusts and infectious agents.

Clinical features

Typical symptoms of IPF include chronic, progressive, exertional breathlessness, accompanied by a non-productive cough. Examination frequently reveals fine end-inspiratory crackles at the lung bases. Up to 50% of patients have finger clubbing and those with advanced disease may develop cor pulmonale.

Investigations

Spirometry can be normal in early disease, but as the disease progresses, the forced expiratory volume in 1 second (FEV_1) and forced vital capacity (FVC) both fall, resulting in a restrictive ventilatory defect. Further tests show reduced lung volumes, impaired gas transfer and O_2 desaturation during exercise.

Chest radiograph may be normal in early IPF, although as the disease progresses changes include reduction in lung volumes with peripheral and basal fibrotic changes. High-resolution CT can estimate disease severity and distribution.

Lung biopsies can be obtained using video-assisted thoracoscopic surgery (VATS).

A strongly positive rheumatoid factor or anti-nuclear antibody raises the possibility of associated connective tissue disease.

Management

Once the diagnosis of IPF is established, it is reasonable to wait for 6 months and decide whether clinical, radiological or physiological deterioration occurs. If so, treatment with steroids and immunosuppressive drugs should be considered.

If the patient is < 60 years of age with no comorbidities, lung transplantation should be considered. Long-term O_2 therapy is often required in hypoxic patients with advanced disease. In end-stage disease, benzodiazepines or opiates can reduce breathlessness.

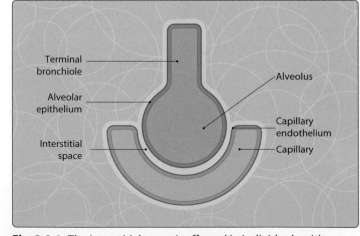

Fig. 3.9.1 The interstitial space is affected in individuals with pulmonary fibrosis.

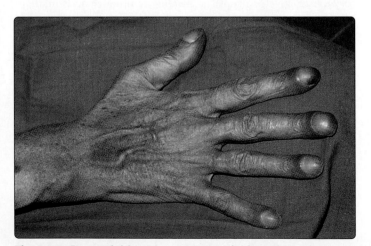

Fig. 3.9.2 Finger clubbing in a patient with idiopathic pulmonary fibrosis.

Prognosis

Untreated IPF follows a relentlessly progressive course in most patients, and median survival is approximately 3 years.

Extrinsic allergic alveolitis

Extrinsic allergic alveolitis (EAA), or hypersensitivity pneumonitis, is caused by inhalation of fine particles, although it is also associated with some oral drugs. The clinical presentations are divided into acute and subacute, with continuous low-level exposure to antigen leading to a chronic form.

Epidemiology

The prevalence of EAA is unknown, although bird fancier's lung and farmer's lung are the two most common forms.

Pathogenesis

The responsible antigen causes an inflammatory response (typically a type III or IV hypersensitivity reaction) affecting the alveoli, lung parenchyma and bronchioles. In the acute form of EAA, the lungs become infiltrated by mononuclear cells and neutrophils, while the subacute form is characterized by infiltration by lymphocytes. In chronic EAA, non-caseating epithelioid granulomas develop with progressive lung fibrosis.

Clinical features

In acute EAA, symptoms typically develop 4–12 h following exposure to the antigen, for example at the workplace. Classic features include flu-like symptoms (fevers, chills, myalgia, malaise) and breathlessness, cough and chest tightness. In subacute and chronic EAA, symptoms have a slow insidious onset. It is important to ask about pets, hobbies, drugs and previous or present occupations as these may be implicated in the development of EAA. Known antigens include:

- thermophilic actinomycetes fungus, e.g. mouldy hay or vegetation, causing farmer's lung
- mushroom compost, causing mushroom worker's lung
- *Aspergillus* sp. on barley, causing maltworker's lung
- proteins on feathers and in excreta, causing bird fancier's lung in those handling or cleaning birds
- *Penicillin casei* on mouldy cheese, causing cheese maker's lung
- *Botrytis* in grape mould, causing wine maker's lung.

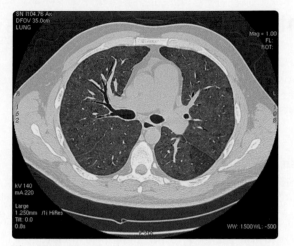

Fig. 3.9.3 Chest high-resolution CT showing classic ground-glass changes in a patient with bird fancier's lung.

Examination frequently reveals tachypnoea and fine inspiratory bibasal crackles. Providing the patient is no longer exposed, the signs and symptoms resolve spontaneously within a couple of days. In chronic EAA, finger clubbing is occasionally found.

Investigations

Spirometry is frequently restrictive in patients with established EAA and the gas transfer also tends to be impaired. Patients with EAA can develop type 1 respiratory failure, and during a 6 min walk the O_2 saturation falls.

Chest radiograph may show reticulonodular changes in the acute and subacute forms, while chronic EAA results in diffuse pulmonary fibrosis with an upper zone predilection. High-resolution CT classically shows ground-glass changes, with fibrosis and honeycombing in advanced disease (Fig. 3.9.3).

IgG antibodies in the blood generally suggest exposure rather than disease.

Lung biopsy may be required to confirm diagnosis.

Management

All patients with EAA should avoid further antigen exposure. In patients where complete avoidance may be difficult, for example farmers with mouldy hay, protective masks with filters are required. In individuals with a combination of functional, radiological and physiological impairment, oral steroids may be required.

10. Interstitial lung disorders II

Questions
- What are the extrapulmonary manifestations of sarcoidosis?
- What treatments are available for sarcoidosis?

Sarcoidosis

Sarcoidosis is a multisystem granulomatous disorder that can affect almost any organ of the body, but most frequently the lungs (Fig. 3.10.1). Other granulomatous disease processes include tuberculosis, extrinsic allergic alveolitis and fungal disease.

Epidemiology

Sarcoidosis can occur at any age but typically affects young adults aged 20–40 years, although a second smaller peak is observed in those aged over 50 years. It is more commonly found in black Americans, who develop more severe disease than whites. In the UK, the prevalence is roughly 20/100 000 population with a slight female preponderance.

Pathogenesis

The characteristic histological feature is a non-caseating granuloma; this consists of accumulations of epithelioid cells, macrophages and T lymphocytes. The genetics of sarcoidosis are not clear, but the risk of being diagnosed with sarcoidosis increases significantly if a family member is affected. The cause is not known, although inhaled or transmissible agents such as Epstein–Barr virus, environmental mycobacteria, fungi and pine tree pollen have all been suggested.

Clinical features

Many patients have non-specific constitutional features such as fever, weight loss and malaise, while many others are asymptomatic and sarcoidosis is only discovered as an incidental chest radiograph finding. Acute sarcoidosis presents with bilateral hilar lymphadenopathy on chest radiography and the rash of erythema nodosum over the shins and forearms (Fig. 3.10.2). Painful red eyes suggestive of uveitis, or the facial skin eruption of lupus pernio are less common features. The combination of erythema nodosum and hilar lymphadenopathy is termed Lofgren's syndrome.

Investigations

ACE activity in serum is frequently raised in patients with sarcoidosis, although this is also seen in leprosy, tuberculosis and histoplasmosis.

Abnormalities in calcium metabolism arise from increased sensitivity to vitamin D, leading to increased absorption of calcium from the gut. This may lead to hypercalcaemia, hypercalcuria and renal stones.

Lung involvement is staged according to the extent of involvement as seen in chest radiographs (Table 3.10.1).

In some patients with sarcoidosis, particularly when atypical features are present, biopsy is required to confirm the diagnosis and exclude other conditions causing lymphadenopathy, such as lymphoma and tuberculosis. Possible biopsy sites include any lymph node (often by means of mediastinoscopy), skin lesions or any scar that has changed in appearance.

Management

In patients with asymptomatic disease, no treatment is required. Constitutional symptoms and arthralgia can be treated with simple analgesics and NSAIDs. Individuals require prolonged treatment with oral steroids if they have progressive parenchymal chest radiographic and pulmonary function abnormalities, cardiac and neurological involvement, hypercalcaemia, disfiguring skin lesions or uveitis.

Patients who present with hilar lymphadenopathy, arthralgia and fever tend to have a good prognosis, while features associated with a poorer prognosis include neurological, bone and cardiac involvement, older age and black race.

Uncommon interstitial lung disorders

Histiocytosis X. This is a rare disease (prevalence of 1 in 50 000) characterized histologically by Langerhan's cell histiocytosis. There is a wide variation in clinical presentation from unifocal bone lesions in older children to chest radiograph showing multiple small cysts (honeycomb lung), fibrosis or widespread nodular shadows. There is an increased risk of pneumothorax.

Lymphangioleiomyomatosis. This is an uncommon condition that affects females of child-bearing age. It is characterized by abnormal proliferation of airway smooth muscle cells and leads to cystic changes in the lung, pneumothoraces and respiratory failure. It can be associated with tuberous sclerosis. High-resolution CT demonstrates thin-walled cysts of variable size throughout both lung fields. There is no specific treatment, although in advanced disease, lung transplantation may be considered.

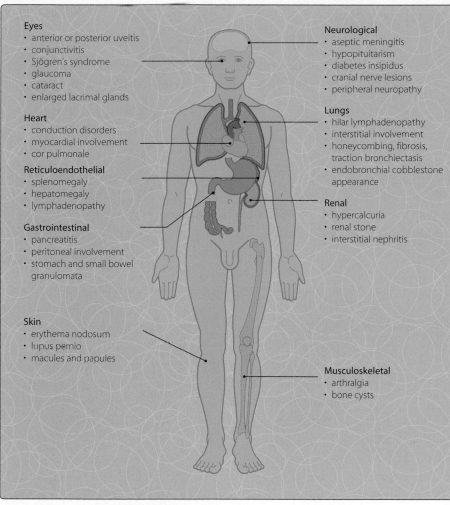

Eyes
- anterior or posterior uveitis
- conjunctivitis
- Sjögren's syndrome
- glaucoma
- cataract
- enlarged lacrimal glands

Heart
- conduction disorders
- myocardial involvement
- cor pulmonale

Reticuloendothelial
- splenomegaly
- hepatomegaly
- lymphadenopathy

Gastrointestinal
- pancreatitis
- peritoneal involvement
- stomach and small bowel granulomata

Skin
- erythema nodosum
- lupus pernio
- macules and papules

Neurological
- aseptic meningitis
- hypopituitarism
- diabetes insipidus
- cranial nerve lesions
- peripheral neuropathy

Lungs
- hilar lymphadenopathy
- interstitial involvement
- honeycombing, fibrosis, traction bronchiectasis
- endobronchial cobblestone appearance

Renal
- hypercalcuria
- renal stone
- interstitial nephritis

Musculoskeletal
- arthralgia
- bone cysts

Fig. 3.10.1 Clinical features of sarcoidosis.

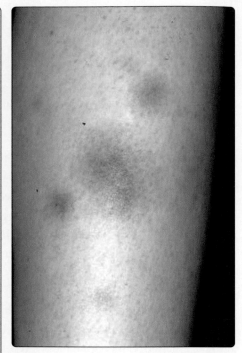

Fig. 3.10.2 A typical rash of erythema nodosum found in the anterior shins.

Table 3.10.1 GRADING OF PULMONARY SARCOIDOSIS ACCORDING TO DEGREE OF CHEST RADIOGRAPH INVOLVEMENT

Grade	Chest radiograph change
0	Normal
1	Bilateral hilar lymphadenopathy
2	Interstitial changes and bilateral hilar lymphadenopathy
3	Interstitial changes alone
4	Fibrosis and traction bronchiectasis

11. Occupational lung disorders

Questions
- What does pneumoconiosis mean and what can cause it?
- How may previous asbestos exposure affect the lungs?

Pneumoconiosis

The term pneumoconiosis refers to interstitial lung disease caused by inhalation of inorganic dusts. Even in the absence of ongoing exposure, the disease frequently progresses. In many cases, individuals have had exposure to the responsible agent over a prolonged period of time during their working life.

Epidemiology

The various pneumoconioses are found throughout the world and occur to differing extents depending on number of workers at risk, legislation, clinical awareness, level of exposure and availability of protective equipment.

Pathogenesis

Inhaled particles of 0.5–5 μm in diameter are able to reach the alveoli and cause damage to host cells. Particles larger and smaller than these tend to be deposited in the upper airways or larger airways of the bronchial tree. In the alveoli, host cells are activated and destroyed, which results in the release of inflammatory mediators, eventually causing lung fibrosis and impaired gas exchange. Several types of pneumoconiosis are shown in Table 3.11.1.

Clinical features

A good history is vital, to identify previous and present occupations and, in particular, exposure to dusts and chemicals. As in many other chronic lung conditions, progressive breathlessness and cough are the main features. Chest examination can be normal, although crackles and wheeze may be heard. In advanced disease, signs of cor pulmonale are present. Coal workers with

Table 3.11.1 TYPES OF PNEUMOCONIOSIS

Disease	Responsible agent	Occupation
Coal worker's pneumoconiosis	Coal dust	Miners
Silicosis	Silicon dioxide	Quarry workers, sandblasters, stonecutters
Stannosis	Tin	Tin workers
Berylliosis	Beryllium	Electronic and nuclear industries

rheumatoid arthritis can develop well-defined rounded lesions that grow to 0.5–5.0 cm in diameter (Caplan's syndrome).

Investigations

Investigations include:
- arterial blood gases: may show type 1 respiratory failure
- spirometry: often restrictive and the SpO_2 (pulse oximetry) may fall during a 6 min walk
- chest radiograph: may show small nodules
- high-resolution CT: shows small nodules throughout both lung fields.

In simple **coal worker's pneumoconiosis,** diffuse bilateral small nodules are evident on the chest radiograph and high-resolution CT of thorax; in its complicated form, upper lobe fibrosis (progressive massive fibrosis) occurs.

Silicosis also causes small nodules, which can be seen on chest radiograph, especially in the upper zones. Hilar or 'eggshell' calcification is classically, although not always, found in silicosis. Tuberculosis is more common in patients with silicosis.

Management

There is no specific treatment available for interstitial lung diseases caused by inhalation of inorganic dusts, and the most important issue is generally prevention and identification. Oxygen and diuretics are used if cor pulmonale is present. Coal dust exposure is a risk factor for the development of chronic obstructive pulmonary disease, and long-acting bronchodilators are used in some individuals with airflow obstruction.

Asbestos-related lung disease

'Asbestos' is used to describe a number of naturally occurring fibrous mineral silicates with fire-resistant properties. During the first six decades of the 20th century, asbestos was widely used to insulate pipes and boilers in ships, power stations, factories and many large buildings. Tradesmen in shipbuilding (e.g. welders, plumbers, electricians and other construction workers) often had considerable exposure to asbestos dust. In the UK, the Control of Asbestos at Work Regulations in 1987 required the use of respirators and protective clothing and the use of asbestos has now virtually ceased in western Europe and North America.

All types of asbestos can cause **asbestosis**, **benign pleural disease**, **lung cancer** and **malignant mesothelioma** (cancer of the pleura). The risk of development of all asbestos-induced diseases increases with exposure, but asbestosis requires much higher doses than that necessary to cause benign pleural disease and mesothelioma. Asbestos-induced lung disease seldom appears less than 20 years after first exposure.

Benign pleural disease

Pleural plaques are circumscribed areas of thickening of the parietal pleura associated with asbestos exposure. They are usually an incidental finding on chest radiograph and do not require any treatment.

Asbestosis

Clinical features and investigations

Patients present with progressive exertional breathlessness and a non-productive cough. Late inspiratory crackles are audible at both lung bases and finger clubbing is often present.

Chest radiograph shows scattered small irregular opacities throughout both lung fields. CT may show basal subpleural shadowing with fibrotic change, often with pleural plaques or thickening. Lung function tests show a restrictive ventilatory defect with low gas transfer. Sputum microscopy may show asbestos bodies and lung biopsy may show fibrosis associated with asbestos fibres.

There is no effective treatment and management relies on prevention of further exposure to asbestos and symptomatic treatment with O_2.

Lung cancer

Lung cancer is significantly more common in those with previous asbestos exposure and approximately 11 times commoner in those who also smoke.

Malignant mesothelioma

Malignant mesothelioma is a tumour arising most commonly from pleura, but also rarely from peritoneum or pericardium. The incidence of mesothelioma in industrialized countries is likely to rise to 2000 male deaths/year until around 2020 (Fig. 3.11.1), reflecting the use of asbestos, largely without protection, until 1970. Females only form 12% of these deaths.

Mesothelioma usually presents with dull chest pain and breathlessness, the latter caused by pleural effusion. There may be signs of pleural effusion.

Chest radiograph may show a pleural effusion or lobulated pleural thickening (Fig. 3.11.2). Pleural biopsy (by means of an Abram's needle or a video-assisted throcoscopy) may confirm the diagnosis.

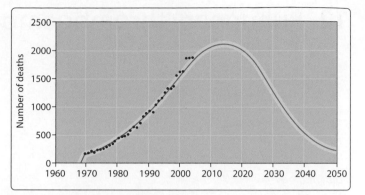

Fig. 3.11.1 Observed deaths (dots) and projected deaths from mesothelioma in the UK; there is often a lag of more than 30 years between exposure to asbestos and development of mesothelioma.

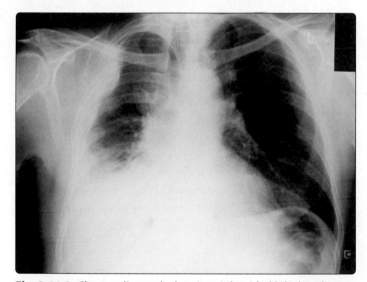

Fig. 3.11.2 Chest radiograph showing right-sided lobulated pleura, pleural effusion and reduced lung volume in a patient subsequently diagnosed with a mesothelioma.

Mesothelioma is usually incurable. However radiotherapy is given to drain or biopsy sites. Chemotherapy is given to fit patients and surgery is considered in a minority. The median survival from mesothelioma is approximately 14 months. Many industrial countries have made arrangements for compensation of workers affected by asbestos-related lung disease, particularly asbestosis and mesothelioma.

12. Pulmonary thromboembolism

Questions
- What are the main risk factors in the development of pulmonary embolism?
- How do you manage acute pulmonary embolism?

Epidemiology

The incidence of symptomatic venous thromboembolism is approximately 117 in 100 000 annually in western Europe. Venous thromboembolism is the second most common acute cardiovascular disease after myocardial infarction, while pulmonary embolism is the third commonest cardiovascular cause of death after myocardial infarction and stroke.

The incidence of pulmonary embolism increases with age and approximately doubles for every decade after 20 years. The mortality from pulmonary embolism is 10–30%, being <5% in those who are haemodynamically stable at presentation, but >20% in those with persistent hypotension.

Pathogenesis

As pulmonary embolism is preceded by deep venous thrombosis (DVT), the factors predisposing to the two conditions are the same. Pathology involves **Virchow's triad** of venous stasis, injury to the vein wall and enhanced coagulability of the blood, possibly also with decreased fibrinolytic activity. A predisposing factor can be identified in approximately 80%.

Clinical features

Deep venous thrombosis. Presentation is with pain in the calf, often with swelling, redness and engorged superficial veins. The affected calf is often warmer and there may be ankle oedema. Homan's sign (pain in the calf on dorsiflexion of the foot) is often present but not diagnostic. Ileofemoral thrombosis presents with severe pain and few physical signs, apart from swelling of the thigh.

Acute minor pulmonary embolism. This is often asymptomatic and approximately 40% of patients with DVT and no other symptoms have evidence of pulmonary embolism on lung scans. Mild breathlessness on exertion is common and occurs because the affected area of lung is still ventilated but not perfused. Some pulmonary emboli cause pulmonary infarction, with localized sharp pleuritic pain and haemoptysis. Patients are usually tachypnoeic and a pleural friction rub may be heard. Fever is common. Minor pulmonary emboli do not compromise the right ventricle; cardiac output is maintained and hypotension does not occur.

Acute massive pulmonary embolism. A far less common event, this occurs when 40% of the pulmonary circulation is suddenly obstructed (volume of clot is approximately 30 ml). The right ventricle suddenly dilates, with marked increase in pulmonary artery systolic pressure, and cardiac output falls; the patient suddenly becoming hypotensive. Death can occur rapidly, but in less-severe cases the patient complains of sudden severe central chest pain or syncope. The patient is pale and sweaty with tachypnoea, tachycardia and hypotension. Jugular venous pressure is markedly raised with a prominent 'a' wave caused by right ventricular dilatation with tricuspid regurgitation. A right ventricular heave may be palpable and a gallop rhythm with widely split second heart sound is heard on auscultation.

Investigations

Clinical diagnosis alone is unreliable but combined with a positive D-dimer has a sensitivity of 80%. Ileofemoral thrombosis can be confirmed by Doppler ultrasound scan, while below knee thromboses can be detected reliably only by venography. Pulmonary embolism is investigated by:

- **arterial blood gases:** hypoxia with a low Pco_2
- **isotope ventilation/perfusion (VQ) lung scan** reveals areas of ventilation–perfusion mismatching (Fig. 3.12.1)
- **spiral CT scan** with i.v. contrast (CT pulmonary angiography; Fig. 3.12.2) has good sensitivity and specificity for medium-sized emboli but does not exclude emboli in small vessels
- **chest radiograph:** may be normal or may show relative absence of pulmonary blood vessels, a wedge-shaped infarct, a raised hemidiaphragm, atelectasis or pleural effusion (Fig. 3.12.3)
- **echocardiography** shows a vigorously contracting left ventricle and dilated right ventricle; thrombus can sometimes be seen in the right ventricular outflow tract
- **ECG** is usually normal or reveals a sinus tachycardia. Less commonly it shows right axis deviation with tall peaked 'p' waves and right ventricular strain. The classical ECG pattern of an S wave in lead I, a Q wave and inverted T wave in lead III (S_1, Q_3, T_3 pattern) is rare.

Management

Deep venous thrombosis. All patients with thrombosis above the knee must receive anticoagulation therapy. Anticoagulation for 6 weeks is also recommended for below knee thrombi, as 30% will have extension of the thrombus proximally.

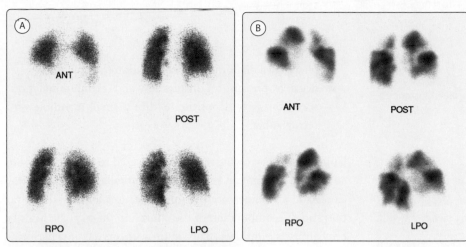

Fig. 3.12.1 Ventilation (A) and perfusion (B) lung scans showing high probability of pulmonary embolism. There are multiple unmatched defects (ventilation or perfusion affected), plus a matched defect at the right base.

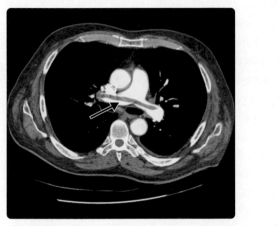

Fig. 3.12.2 CT pulmonary angiogram showing a saddle embolism (arrow).

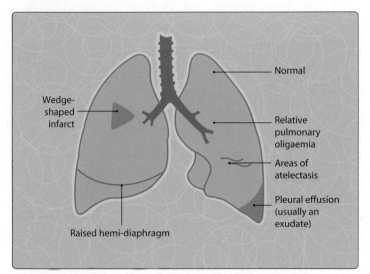

Fig. 3.12.3 Chest radiograph features of pulmonary embolism.

Bed rest is advised until anticoagulation is fully established, and elastic stockings giving graduated pressure over the leg are helpful. Low-molecular-weight heparin (LMWH) has replaced unfractionated heparin as no monitoring is required and there is less risk of bleeding. Warfarin is started immediately and heparin discontinued when the 'international normalized ratio' (INR) is in the target range. Warfarin treatment is usually for 3 months, but may be longer if there is recurrent DVT.

Pulmonary embolism. All hypoxic patients should receive high-flow O_2 (60–100%). Patients with pulmonary infarction require bed rest and analgesia. In severe cases, i.v. fluids and inotropic agents may be required. Anticoagulation with LMWH is started immediately and continued for 7 days. Warfarin will be required for at least 3 months. Occasionally, a filter is inserted into the inferior vena cava to prevent further emboli in patients at high risk. In acute massive pulmonary embolism, fibrinolytic therapy or surgical embolectomy may be life saving.

Prevention

Patients immobilized in hospital or following surgery to the leg or pelvis, or with heart failure, should receive low-dose subcutaneous LMWH. Early mobilization should be encouraged as most thrombi occur within 72 h following surgery. Elastic support stockings should be given to patients at high risk.

Risk factors for venous thromboembolism include:

- **major:** hip, pelvis, or leg fracture; hip or knee replacement; major general surgery; major trauma
- **moderate:** arthroscopic knee surgery, malignancy, congestive heart or respiratory failure, hormone replacement therapy, oral contraceptive use, stroke, postpartum, previous venous thromboembolism, thrombophilia
- **minor:** immobile for more than 3 days, immobility from sitting, increasing age, laparoscopic surgery, obesity, antepartum period, varicose veins.

13. Sleep apnoea

Questions
- What are the clinical features of sleep apnoea/hypopnoea syndrome (SAHS)?
- What is the management of SAHS?

An apnoea is defined as absence of respiration for 10 seconds. Sleep apnoea is defined as excessive daytime sleepiness with more than five apnoeic periods per hour during sleep.

Epidemiology
Snoring is very common and community studies suggest that approximately 32% of males and 21% of females snore regularly during sleep. Some of these individuals will also have obstructive sleep apnoea, which occurs in approximately 4% of males and 2% of females. The risk of sleep apnoea increases with age and with obesity, particularly in individuals with an increased neck circumference of > 43 cm (> 17 inches).

Pathogenesis
Snoring results from recurrent narrowing of the supraglottic airway during sleep (Fig. 3.13.1). Patency of the upper airway depends on a balance between:

- pharyngeal dilator muscle contraction (genioglossus)
- negative pressure of inspiration and extraluminal pressure from fatty deposition and/or a small mandible with retrognathia.

Upper airway narrowing results in increased respiratory effort in an attempt to maintain ventilation. Eventually, the upper airway closes and an apnoea occurs. Apnoea causes hypoxic desaturation and the combination of the effort and the hypoxia leads to brief arousals from sleep. This, in turn, affects daytime performance, producing excessive sleepiness.

Clinical features
Patients typically snore loudly, sometimes with witnessed prolonged periods of apnoea and restlessness. It is important to obtain a history from the patient's bed partner. Patients complain of excessive daytime sleepiness, poor concentration, night-time 'choking', morning lethargy, reduced libido and drowsiness while driving long distances. Falling asleep at the wheel probably accounts for approximately 15% of road traffic accidents.

Approximately 50% of patients with obstructive sleep apnoea are obese (body mass index > 30), often with collar size 17 or more. The pharynx may appear narrowed with a large uvula. There is an association with hypertension.

Investigations
Daytime sleepiness can be assessed using the Epworth Sleepiness Scale, which should be given to patients suspected of having sleep apnoea/hypopnoea syndrome. A score of ≥ 11 is considered abnormal (Table 3.13.1).

Overnight oximetry showing episodes of desaturation will confirm approximately 60% of cases. Other more complex respiratory sensor devices or full polysomnography may be required in more difficult cases. Less than five apnoeic periods per hour is considered normal, 15–30/h is moderate and > 30/h is severe sleep apnoea.

Management
Obese patients should be strongly advised to lose weight and there is evidence that weight loss of 15% can reduce apnoeas. Alcohol, sedatives and other hypnotics should be avoided in the evening, as these all decrease airway dilator function. Similarly, stimulants such as caffeine should be avoided in the evening as this may reduce the quality of sleep. Car drivers, particularly holders of heavy goods vehicle licences should inform the licensing authority (DVLA in the UK) of their diagnosis.

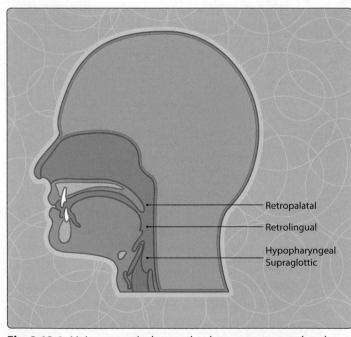

Retropalatal

Retrolingual

Hypopharyngeal
Supraglottic

Fig. 3.13.1 Main anatomical areas that become narrowed and cause snoring and sleep apnoea/hypopnoea syndrome. Upper airway narrowing can be exacerbated by the supine position, reduced oropharyngeal muscle tone (e.g. caused by alcohol), adipose tissue around the throat and a short mandible.

Table 3.13.1 EPWORTH SLEEPINESS QUESTIONNAIRE
How likely are you to doze off or fall asleep in the following situations in contrast to just feeling tired? This refers to your usual way of life over the last few weeks. Even if you have not done some of these things, try to work out how they would have affected you. Use the following scale to choose the most appropriate number for each situation. Tick one box on each line.
0, would never doze
1, slight chance of dozing
2, moderate chance of dozing
3, high chance of dozing

Situation	0	1	2	3
Sitting and reading				
Watching television				
Sitting inactive in a public place (e.g. theatre or meeting)				
As a passenger in a car for an hour without a break				
Lying down in the afternoon when circumstances permit				
Sitting and talking to someone				
Sitting quietly after lunch without alcohol				
In a car when stopped for a few minutes in traffic				

Continuous positive airway pressure (CPAP) is the treatment of choice for patients with moderate or severe sleep apnoea (i.e. >15/h associated with O_2 desaturation). CPAP therapy involves wearing an airtight face or nasal mask during sleep, through which positive pressure is applied to maintain the upper airway (Fig. 3.13.2). This often results in rapid improvement in quality of sleep and resolution of excessive daytime sleepiness.

For those with milder forms of sleep apnoea (5–15 apnoeic episodes/h) and who also snore, fitting of a mandibular advancement device may also be helpful.

Other sleep disorders

Central sleep apnoea. A small minority of patients who do not respond to CPAP may have central sleep apnoea, with abnormality of central control of sleep pattern. This is typically seen in the non-obese with no history of snoring and is thought to be caused by brainstem pathology.

Narcolepsy. Narcolepsy occurs in 1 in 2–3000 individuals aged between 10 and 30 years, whereas those with sleep apnoea tend to present in middle age. Its main features include:

- irresistible daytime sleepiness
- cataplexy (sudden onset of muscle weakness when awake, often in response to amusement or strong emotion)

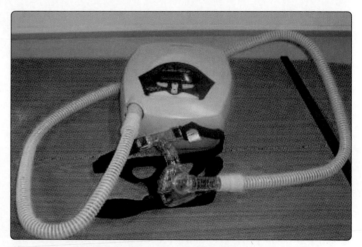

Fig. 3.13.2 A CPAP (continuous positive airway pressure) machine should be used in most patients diagnosed with sleep apnoea syndrome; individuals may use a face or nose mask.

- hypnagogic hallucinations (vivid dreams at the onset of sleep)
- sleep paralysis.

Narcolepsy can be familial and has been associated with abnormalities in the short arm of chromosome 6 (HLA type *DQB10602*). Modafinil can be used to reduce excessive daytime sleepiness, while sodium oxybate and various antidepressants can be used to suppress cataplexy.

14. Pulmonary hypertension

Questions
- What are the causes of pulmonary hypertension?
- What investigations are carried out in the diagnosis of pulmonary hypertension?

Pulmonary hypertension is present when mean pulmonary artery pressure >25 mmHg at rest or >30 mmHg on exercise. Resting pulmonary hypertension implies that more than 70% of the pulmonary vascular bed has been damaged. The prevalence of both primary (idiopathic, familial) and secondary pulmonary hypertension is unknown.

Pathogenesis
Primary pulmonary hypertension may be familial, with autosomal dominant inheritance and at least two genes involved. Up to 10% will have Raynaud's phenomenon. Patients with connective tissue disease are at risk of secondary pulmonary hypertension, particularly those with the 'CREST' variant of systemic sclerosis. Appetite suppressants, particularly aminorex, fenfluramine and dexfenfluramine, have been implicated. Pulmonary hypertension also results from left-to-right cardiac shunt (e.g. atrial septal defect). Other common causes of secondary pulmonary hypertension include thromboembolic disease and severe COPD, which is usually associated with hypoxia and CO_2 retention.

Clinical features
Patients with primary pulmonary hypertension present with breathlessness with no obvious cause. Symptoms and signs of severe pulmonary hypertension are often enigmatic, delaying diagnosis for up to 2 years:
- cardiac signs: right ventricular heave, loud pulmonary component to the second heart sound, tricuspid regurgitation and a pulmonary flow murmur
- cor pulmonale may develop: elevated jugular venous pressure with prominent V waves in the neck, liver changes (hepatomegaly, ascites, hepatic pulsation) and sacral and peripheral oedema (pitting ankle oedema).

There may also be signs of the underlying cause.

Investigations
Chest radiograph may show cardiomegaly with enlarged main pulmonary arteries and peripheral pruning of vessels.

Echocardiography may show a dilated right heart, tricuspid regurgitation and pulmonary artery hypertension. ECG will show right ventricular hypertrophy (Fig. 3.14.1). Cardiopulmonary exercise testing and MRI confirms changes in the right heart.

Right-heart catheterization is required for direct pulmonary artery pressure measurement.

Management
Management depends on the underlying cause, although oxygen is indicated in most patients. Warfarin should be given in primary pulmonary hypertension and when chronic thromboembolic pulmonary hypertension is responsible. Surgical thromboendarterectomy may be effective in the latter. Other forms of treatment include vasodilators such as prostacyclin, nitric oxide, phosphodiesterase inhibitors (e.g. sildenafil) or endothelin-1 antagonists (e.g. bosentan). Lung transplantation may be necessary in symptomatic advanced primary pulmonary hypertension. Pulmonary hypertension shortens life and the untreated 3-year survival after diagnosis is less than 35%.

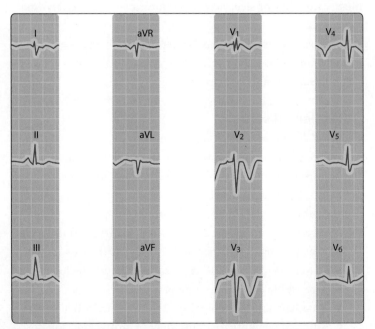

Fig. 3.14.1 ECG features in pulmonary hypertension: right axis deviation, partial right bundle branch block, inverted T waves in anterior chest leads.

15. Acute respiratory distress syndrome

Questions
- What are the causes of acute respiratory distress syndrome?
- How is it managed?

Acute lung injury is used to describe the widespread pulmonary injury that occurs as a consequence of direct and indirect insults to the lung. Acute respiratory distress syndrome (ARDS) represents the more severe end of this spectrum and is characterized by bilateral pulmonary infiltrates, hypoxaemia and fibrosis. Clinically, ARDS is diagnosed when gas exchange is severely impaired in conjunction with widespread chest radiograph infiltrates in the absence of cardiogenic pulmonary oedema.

Epidemiology
The prevalence of ARDS is unknown.

Pathogenesis
ARDS can be caused by a variety of direct pulmonary and non-pulmonary insults but overwhelming sepsis is the most common cause (Table 3.15.1). In ARDS, the normal barrier between the pulmonary capillaries that prevents fluid leaking into the lung parenchyma is damaged. As a result, the lungs become oedematous, lose compliance and become 'stiff'. A number of inflammatory mediators and cells (especially neutrophils) are involved in the development of ARDS. Pulmonary hypertension is a relatively common finding; it is caused by a combination of hypoxia, thrombosis and vasoconstriction by circulating mediators. After several days, lung fibrosis and remodelling occurs.

Clinical features
Patients report progressive breathlessness often in the context of severe underlying illness. Clinical examination reveals bilateral fine inspiratory crackles and progressive hypoxia in an unwell individual.

Investigations
Chest radiograph shows bilateral infiltrates, which can progress to complete opacification of both lung fields (Fig. 3.15.1).

Some patients with suspected ARDS have a cannula inserted into the pulmonary artery through a peripheral vein (a Swan–Ganz catheter). This can indirectly estimate the pressure in the pulmonary capillaries, which is normal in ARDS but elevated in cardiogenic pulmonary oedema.

Management
Management involves treatment of the underlying condition (with antibiotics, removal of infected tissue, etc.), respiratory support, adequate nutrition and an attempt to halt the capillary leak of fluid. Most patients with ARDS require intubation and mechanical ventilation. Strategies tried with varying success include prone positioning, high CO_2 levels, high-frequency ventilation, high-dose steroids and drugs to lower pulmonary artery pressure.

The mortality from ARDS has fallen over the past few years but remains high, at approximately 30%.

Table 3.15.1 CAUSES OF ACUTE RESPIRATORY DISTRESS SYNDROME

Type	Causes
Infective	Viral or bacterial pneumonia; septicaemia
Aspiration	Near drowning; gastric contents
Embolic	Fat; amniotic fluid
Gas inhalation	Smoke, nitrogen dioxide
Drugs	Opioids, benzodiazepines
Neurogenic	Head injury, seizures
Haematological	Disseminated intravascular coagulation, after blood transfusion
Miscellaneous	Pancreatitis, lung contusion, high altitude

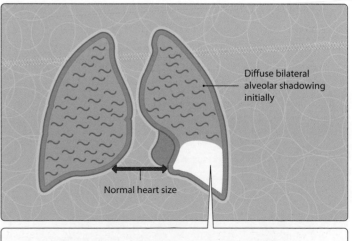

Diffuse bilateral alveolar shadowing initially

Normal heart size

Air bronchograms show progression to complete 'white out'

Fig. 3.15.1 Radiograph features of acute respiratory distress syndrome.

16. Drugs and systemic diseases affecting the lungs

Questions
- What drugs can cause bronchospasm?
- How can rheumatoid arthritis affect the lung?

Drugs and the lung

The lung can be damaged by drugs taken by inhalation or orally.

Tobacco is the most commonly used drug producing lung disease; it contains tars with carcinogens and the smoke contains carbon monoxide and particulates. **Cannabis** causes very similar reactions to tobacco and may be even more carcinogenic. **Heroin** can cause severe bullous lung disease similar to chronic obstructive pulmonary disease when smoked.

Bronchoconstriction

- **beta-blockers:** used in the treatment of angina or glaucoma constrict airway smooth muscle
- **aspirin and other NSAIDs:** inhibit cyclooxygenase thus producing leukotrienes, which cause symptoms of asthma
- **penicillin and other antibiotics:** classic type I hypersensitivity results in wheeze and anaphylaxis
- **tartrazine:** a yellow dye, also causes type I hypersensitivity.

Cough. ACE inhibitors cause cough in up to 20% of patients owing to bradykinin accumulation. Angiotensin II receptor antagonists may be used instead.

Bronchiolitis obliterans. Penicillamine can produce this rare syndrome of progressive breathlessness associated with increasing airflow obstruction. On auscultation, the typical finding is of late inspiratory crackles with a mid-inspiratory squeak.

Alveolitis. Diffuse alveolitis presents with slowly increasing breathlessness, cough, lung crackles and diffuse patchy infiltration on chest radiograph (Table 3.16.1, Fig. 3.16.1).

Pulmonary oedema. Overdoses of aspirin or opiates can cause pulmonary oedema. Oral steroids occasionally exacerbate preexisting pulmonary oedema.

Pulmonary thromboembolism. Oral contraceptives, particularly oestrogens, can increase the risk in women approximately six-fold.

Pulmonary hypertension. The slimming agents fenfluramine, dexfenfluramine and aminorex can cause this severe reaction, which may only become apparent several years later.

Pleural and mediastinal fibrosis. Methysergide, used in the treatment of migraine, can induce this severe but rare reaction.

Pleural effusion. Drug-induced pleural effusion are uncommon but amiodarone, nitrofurantoin, phenytoin, methotrexate and pergolide have all been implicated (Fig. 3.16.1).

Acute lung injury. The weedkiller paraquat causes this severe progressive and often fatal reaction, often several days following ingestion.

Systemic diseases and the lung

Many systemic diseases present with symptoms and signs of lung involvement. Some disorders, such as motor neuron disease, that affect neuromuscular transmission can lead to respiratory failure through muscle weakness.

Autoimmune disorders and vasculitis
Rheumatoid arthritis

Rheumatoid arthritis can affect the lung in a variety of ways (Fig. 3.16.2).

Table 3.16.1 DRUGS CAUSING ALVEOLITIS

Group	Drugs
Antibiotics	Nitrofurantoin
Anticonvulsants	Phenytoin, carbamazepine
Anti-inflammatory drugs	Sulfasalazine, penicillamine, gold
Cytotoxic drugs	Bleomycin, busulfan, cyclophosphamide, methotrexate
Antiarrhythmic drugs	Amiodarone
Hypotensive agents	Hydralazine

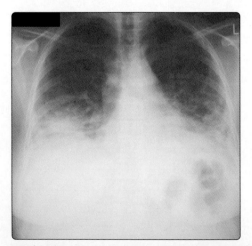

Fig. 3.16.1 Chest radiograph showing bilateral mid and lower zone shadowing secondary to amiodarone lung toxicity.

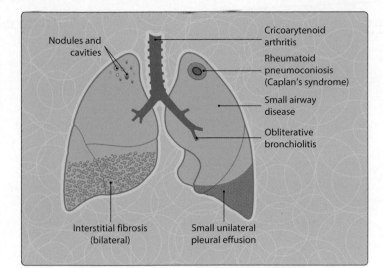

Fig. 3.16.2 The effect of rheumatoid arthritis on the lungs.

Interstitial disease. Some patients develop features identical to idiopathic pulmonary fibrosis, with progressive exertional breathlessness, finger clubbing, fine late inspiratory crackles at both lung bases, restrictive ventilatory defect on spirometry, reduced gas transfer and bilateral peripheral basal interstitial change on high-resolution CT.

Pleural involvement. Some patients develop pleuritic chest pain caused by pleuritis, while others develop unilateral pleural effusions containing inflammatory exudate (protein >30 g/l) with high LDH (>700 IU/l), low pH, low glucose (<2.5 mmol/l) and high rheumatoid factor titre.

Airway involvement. Rarely small airways are involved in an inflammatory process termed bronchiolitis obliterans. Some patients develop bronchiolitis obliterans organizing pneumonia (BOOP).

Rheumatoid nodules. Nodules are sometimes found within the lung in patients seropositive for rheumatoid factor. These nodules are typically 1–2 cm in diameter, positioned subpleurally and biopsy may be needed to exclude malignancy.

Infection. Patients with rheumatoid arthritis are susceptible to lung infection. Those receiving immunosuppressive drugs (e.g. methotrexate, azathioprine) have an increased risk of opportunistic infection such as *Pneumocystis jirovecii* and chickenpox. Treatment with anti-tumour necrosis factor alpha is associated with increased reactivation of tuberculosis.

Systemic lupus erythematosus (SLE)

Interstitial disease. Although this is uncommon in SLE, it may be associated with diffuse alveolar haemorrhage.

Pleural involvement. Pleuritic chest pain is more common in active SLE and is a presenting symptom in 10% of patients.

Pulmonary hypertension. A rare feature of SLE but may relate to pulmonary vasculitis or thrombosis.

Anti-phospholipid syndrome. Patients with SLE are at increased risk of venous and pulmonary thromboembolism because of circulating lupus anticoagulant and anti-phospholipid antibodies. Approximately 8% of those with SLE develop anti-phospholipid syndrome and require lifelong anticoagulation.

Systemic sclerosis

Interstitial disease. Systemic sclerosis may also produce pulmonary fibrosis, which often affects the lung bases. There is also an association with bronchiectasis.

Pulmonary hypertension. Pulmonary artery involvement may cause severe pulmonary hypertension.

Other disorders

Ankylosing spondylitis is associated with reduced chest wall movement and a restrictive ventilatory defect. Bilateral upper lobe fibrosis and upper lobe cavitation can occur.

Sjögren's syndrome is characterized by hypergammaglobulinaemia, multiple organ-specific and non-organ-specific antibodies and lymphocytic infiltration of various tissues. Lung involvement occurs in up to one-third of patients and includes chronic bronchitis, mucus plugging and lymphocytic interstitial pneumonitis.

Behçet's syndrome is characterized by arthritis, recurrent oral and genital ulceration and pulmonary vascular involvement in 5%. Patients present with haemoptysis, and pulmonary angiography may reveal pulmonary arterial aneurysms.

Vasculitides affecting lung and kidney

Wegener's granulomatosis is characterized by upper respiratory tract, lung and renal involvement, and by anti-neutrophil cytoplasmic antibodies (ANCA); these stain in a diffuse cytoplasmic pattern (c-ANCA) mainly against neutrophil enzyme proteinase 3. Symptoms include cough, haemoptysis, breathlessness or pleuritic chest pain. Life-threatening alveolar haemorrhage is the most serious complication. Chest radiograph shows asymptomatic pulmonary infiltrates and the treatment is long-term immunosuppression.

Anti-glomerular basement (anti-GBM) antibody disease is rare (30 cases per year in the UK). Lung haemorrhage is common, particularly in smokers, and patients often progress to renal failure. The presence of anti-GBM antibodies is diagnostic.

Microscopic polyangiitis is a necrotizing small vessel vasculitis associated with ANCA showing a perinuclear staining pattern (pANCA; or MPO-ANCA as it is mainly myeloperoxidase that is stained). Patients may present with haemoptysis or alveolar haemorrhage.

17. Eosinophilic lung diseases

Questions
- What pulmonary conditions are associated with an eosinophilia?
- How may *Aspergillus fumigatus* affect the lung?

In normal airways, eosinophils are not usually present. However, the presence of eosinophils in lung tissue indicates a cellular response of the host to an exogenous or endogenous agent. Blood eosinophils account for 1–3% of peripheral blood white cells and in most cases, pulmonary eosinophilia is associated with blood eosinophilia. Asthma is the most common cause of peripheral blood and airway eosinophilia in the UK, although regular use of adequate anti-inflammatory treatment usually suppresses eosinophils. Eosinophils can be detected in sputum in poorly controlled asthma (Fig. 3.17.1).

Infective causes

Tropical eosinophilic pneumonia
Pulmonary and blood eosinophilia is a common response to worm infestation, particularly with *Wucheria bancrofti* or *Brugia malayi*. Other less common causative parasites include *Ascaris, Toxocara* (visceral lava migrans), *Ancylostoma*, *Schistosoma* and *Strongyloides* spp. The parasite eggs are ingested and larvae migrate through the body and into the lungs. This causes an allergic reaction in the lungs. Pathogenesis involves production of interleukin-4 and specific IgE directed against the parasite. Patients present with tiredness, cough, wheeze, breathlessness, chest pain, fever

and weight loss. Blood eosinophilia is present and chest radiograph shows fine nodular infiltrates. The diagnosis is confirmed by detecting ova, larvae or adult worms in the stool. For some parasites such as schistosoma, IgG serology is helpful. Management includes specific treatment for the parasites, such as diethylcarbamazine for filariae, thiabendazole for strongyloides and ancylostomas and mebendazole for ascarides. *Toxocara canis* (the dog roundworm) infestation does not usually require treatment.

Allergic reactions

Drug-induced pulmonary eosinophilia
Pulmonary eosinophilia induced by drugs (e.g. penicillin, sulphonamides, chlorpropamide and carbamazepine) is an allergic reaction in the lungs and can cause diffuse chest radiograph shadowing. Clinical features include breathlessness, cough and fever. Symptoms rapidly improve on withdrawal of the drug. Oral steroids may be necessary in more severe events.

Allergic bronchopulmonary aspergillosis
Allergic bronchopulmonary aspergillosis is an uncommon complication of allergic asthma and causes symptoms of poorly controlled asthma. Pathogenesis involves an intense hypersensitivity reaction to the fungus *Aspergillus fumigatus* together with mucus plugging of proximal airways (Figs 3.17.2 and 3.17.3). Patients often develop proximal bronchiectasis. Diagnosis requires a positive skin prick test to aspergillus, aspergillus IgG precipitating antibodies, raised eosinophil count, raised ESR and chest radiograph abnormalities. Management involves improving asthma control with high doses of inhaled steroid and long-term oral steroids. Antifungal drugs (e.g. voriconazole) can also be given but are of uncertain overall benefit.

Autoimmune eosinophilia

Churg–Strauss syndrome
Churg–Strauss syndrome is an uncommon small-vessel vasculitis found in association with moderate to severe asthma. Other features include eosinophil count $>1.5\times10^9$ cells/l, pulmonary infiltrates, sinus disease, signs of a systemic vasculitis and high IgE. Organ involvement is variable and it can affect the skin (purpura), nervous system (peripheral neuropathy or mononeuritis multiplex), cardiovascular system (pericarditis and heart failure), kidneys (renal failure) and GI system (abdominal pain and bleeding). Tissue diagnosis is preferable and serum pANCA is positive in approximately 70% of

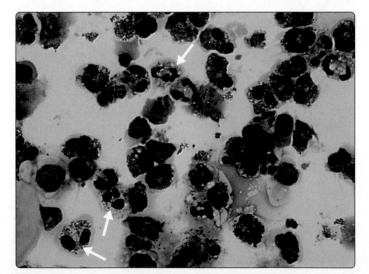

Fig. 3.17.1 Sputum eosinophils in a patient with poorly controlled asthma (arrows).

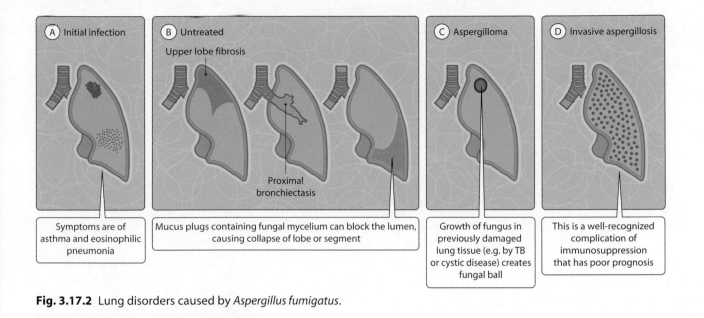

Fig. 3.17.2 Lung disorders caused by *Aspergillus fumigatus*.

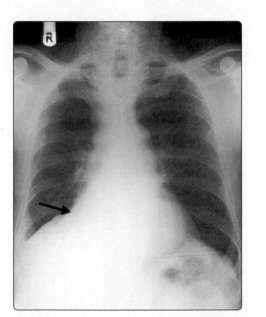

Fig. 3.17.3 Chest radiograph showing right lower lobe collapse (arrow) in a patient with allergic bronchopulmonary aspergillosis.

cases. Treatment consists of high-dose oral steroids along with immunosuppressive drugs such as cyclophosphamide.

Idiopathic pulmonary eosinophilia

Acute eosinophilic pneumonia (Löffler's syndrome)

Acute eosinophilic pneumonia is a mild disorder that may occur at any age and presents with fever, cough, breathlessness, muscle aches, fleeting pulmonary infiltrates on chest radiograph and airway eosinophilia. The cause is unknown. Oral steroids result in immediate improvement in symptoms.

Chronic eosinophilic pneumonia

Chronic eosinophilic pneumonia occurs more commonly in middle age, with a slight female preponderance, although the cause is unknown. Clinical features include cough, breathlessness, weight loss, fever and night sweats. The chest radiograph shows peripheral consolidation. Airway eosinophils are found, although blood eosinophilia may not occur. Treatment is with tapering high-doses of oral steroids over several months. Clinical response is rapid but relapse may occur if steroids are discontinued too early.

Hypereosinophilic syndrome

The hypereosinophilic syndrome is an uncommon leukoproliferative disorder characterized by an overproduction of eosinophils resulting in organ damage. It is characterized by a persistently elevated blood eosinophil count ($>1.5 \times 10^9$ cells/l) over at least 6 months, with no recognizable cause. Fever, breathlessness, weight loss and night sweats are common. It is caused by eosinophilic infiltration of different organs and can cause pulmonary infiltrates, pleural effusions, neuropathy, cardiomyopathy, and GI upset. Treatment is with high-dose oral steroids. The differential diagnosis includes eosinophilic leukaemia.

PART IV

Gastrointestinal disorders

IV

Lindsay McLeman

The big picture

The functions of the gastrointestinal (GI) tract system are diverse. Consequently, malfunction can result in a broad spectrum of symptoms and diseases. The oesophagus, stomach, small and large bowel are subject to disorders of secretion, motility, digestion and absorption.

Mortality

In luminal gastroenterology, cancer is the leading cause of death. Colorectal cancer is the second commonest cause of cancer death in the UK, with a 5-year survival of around 50%. Cancer of the oesophagus, pancreas and stomach are the fifth, sixth and seventh commonest causes of cancer death, respectively, with a 5-year survival of 5–15%. In recent years, however, mortality rates have been falling. Mortality linked to peptic ulcer disease is also declining.

Morbidity

Gastro-oesophageal reflux disease, peptic ulcer disease and dyspepsia are the cause of 1 in 10 primary care consultations. Although mortality from peptic ulcer disease is falling, hospital admission with complications (e.g. bleeding or perforation) is not. Inflammatory bowel disease has a low mortality but high morbidity; it runs a relapsing and remitting course and affects young people. The majority of patients do manage a near normal lifestyle with the aid of medical or surgical therapy.

Prevalence and incidence

Peptic ulcer disease affects 10% of the adult population at some point in their lives. The annual incidence of peptic ulcers is approximately 0.1–0.3% in the population. Dyspepsia and gastro-oesophageal reflux disease are far more common and are thought to affect 20–40% of adults in the developed world.

Coeliac disease has an estimated prevalence of 1 in 250 people. It is more common in northern Europe and normally presents in teenage years, with a second peak in the sixth decade. There is a genetic influence as around one in four patients have a first-degree relative with the disease. Other disorders of the small intestine are rare in the UK.

Inflammatory bowel disease affects around 1 in 400 people in the UK. The peak incidence is 20–40 years, with around a quarter of patients presenting before the age of 20 years. Crohn's disease has a female preponderance and is more common in smokers, while ulcerative colitis has a male preponderance and is less common in smokers.

Colorectal cancer is the third most common cancer in the UK. Cancer Research UK estimates that 100 new cases of colorectal cancer are diagnosed each day in the UK. Around 80% of cases occur in patients >60 years. However the incidence is falling in the UK and it is becoming more prevalent in countries undergoing 'Westernization'. The majority of squamous cell oesophageal cancers occur in developing countries. The incidence of adenocarcinoma of the oesophagus is rising in the UK, especially amongst men. Gastric cancer represents 3% of all cancers in the UK and again it is more prevalent amongst men; however, the incidence is falling.

Helicobacter pylori

The discovery of the role of *Helicobacter pylori* in peptic ulceration in the 1980s radically changed ulcer treatment. It is thought to be the underlying cause of ulceration in 90% of duodenal ulcers and 70% of gastric ulcers (the remaining 30% are linked to use of NSAIDs). It is contracted in childhood by faecal–oral or oral–oral spread but lies dormant in the gastric mucosa. It is detected in patients with peptic ulcer disease or dyspepsia by antigen testing, urease breath testing or endoscopic biopsy and eradicated by a short course of multiple antibiotics and acid suppression.

Diet

Diet plays a central role in managing diseases such as gluten enteropathy in coeliac disease or food intolerance in irritable bowel syndrome. The role of diet in the development of other GI diseases is not as clearly understood. Studies have shown that the prevalence of inflammatory bowel disease and colorectal cancer are increasing in the Far East, perhaps because of the introduction of a Westernized diet of increased dairy products and red meat.

Table 1.1 PRESENTATION AND PREVALENCE OF SOME COMMON GASTROINTESTINAL DISORDERS

Site and disorder	Who gets it	Symptom	Prevalence UK	Comment
Oesophagus				
Achalasia	Any	Dysphagia	1 in 100 000	Requires surgery
Gastro-oesophageal reflux	Common in obesity, pregnancy	Dyspepsia, cough	Affects 30% of UK population	Recurrent, difficult to treat
Oesophageal cancer	> 60 years	Progressive dysphagia, bleeding	4 in 100 000	More common in Iran, China and Africa
Stomach				
Peptic ulcer	10% of adults	Dyspepsia, bleeding	Duodenal 1:8; gastric less common	*H. pylori* in 90% duodenal and 70% gastric
Non-ulcer dyspepsia	< 40 years	Chronic dyspepsia	Unknown	Associated with irritable bowel
Gastric cancer	> 50 years	Weight loss, dyspepsia	15 in 100 000	More common in Far East and Chile
Small intestine				
Coeliac disease	Any age	Asymptomatic, diarrhoea, weight loss	1 in 250	More common in northern Europe
Crohn's disease	Young adults, average age 26 years	Abdominal pain, diarrhoea, weight loss	~75 in 100 000; more common in females	Can occur anywhere from mouth to anus
Large intestine				
Ulcerative colitis	Young adults, average age 34 years	Bloody diarrhoea	~110 in 100 000; more common in males	Less common in non-white races
Diverticular disease	> 50 years	Asymptomatic, left iliac fossa pain	Found in 50% aged > 70 years	Rare in Asia
Irritable bowel syndrome	Any age	Abdominal discomfort, stools vary	Probably 20% of the population	Important to make a positive diagnosis
Colorectal cancer	> 50 years	Rectal bleeding, altered bowel habit	55 in 100 000; 68% colon, 32% rectal	Less common in Africa and Asia

High-return facts

1 **Achalasia**, the most common oesophageal motility disorder, is failure of the gastro-oesophageal junction to open properly following food ingestion. Endoscopy will show a dilated oesophagus filled with food residue and a contracted lower oesophageal sphincter. **Oesophageal varices** are dilated collateral blood vessels found in the distal oesophagus as a result of portal hypertension. They commonly occur in individuals with chronic liver disease. Spontaneous rupture causes major haemorrhage. Acute management involves replacement of blood loss and measures to stop bleeding. Early endoscopy allows varices to be injected or banded. Patients with known varices are sometimes treated with non-selective beta-blockers (e.g. propanolol) to reduce the risk of bleeding. **Gastro-oesophageal reflux disease** is mucosal damage (oesophagitis) resulting from reflux of gastric contents into the distal oesophagus, which causes burning retrosternal discomfort. A hiatus hernia may contribute to the symptoms through displacement of the lower oesophageal sphincter to above the diaphragm. Symptoms are relieved by reducing the acidity of gastric contents and improving lower oesophageal sphincter function. Persistent symptoms can be treated with surgery.

2 Dyspepsia is epigastric discomfort arising from underlying inflammation (gastritis) or ulceration of the stomach or duodenum. **Oesophageal cancer** presents with progressive dysphagia and weight loss. Adenocarcinoma arises in a segment of Barrett's oesophagus in the lower third and squamous cell cancer arises in the middle third. Biopsies taken during endoscopy confirms the diagnosis. Treatment options include surgery (oesophagectomy), chemotherapy, radiotherapy and stenting. A **Mallory–Weiss tear** is a longitudinal tear in the mucosa at the oesophago-gastric junction caused by severe vomiting. Patients present with haematemesis after an episode of retching. Bleeding usually settles spontaneously and management is usually with antiemetic drugs and i.v. fluids.

3 **Ulcers** normally present with dyspeptic symptoms over a number of days or weeks. The majority of ulcers are caused by *Helicobacter pylori* infection or the use of aspirin or NSAIDs. Diagnosis is made at endoscopy and treatment is with acid suppression, discontinuing exacerbating medications and eradicating *H. pylori*. Patients with peptic ulcers may also present more acutely with haematemesis or melaena, or with symptoms and signs of peritonitis due to perforation. **Gastric cancer** presents with early satiety, anorexia, weight loss, anaemia or upper GI bleeding. Appearances at endoscopy are those of a non-healing gastric ulcer with rolled edges and the diagnosis is confirmed by biopsy. If diagnosed early, the prognosis is good following partial or total gastrectomy. Patients who present in later stages are offered palliative chemotherapy.

4 Disease of the small intestine causes malabsorption and maldigestion of food, resulting in nutrient, electrolyte, vitamin and mineral deficiencies. The most common disorder is **coeliac disease**, which is an autoimmune disorder in which dietary gluten stimulates an inappropriate immune-mediated response. Atrophy of small intestinal villi leads to loss of the absorptive surface area. Endomysial antibodies are present. Patients are treated with lifelong dietary exclusion of gluten. **Bacterial overgrowth** by colonic bacteria can occur if there are structural or motility abnormalities of the small bowel. Treatment is with broad-spectrum antibiotics and if possible correction of the small bowel abnormality. **Short bowel syndrome** occurs with loss of absorptive surface area and can follow either physical reduction in the bowel (e.g. small bowel resections for Crohn's disease) or functional impairment of the bowel by disease. Management aims to achieve adequate hydration, replacement of electrolytes and treatment of the underlying cause. Small bowel malabsorption can also rarely be caused by infections.

5 **Inflammatory bowel disease** includes **Crohn's disease** and **ulcerative colitis**. Both are chronic inflammatory disorders of the GI tract and follow a relapsing and remitting course that can be associated with extra-intestinal complications. Although Crohn's disease and ulcerative colitis share some clinical features, many important differences exist. Crohn's disease may affect the mucosa anywhere from mouth to anus and involves the full thickness of the bowel wall with deep ulcers, fissures and granulomata with patches of normal mucosa between areas of inflammation (skip lesions). By comparison, ulcerative colitis affects solely the colon proximally from the rectum; the inflammation is continuous, with friable and ulcerated mucosa but no involvement of the deeper layers of the bowel wall. Inflammatory bowel disease is diagnosed by sigmoidoscopy or colonoscopy with biopsies and small bowel barium studies. Treatment is with dietary supplements and drugs. Surgical intervention may be required in some patients.

6 **Irritable bowel syndrome** is a common functional disorder with poorly understood pathogenesis. Symptoms include abdominal discomfort and bloating relieved by defaecation with or without alteration in bowel habit. It is important to exclude colorectal cancer in patients with other risk factors. The majority of patients are managed in primary care with dietary change, antispasmodics and antidepressants.

7 **Antibiotic-associated diarrhoea** is caused by overgrowth in the colon of *Clostridium difficile*. Patients at risk are the elderly, those with prolonged hospital stay and those who have had multiple or prolonged courses of antibiotics. **Pseudomembranous colitis** is a more severe form in which a 'membrane' forms over the rectal mucosa. Treatment is with rehydration, withdrawal of broad-spectrum antibiotics and oral vancomycin or metronidazole.

8 **Diverticular disease is** common in those >50 years and usually asymptomatic. Diverticulae within the large bowel are mucosal out-pouchings in the bowel lumen. Patients present with constipation or complications (e.g. rectal bleeding, perforation or infection). Management includes a high-fibre diet and laxatives for constipation. Diverticulitis is infection within a diverticulum and presents with pyrexia and abdominal pain. Treatment is with broad-spectrum antibiotics. **Ischaemic colitis** results from temporary occlusion of blood supply to a segment of the colon. Causes include venous thrombosis, arterial or fat embolism, small vessel vasculitis or following intra-abdominal surgery. Patients present with sudden-onset severe abdominal pain and bloody diarrhoea. Most episodes resolve with conservative management and i.v. fluids, although some may require colectomy.

9 A **polyp** is a protuberance of the colonic mucosa into the lumen, which can be sessile (flat) or polypoidal (on a stalk). The most common polyps are adenomatous and have malignant potential. Patients may be asymptomatic or present with altered bowel habit or bleeding. **Colorectal cancer** is the third commonest cause of cancer. Most occurs in patients > 50 years but the risk is greater in those with a long history of ulcerative colitis, strong family history or who have syndromes that predispose to cancer. Clinical features include altered bowel habit, chronic anaemia, a feeling of incomplete evacuation (tenesmus) and rectal bleeding. Cancer of the caecum presents with weight loss and anaemia. Management depends on disease stage. Early disease is treated with surgical resection and adjuvant chemotherapy. Later disease may require palliative chemotherapy, colonic stenting or resection of an obstructing tumour.

1. Oesophageal disorders I

Questions
- What are the causes of dysphagia?
- What is the management of oesophageal varices?
- What is the management of gastro-oesophageal reflux disease?

Dysphagia (difficulty swallowing) is often the presenting complaint of an oesophageal disorder but may be caused by a wide variety of other conditions (Fig. 3.1.1).

Achalasia

Achalasia means 'without relaxation'. It is characterized by lack of peristalsis of the oesophagus and failure of the oesophago-gastric junction to relax and open following ingestion of food. Patients present with a long history of dysphagia for liquids and solids, vomiting, aspiration of gastric contents, regurgitation or chest discomfort. Achalasia is associated with an increased risk of squamous cancer of the oesophagus.

Investigations

Chest radiograph shows a dilated oesophagus with retrocardiac fluid. A barium swallow shows a dilated oesophagus with lack of peristalsis and a smooth tapered distal oesophageal stricture ('birds beak' appearance). At endoscopy, a dilated oesophagus may be seen and oesophageal manometry shows failure of the lower oesophageal sphincter to relax on swallowing.

Management

For elderly patients or those with mild symptoms, calcium channel blockers promote smooth muscle relaxation. Moderate to severe symptoms may need balloon dilatation under radiological or endoscopic control or botulinum toxin injection into the oesophago-gastric junction at endoscopy. Surgery (laparoscopic myotomy) may provide more permanent relief.

Oesophageal varices

Oesophageal varices are collateral blood vessels that occur in the wall of the oesophagus as a result of portal hypertension. Spontaneous rupture causes life-threatening haemorrhage. The incidence is unknown. Approximately one-third of patients with compensated liver cirrhosis have varices, but only one-third with varices will have an episode of haemorrhage.

Pathogenesis

The portal vein drains towards the liver and may become obstructed by distortion of the liver architecture or by occlusion of the hepatic veins. Obstruction causes high pressure (portal hypertension) and blood is diverted into portosystemic collaterals. Collaterals that form at the gastro-oesophageal junction are known as oesophageal varices. Portal hypertension is usually a result of liver cirrhosis. Other causes include portal vein thrombosis, Budd–Chiari syndrome (hepatic vein thrombosis),

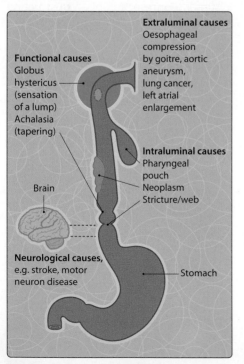

Functional causes
Globus hystericus (sensation of a lump)
Achalasia (tapering)

Brain

Neurological causes, e.g. stroke, motor neuron disease

Extraluminal causes
Oesophageal compression by goitre, aortic aneurysm, lung cancer, left atrial enlargement

Intraluminal causes
Pharyngeal pouch
Neoplasm
Stricture/web

Stomach

Fig. 3.1.1 Causes of dysphagia.

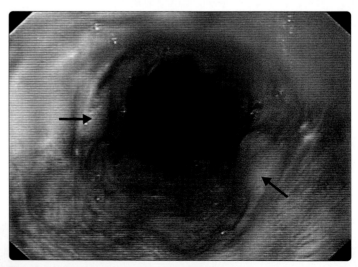

Fig. 3.1.2 Low-tension varices (arrows).

sickle cell disease, amyloidosis, inferior vena caval thrombosis and Banti syndrome (chronic congestion of the spleen).

Clinical features

Varices are asymptomatic until they bleed. Variceal haemorrhage may present with fresh haematemesis, melaena (black tarry stool) and/or hypovolaemic shock. Blood pressure and heart rate provide an indication of the degree of blood loss. (Signs of chronic liver disease may be present.)

Investigations

Low haemoglobin and raised urea are suggestive of upper GI bleeding. Endoscopy confirms the site of bleeding (Fig. 3.1.2).

Management

Urgent resuscitation with fluids and blood should be followed by endoscopy with variceal band ligation or sclerotherapy. Vasopressor agents (e.g. terlipressin) aid control of haemorrhage by causing splanchnic vasoconstriction and reduction in portal venous pressure. When bleeding cannot be controlled through endoscopy, a shunt inserted radiologically between the right hepatic vein and the right portal vein can reduce portal pressure (transjugular intrahepatic portosystemic shunt).

Patients with liver cirrhosis should undergo screening endoscopy of the upper GI tract to look for varices every few years. Patients with moderate to large varices should take non-selective beta-blockers prevent to haemorrhage.

Gastro-oesophageal reflux disease

Gastro-oesophageal reflux disease (GORD) occurs when the distal oesophageal mucosa is damaged by refluxed gastric contents. It is common in developed countries, with 20–40% of adults experiencing symptoms. The incidence increases with age.

Pathogenesis

The lower oesophageal sphincter is designed to prevent reflux of gastric contents into the distal oesophagus. Factors such as cigarette smoking and drugs such as calcium channel blockers can cause relaxation of the sphincter, encouraging reflux. As the junction normally sits below the diaphragm, the sphincter is reinforced by intra-abdominal pressure. Factors that raise intra-abdominal pressure (e.g. pregnancy, constipation, ascites or obesity) predispose to GORD. In hiatus hernia, the sphincter sits above the diaphragm, predisposing to reflux (Fig. 3.1.3). Repeated or severe reflux can cause ulceration to the distal oesophagus (oesophagitis).

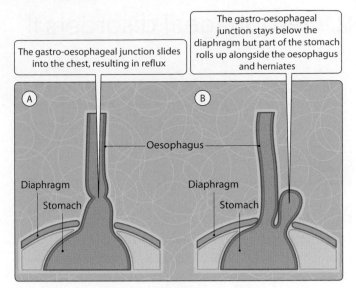

Fig. 3.1.3 Sliding (A) and rolling (B) hiatus hernia.

Clinical features

Typical symptoms include retrosternal burning or discomfort (heartburn), an unpleasant watery taste in the mouth (waterbrash), caused by regurgitation of gastric contents, and nocturnal coughing. Symptoms are often worse on lying flat, bending forward or straining. Examination is usually unremarkable. It is important to identify alarm features such as weight loss, early satiety or anaemia as they may indicate underlying oesophageal malignancy.

Investigations

Patients with alarm symptoms or symptoms significantly affecting their quality of life should be referred for further investigation:

- endoscopy may show oesophagitis or a hiatus hernia
- barium swallow and meal can diagnose reflux and help to exclude malignancy in patients not fit for endoscopy
- oesophageal pH studies and manometry assesses the correlation between the degree of reflux and symptoms.

Management

Simple measures such as avoiding large evening meals, exacerbating foods and tight clothing, plus raising the head of the bed, can be effective. Weight loss, smoking cessation, minimal alcohol and avoiding exacerbating drugs (anticholinergic drugs and calcium channel blockers) can also be effective.

Those with persistent symptoms should have a trial of acid suppression with a proton pump inhibitor (PPI). If this offers relief, patients should be maintained on the lowest dose that controls symptoms. Patients who cannot be controlled with drugs and have evidence of reflux on oesophageal manometry, may benefit from anti-reflux surgery (fundoplication).

2. Oesophageal disorders II

Questions
- What are the presenting features of oesophageal cancer?
- What is Barrett's oesophagus?

GI symptoms of dyspepsia and bleeding have several causes and often require further investigation (Figs 3.2.1 and 3.2.2).

Oesophageal cancer
Oesophageal cancer presents with progressive dysphagia. It has a relatively poor prognosis, as patients tend to present at a late stage.

Epidemiology
The UK incidence of oesophageal cancer is rising. Incidence increases with age and is rare in those <45 years. Squamous cell cancer is more common in the Far East and parts of Africa.

Pathogenesis
Oesophageal cancers are either squamous cell or adenocarcinoma. Squamous cell cancer accounts for 30% and usually occurs in the middle third of the oesophagus. Risk factors for oesophageal cancer include obesity, poor diet, excessive alcohol intake, smoking, achalasia, coeliac disease and Barrett's oesophagus. Smoking, alcohol abuse, achalasia and tylosis (an autosomal dominant disorder characterized by hyperkeratinization of the palms and soles) predispose to squamous cell cancer. Cigarette smoking also predisposes to adenocarcinoma of the oesophagus.

Most adenocarcinomas arise in the lower third of the oesophagus, often within Barrett's metaplasia.

Clinical features
Patients describe progressive dysphagia, initially for solids and subsequently for liquids, often associated with weight loss, lethargy and symptoms of anaemia (tiredness and breathlessness). Patients may have a history of gastro-oesophageal reflux disease. Occasionally oesophageal cancer presents with sudden dysphagia owing to impaction of a food bolus within the tumour.

Investigations
Endoscopy permits direct visualization and biopsy. Barium swallow can identify an oesophageal cancer, although endoscopy is required to obtain histological evidence. CT of chest and abdomen allows staging.

Management
Surgery. Disease in the early stages is treated surgically by oesophagectomy. Patients with evidence of spread to lymph nodes may undergo neoadjuvant chemotherapy or radiotherapy prior to surgery. Only 20% of surgery is curative and the operative mortality is significant, at 5–10%.

Palliative treatment. Patients with full-wall thickness tumours or metastases should be offered palliative chemotherapy. Oesophageal stenting (Fig. 3.2.3) and thermal laser tumour ablation can alleviate symptoms.

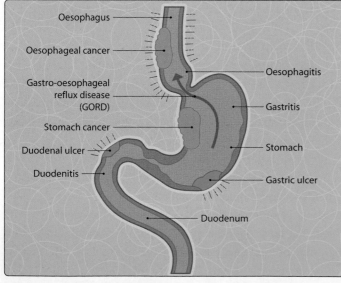

Fig. 3.2.1 Causes of dyspepsia.

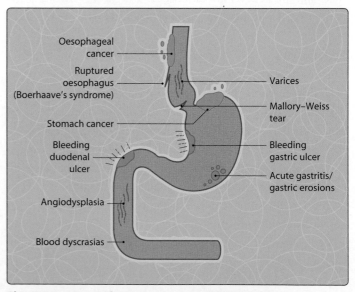

Fig. 3.2.2 Causes of upper gastrointestinal bleeding.

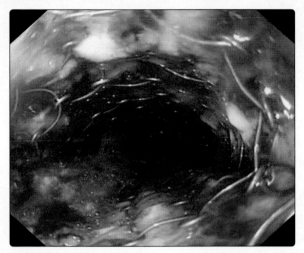

Fig. 3.2.3 A stent in place in a patient with advanced oesophageal cancer.

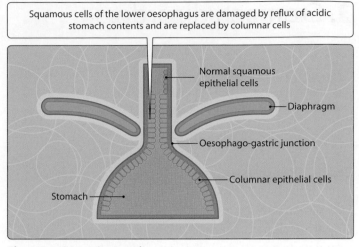

Squamous cells of the lower oesophagus are damaged by reflux of acidic stomach contents and are replaced by columnar cells

Normal squamous epithelial cells

Diaphragm

Oesophago-gastric junction

Columnar epithelial cells

Stomach

Fig. 3.2.4 Barrett's oesophagus.

Miscellaneous disorders of the oesophagus

Barrett's oesophagus. This is gastric metaplasia of the squamous epithelium in the distal oesophagus (Fig. 3.2.4). The distal oesophageal mucosa becomes lined with columnar epithelium to protect it from gastric acid. It affects 5% of the population, predominantly men >65 years. Barrett's oesophagus is a premalignant condition, with an increased risk of adenocarcinoma (0.5–1% develop cancer). It is diagnosed by biopsy at endoscopy. Surveillance endoscopy on a 2-yearly basis aims to detect high-grade dysplasia within the Barrett's segment before malignant change.

Diffuse oesophageal spasm. This is caused by abnormal oesophageal motility. Patients give a long history of retrosternal chest discomfort or dysphagia. It is important to identify alarm features (e.g. weight loss, anaemia or early satiety) that suggest oesophageal cancer. Dysphagia is usually intermittent with variable consistencies of food; severity does not change with time. Treatment is often unsatisfactory, although oral nitrates, calcium channel blockers or endoscopic dilatation can be considered.

Mallory–Weiss tear. A mucosal tear in the gastro-oesophageal junction can occur, following severe vomiting or retching. Patients present with haematemesis. In most patients bleeding stops spontaneously, although some may require endoscopic therapy or even surgery to control bleeding.

Schatzki ring. A mucosal ring forms a shelf around the wall of the lower oesophagus and sometimes this can cause dysphagia, especially after ingestion of a large food bolus. Dietary advice is required, but if symptoms are frequent or severe, the ring can be dilated at endoscopy.

Oesophageal web. This is a thin membrane that forms in the oesophagus above the level of the aortic arch and causes dysphagia. If associated with iron-deficiency anaemia, angular stomatitis and glossitis, it is known as Plummer–Vinson syndrome. Balloon dilatation endoscopy can be helpful. Iron replacement should be considered.

Pharyngeal pouch. This diverticulum occurs at the level of the cricopharyngeus. Symptoms include regurgitation of food and dysphagia. It is more common in elderly men. A palpable neck swelling, with gurgling, may be present. It is confirmed by barium swallow and may require surgical resection.

Oesophageal infection. Those who are immunosuppressed, malnourished, using antibiotics or taking oral or inhaled steroids are vulnerable to oesophageal infection. Patients may be asymptomatic or complain of dysphagia or odynophagia (pain on swallowing). Common infections are *Candida albicans*, herpes simplex or cytomegalovirus, all of which can cause mucosal ulceration. Oesophageal candidiasis causes white, patchy ulcerated slough. Diagnosis is confirmed by oesophageal biopsy and treatment is usually with oral antifungal or antiviral drugs.

Oesophageal perforation. This may occur following a sudden increase in intraluminal oesophageal pressure (e.g. during severe vomiting or retching). This causes transmural oesophageal perforation and sometime mediastinitis. Patients complain of lower chest or upper abdominal pain (worse on swallowing) and breathlessness. A chest radiograph may show a small left pleural effusion. Diagnosis is confirmed by a contrast swallow or CT of chest and abdomen. Treatment is with i.v. antibiotics, and thoracic surgery (especially if diagnosed within 24 h). Mortality is high.

3. Stomach disorders

Questions
- What is the management of peptic ulcer disease?
- What are the presenting features of stomach cancer?

Peptic ulcer disease

Peptic ulcer disease encompasses both gastric and duodenal ulceration. An ulcer is a break in the mucous membrane and may be acute or chronic. The most common causes are *Helicobacter pylori* infection (70%) and NSAID use (30%) (Fig. 3.3.1).

Epidemiology

Although the prevalence of peptic ulcer disease is falling in developed countries, 10% of adults will develop a peptic ulcer. Incidence of duodenal and gastric ulcers increases with age.

Pathogenesis

H. pylori infection is acquired in childhood through oral–oral or faecal–oral spread. The organism lives within the gastric epithelium and is not detected by the host immune system. *H. pylori* produce the enzyme urease, which converts urea to ammonia. This raises the surrounding pH and provides protection against gastric acid. *H. pylori* infection causes chronic gastritis

in adulthood, which may or may not be symptomatic. In some patients, the infection causes peptic ulceration.

Other factors associated with peptic ulceration are aspirin and NSAIDs, which deplete mucosal prostaglandins. Smoking increases the risk of gastric and, to a lesser extent, duodenal ulceration.

Clinical features

The most common symptom is epigastric discomfort or indigestion (dyspepsia). Patients may report temporary relief from taking antacids or after eating. Chronic ulceration can cause weight loss, anorexia and anaemia, and in these cases malignancy must be excluded. Some patients present with complications of peptic ulcer disease, such as bleeding (Fig. 3.3.2) or perforation. Patients with uncomplicated peptic ulcer disease may have epigastric tenderness.

Investigations

Upper GI endoscopy (UGIE) allows direct visualization and biopsy. Barium meal is a useful alternative.

Testing for *H. pylori* can be by:
- biopsy of an ulcer: histology or an agar-based urease test (CLO test for '*Campylobacter*-like organisms'); false negatives can be found in patients with blood in their stomach or who are using proton pump inhibitors (PPIs)
- serology (IgG antibody) is used when patients are taking PPIs but is unable to differentiate between recent past and current infection
- urea breath tests: high sensitivity and specificity but PPIs need to be discontinued for 4 weeks prior to the test.

Management

High-dose acid suppression with a PPI is given for 4 to 6 weeks. NSAIDs and aspirin should be stopped where possible. If patients need to continue these drugs, a long-term PPI should be considered. Eradication of *H. pylori* is achieved in 80% with a 7-day course of a PPI with a combination of antibiotics (amoxicillin or metronidazole with clarithromycin). It is rare for patients to become reinfected.

Patients with gastric ulcers should have repeat endoscopy at 6 weeks to ensure healing, since chronic ulcers may be malignant.

Bleeding. Individuals may vomit fresh or altered blood (haematemesis) or pass loose, black, tarry stool (melaena). Treatment is resuscitation with blood or i.v. fluids, acid suppression and UGIE. If active bleeding persists, ulcers

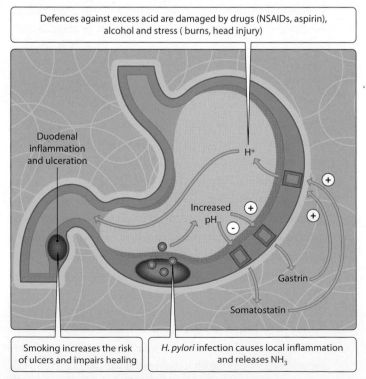

Fig. 3.3.1 Pathophysiology of peptic ulcer disease.

can be treated with epinephrine (adrenaline) injection, heater probe coagulation or clip placement. If bleeding cannot be controlled, surgery may be required.

Perforation. Peritonitis occurs with significant abdominal tenderness, rebound and guarding. An erect chest radiograph shows free air under the diaphragm. Broad-spectrum antibiotics and emergency surgery are needed.

Non-ulcer ('functional') dyspepsia

Non-ulcer dyspepsia is a functional disorder, similar to irritable bowel syndrome, thought to result from dysmotility and influenced by psychological factors.

Clinical features

Patients describe a long history of epigastric discomfort or pain, sometimes associated with bloating or belching. Patients appear well and have no weight loss.

Investigations

Investigation with UGIE is only required for alarm symptoms or >55 years of age with symptoms not responding to treatment.

Management

The condition is benign and lifestyle changes, (e.g. regular meals, weight loss, reducing alcohol intake and smoking cessation) may help. Eradication of *H. pylori* infection, if present, may relieve symptoms. If there is no improvement a PPI should be considered. Tricyclic antidepressants and prokinetic agents may offer symptomatic benefit.

Gastric cancer

Gastric cancer is the second most common cause of cancer death worldwide and is more common in the Far East and developing countries. It is more common in men and the incidence increases with age. The incidence of gastric cancer is falling, possibly through greater awareness of risk factors.

Pathogenesis

Gastric cancer is usually an adenocarcinoma. Risk factors include smoking, long-standing *H. pylori* infection, previous gastric surgery, family history and gastric atrophy. Approximately 1% of gastric cancers are hereditary, with an autosomal dominant pattern. A diffuse type of gastric cancer, linitus plastica, may occur with extensive submucosal spread.

Clinical features

Patients present with persistent dyspepsia, early satiety, weight loss and anaemia. Some present acutely, with either haematemesis

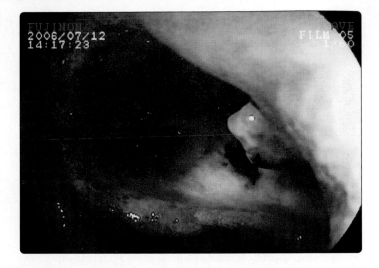

Fig. 3.3.2 A bleeding duodenal ulcer with visible vessel (arrow).

or melaena, caused by bleeding from an ulcerating tumour. Cancers in the distal part of the stomach cause vomiting secondary to outflow obstruction, while proximal tumours cause dysphagia. Examination may reveal weight loss, pallor or lymphadenopathy. An epigastric mass or enlargement of a left supraclavicular lymph node (Virchow's node) may be present.

Investigations

FBC may show iron-deficiency anaemia. UGIE will show a non-healing gastric ulcer, often with thickened, rolled edges. Diagnosis is confirmed by biopsy. Endoscopic ultrasound can show the depth of tissue invasion and local lymph node involvement and may aid staging prior to surgery. CT allows accurate staging.

Management

Patients with disease confined to the stomach should undergo partial or total gastrectomy. Chemotherapy can improve the prognosis of patients with advanced gastric cancer. Bypass surgery and endoscopic stenting for lesions obstructing the pylorus can improve symptoms.

Other gastric tumours

Lymphomas associated with *H. pylori* infection (maltomas) can be managed by eradication of the organism. High-grade lymphomas are treated with chemotherapy.

Gastrointestinal stromal tumours arise from gastric subepithelial tissue and may be benign or malignant. They appear as a mass during endoscopy and the diagnosis is confirmed by endoscopic ultrasound and biopsy. Small benign tumours are followed up with regular ultrasound and large or malignant tumours can be treated with chemotherapy and/or surgery.

4. Disorders of the small intestine

Questions
- What are the symptoms of coeliac disease?
- How is coeliac disease managed?

The small bowel plays an important role in nutrient and electrolyte absorption, acid–base balance and digestion. Disorders present with malabsorption, which results in chronic diarrhoea and weight loss (Fig. 3.4.1). Causes of malabsorption include:

- **structural**: small bowel lymphoma, coeliac disease, Crohn's disease, short bowel syndrome, bacterial overgrowth
- **infections**: giardiasis, Whipple's disease, tropical sprue
- **other**: chronic pancreatitis, cirrhosis, biliary obstruction.

Coeliac disease

Coeliac disease is an autoimmune disorder of the small intestine that causes maldigestion and malabsorption.

Epidemiology

Coeliac disease occurs in 1 in 250 people. It is more common in northern Europe and is equally common in males and females. In 25% of patients there is a family history.

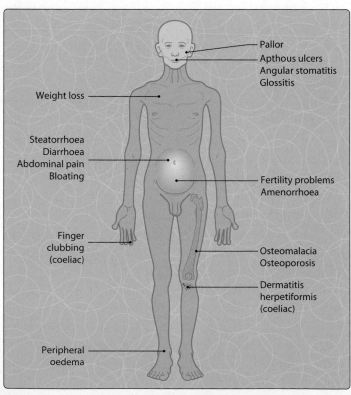

Fig. 3.4.1 Clinical features of malabsorption.

Pathogenesis

Gluten (protein in wheat, barley and rye) reacts with small intestinal mucosa causing an inappropriate T cell-mediated immune response in genetically susceptible individuals. This results in abnormalities of the mucosa of the duodenum and jejunum that impairs its absorptive surface. Villi become short and wide (subtotal villous atrophy) or disappear (total villous atrophy) (Fig. 3.4.2).

Clinical features

Coeliac disease can present at any age. Children present with impaired growth, pubertal delay, diarrhoea or abdominal pain. Adults present with weight loss, pallor, lethargy and diarrhoea caused by malabsorption. Women may present with subfertility that resolves with dietary gluten exclusion.

Investigations

FBC shows iron-deficiency (reduced mean cell volume (MCV)) or folate-deficiency (raised MCV). Blood film may show target cells and Howell–Jolly bodies indicative of hyposplenism. Endomysial antibody has a high sensitivity and specificity (Fig. 3.4.3). Duodenal biopsy show subtotal or total villous atrophy.

Management

Patients should start a gluten-free diet for life. By 2 weeks, 70% of patients will have symptomatic improvement and 6 to 12 months later, endomysial antibody will be negative. Recurring symptoms may indicate gluten inadvertently entering the diet or development of small-bowel T cell lymphoma.

Bacterial overgrowth

In the presence of structural abnormality, decreased intestinal motility or depressed immunity, the small intestine may become colonized with bacteria that normally reside in the large intestine.

Clinical features

Patients present with features of malabsorption in the presence of structural small bowel disease. Non-invasive breath tests may be helpful but have a low sensitivity and specificity.

Management

Treatment is aimed at eliminating any underlying small intestinal disease and using broad-spectrum antibiotics. Patients may respond to a 10-day course of antibiotics, but some require longer rotational courses to control symptoms.

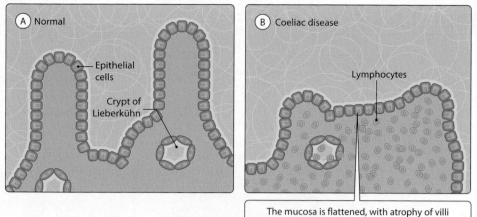

Fig. 3.4.2 Histological features of coeliac disease.

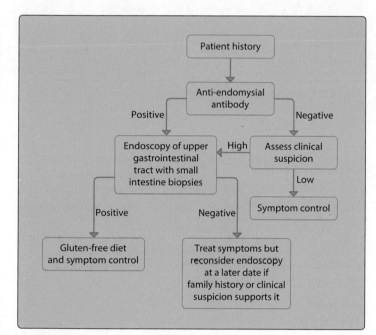

Fig. 3.4.3 Diagnosis of coeliac disease.

Short bowel syndrome

Short bowel syndrome occurs either after surgery (small bowel resection) or in the presence of severe malabsorption (functional short bowel syndrome). The reduction in absorptive capacity results in loss of fluid, electrolytes, fat, bile salts and vitamins, depending on the site of small intestinal resection. This causes diarrhoea or high stoma output, malnutrition and electrolyte imbalance.

Management
Oral rehydration solutions help to replenish water, sodium chloride and glucose. Subcutaneous octreotide, a synthetic analogue of the hormone somatostatin, suppresses the endocrine secretions of the small intestine, and high-dose loperamide or codeine slows intestinal motility. Total parenteral nutrition is occasionally required. The prognosis of short bowel syndrome depends on the underlying cause, length of remaining bowel, age and comorbidities.

Small bowel infections
Whipple's disease is rare and caused by the Gram-positive bacillus, or actinobacterium, *Tropheryma whippelii*. It affects middle-aged men (40–50 years) and presents with low-grade fever, steatorrhoea and abdominal pain in addition to pleuritic pain, migratory arthritis, pericarditis, finger clubbing and occasionally myoclonus, dementia and ophthalmoplegia. Jejunal biopsies show stunted villi with infiltration of the lamina propria by foamy macrophages that are positive for periodic acid–Schiff (PAS) stain. There is usually a good response to cotrimoxazole, which should be continued for 1 year. Long-term follow-up is required and relapse is common.

Giardiasis is caused by the flagellated protozoan *Giardia lamblia*. Infection occurs through contaminated drinking water. The incubation period is 1–3 weeks and patients present with chronic diarrhoea and weight loss, which can persist for many months. Microscopy of stool or jejunal aspirate confirms cysts. Treatment is with metronidazole.

Tropical sprue is a rare postinfective malabsorptive syndrome occurring in adults who have visited India, Asia or Central America. The cause is unknown. Patients present with diarrhoea, abdominal distension, anorexia, fatigue and weight loss. Duodenal biopsies show partial villous atrophy. Treatment is with tetracycline.

5. Inflammatory bowel disease

Questions
- What are the differences between Crohn's disease and ulcerative colitis?
- What parts of the bowel are affected by Crohn's disease and ulcerative colitis?

Crohn's disease and ulcerative colitis are collectively known as inflammatory bowel disease.

Pathogenesis

The causes of Crohn's disease and ulcerative colitis are not known. Twin studies suggest a genetic influence, particularly in Crohn's disease. While the two conditions have common features, they are also quite distinct (Fig. 3.5.1).

Crohn's disease

Crohn's disease is more common in developed countries, affecting approximately 1 in 1500. It usually presents in those aged 20–40 years and is more common in smokers.

Clinical features

Crohn's disease may affect any part of the GI tract from the mouth to the anus and symptoms depend on the area affected:

- colon: bloody diarrhoea (Crohn's colitis) similar to ulcerative colitis
- small bowel: malabsorption (e.g. weight loss, diarrhoea and vitamin deficiencies); abdominal pain is common particularly in the right iliac fossa if the disease affects the terminal ileum; healing of an inflamed segment of small bowel can cause scarring and strictures, resulting in intermittent obstruction
- rectum and anus: anal fissures, abscess formation and perianal discharge from fistulae (enterovesiculae, enterovaginal or cutaneous)
- an abnormal communication (fistula) between structures may arise in inflamed tissue (enterovesicle, enterovaginal or enterocutaneous).

Investigations

In active disease, CRP, ESR, white cell count and platelets are raised, often with anaemia.

Colonoscopy shows inflammation (fissures, deep ulcers and a cobblestone mucosa) with normal mucosa between inflamed areas ('skip lesions'). Small bowel studies can show areas of narrowing ('string sign'), 'rosethorn' ulcers (fissuring) or fistulae. Histology typically shows non-caseating granulomatous inflammation.

Radioisotope-labelled white cell scans can highlight areas of inflammation.

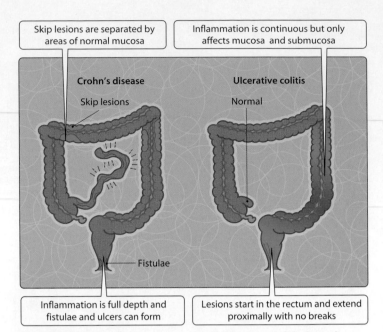

Skip lesions are separated by areas of normal mucosa

Inflammation is continuous but only affects mucosa and submucosa

Crohn's disease

Skip lesions

Ulcerative colitis

Normal

Fistulae

Inflammation is full depth and fistulae and ulcers can form

Lesions start in the rectum and extend proximally with no breaks

Fig. 3.5.1 Distribution and pathological features of Crohn's disease and ulcerative colitis.

Ulcerative colitis

The prevalence of ulcerative colitis in developed countries is 1 in 1000, usually affecting those 20–40 years of age. It is more common in women and less common in smokers.

Pathogenesis

Ulcerative colitis only affects the colon. It may affect the entire colon and rectum (pancolitis), the left side of the colon and rectum (distal colitis) or the rectum alone (proctitis). Macroscopically, there is continuous involvement of the mucosal surface (no skip lesions). The mucosa is red and friable and in severe disease there may be ulcers and pseudopolyps (islands of regenerating mucosa). Biopsy of the colon shows mucosal inflammation and goblet cell depletion but no granulomata.

Clinical features

Patients usually present with diarrhoea mixed with blood and mucous. Features that suggest a severe exacerbation of ulcerative colitis include bloody diarrhoea occurring more than six times/day, fever (>37.5°C), tachycardia >90 beats/min, ESR >30 mm/h, anaemia (haemoglobin <100 g/l) and albumin <30 g/l. Finger clubbing and apthous oral ulceration may be present. In moderate disease, hypotension, signs of dehydration and abdominal tenderness may be present. In severe acute attacks, rebound tenderness, suggesting peritonism, and abdominal guarding occur.

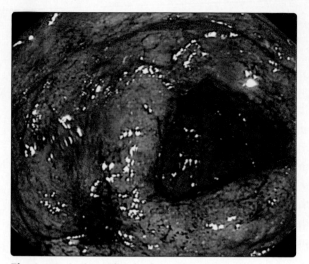

Fig. 3.5.2 Active colitis in the transverse colon.

Investigations

In acute disease, the ESR is elevated, serum albumin is low and anaemia is present. Plain abdominal radiograph can show features of mucosal oedema (thumb-printing), empty distal colon, proximal faecal loading. and colonic dilatation in toxic megacolon. Colonoscopy or flexible sigmoidoscopy reveals red, ulcerated and friable mucosa (Fig. 3.5.2). Histology typically shows chronic inflammation of the mucosa with crypt abscesses. Radioisotope-labelled white cell scans can highlight areas of inflammation.

Extra-intestinal manifestations of inflammatory bowel disease

Table 3.5.1 lists extra-intestinal manifestations of inflammatory bowel disease. Finger clubbing and recurrent apthous ulcers within the oral cavity occur in both Crohn's disease and ulcerative colitis. Nephrolithiasis (5–10 oxalate stones) can occur with small-bowel Crohn's disease.

Management of inflammatory bowel disease

Inflammatory bowel disease is often relapsing and remitting. Treatment is prolonged and dependent on disease severity. Aminosalicylates are used in mild-to-moderate colitis and help to maintain remission. Oral or i.v. steroids are thought to suppress the immune response and are important during acute exacerbations. Steroid-sparing agents (azathioprine, methotrexate or ciclosporin) can also be used to suppress the immune system. Topical steroids and aminosalicylic acid can be given as enemas to induce remission and limit systemic absorption. Infliximab (monoclonal antibody against tumour necrosis factor alpha) may be useful in severe Crohn's disease.

Adequate nutrition is important in patients with malabsorption secondary to small-bowel Crohn's disease. A high-calorie diet, vitamin replacement and enteral or parenteral feeding may be necessary in patients with severe disease.

Patients with severe ulcerative colitis unresponsive to medical therapy may require total or partial colectomy to control symptoms; total colectomy is curative. Patients with Crohn's disease and small-bowel strictures may require surgery to avoid obstruction. Fistulae may require surgical excision and perianal abscesses need draining.

Toxic megacolon is a medical emergency and may result in colonic perforation and peritonitis. It should be considered in patients with ulcerative colitis who develop abdominal pain, distension, guarding or rebound tenderness. Plain abdominal radiograph may confirm dilatation of the colon to >5 cm in diameter. Emergency colectomy is often required.

Inflammatory bowel disease and cancer

Depending on the extent and duration of disease, there is increased risk of colorectal cancer (approximately 1–2% after 10 years of pancolitis). Individuals with pancolitis should be offered screening colonoscopy every 10 years.

Table 3.5.1 EXTRA-INTESTINAL FEATURES

Features	Percentage	
	UC	CD
Eyes		
Uveitis, episcleritis	2	5
Conjunctivitis	5–8	3–10
Joints		
Synovitis	10–20	10–20
Type I arthropathy (pauci-articular)	4	6
Type II arthropathy (polyarticular)	2.5	4
Arthralgia	5	14
Ankylosing spondylitis	1	1.2
Inflammatory back pain	3.5	9
Skin		
Erythema nodosum	1	4
Pyoderma gangrenosum	1	2
Liver and biliary tree		
Sclerosing cholangitis	2.5–7.5	1–2
Fatty liver	C	C
Chronic hepatitis, cirrhosis	U	U
Gallstones	N	15–30
Vascular: venous thrombosis	5	1

UC, ulcerative colitis; CD, Crohn's disease; C, common; U, uncommon; N, normal.

6. Irritable bowel syndrome

Questions
- What are the symptoms of irritable bowel syndrome?
- How is it managed?

Irritable bowel syndrome describes a range of functional bowel disorders and it is one of the most common GI disorders.

Epidemiology

Irritable bowel syndrome is common in developed countries, with as many as 1 in 5 people experiencing symptoms. It is more common in women of child-bearing age.

Pathogenesis

The cause is not fully understood but it may result from disturbance of colon motility. Factors such as visceral hypersensitivity, neuromuscular dysfunction, psychological conflicts and diet may play a role. The illness often starts following an episode of gastroenteritis or stress. Other potential triggers are:

- antibiotic therapy
- pelvic surgery
- psychological stress or trauma
- mood disturbance, anxiety, depression
- sexual, physical or verbal abuse
- food intolerance
- eating disorders.

Clinical features

The main symptom is abdominal discomfort relieved by defaecation (Fig. 3.6.1). Other symptoms include altered stool frequency or consistency, the passage of mucous, incomplete defaecation, audible borborygmi (bowel sounds), excess flatus or abdominal distension, sometimes associated with dyspepsia. Rectal bleeding should never be attributed to irritable bowel syndrome. Examination is usually normal. Non-GI features include:

- gynaecological symptoms: dysmenorrhoea, dyspareunia, premenstrual tension
- urinary symptoms: frequency, urgency, nocturia, incomplete bladder emptying
- other: back pain, headaches, bad breath, unpleasant taste in the mouth, poor sleeping, fatigue, anxiety, depression.

Investigations

Some patients require investigation (barium enema or colonoscopy) to exclude colon cancer or inflammatory bowel disease, particularly those

- aged > 45 years with a change in bowel habit
- with a strong family history of GI malignancy
- with rectal bleeding
- with anaemia
- with weight loss.

Most other patients do not need invasive investigation.

Management

Many patients benefit from an explanation of their illness. They should be made aware that, although it is a chronic condition, it is benign.

Dietary change

A high-fibre diet is often recommended. Although irritable bowel syndrome is not caused by a food allergy, many patients find that excluding certain food types (e.g. dairy or wheat produce) relieves symptoms.

Pharmacological measures

The pain caused by colonic spasm associated with visceral hypersensitivity may respond to antispasmodics (e.g. peppermint oil, hyoscine or mebeverine). Patients with diarrhoea may benefit from antidiarrhoeal drugs (e.g. loperamide) and those with constipation may improve with bulking agents (e.g. ispaghula husk). Low-dose tricyclic antidepressants can raise the pain threshold, decrease intestinal spasm and reduce anxiety. Probiotics containing lactobacilli may help to relieve symptoms.

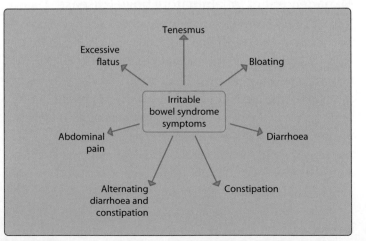

Fig. 3.6.1 Intestinal symptoms of irritable bowel syndrome.

7. Antibiotic-associated diarrhoea

Questions
- Who is at risk of *Clostridium difficile* infection?
- How is *C. difficile* managed?

Diarrhoea is a common adverse effect of antibiotics. In some cases this is a result of overgrowth with the anaerobic organism *Clostridium difficile*. If severe, this infection can result in acute colitis or pseudomembranous colitis.

Epidemiology
The incidence of antibiotic-associated diarrhoea is unknown, but it is more common in the very young and elderly.

Pathogenesis
C. difficile is part of the normal bowel flora in 3–5% of the population. Broad-spectrum antibiotics eliminate intestinal commensal organisms, thus allowing *C. difficile* to overgrow. *C. difficile* produces two toxins: toxin A is an enterotoxin and toxin B is cytotoxic and causes bloody diarrhoea. These toxins cause secretion of fluid into the gut and focal inflammation and ulceration of the mucosa (colitis). Ulcerated areas may become covered by a creamy-white adherent 'pseudomembrane' (Fig. 3.7.1). Diarrhoea can develop from 2 days to 4 weeks after taking antibiotics. Factors such as prolonged hospital stay, multiple or prolonged antibiotic therapy, GI surgery and proton pump inhibitor use increase the risk of diarrhoea.

C. difficile spores occur in hospital wards, nurseries and bathrooms and are spread by the faecal–oral route. They can be carried from patient to patient on stethoscopes, clothing or hands.

Clinical features
Patients present with watery diarrhoea and lower abdominal pain. Others present with fulminant colitis (bloody diarrhoea), which may progress to toxic megacolon and perforation. Signs of dehydration, low-grade fever and abdominal tenderness often occur. Those with more severe infections present with abdominal distension and hypotension.

Investigations
In most cases, *C. difficile* toxins A and B can be detected in stools by ELISA (enzyme-linked immunosorbent assay) and *C. difficile* can be isolated from stool cultures in 30%.

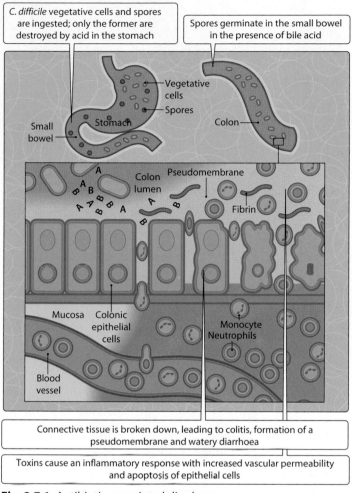

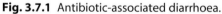

Fig. 3.7.1 Antibiotic-associated diarrhoea.

Sigmoidoscopy may show ulceration and an adherent pseudomembrane.

Management
Antibiotics should be stopped and dehydration treated with oral or i.v. fluids. Infection control measures (e.g. barrier nursing and hand washing) prevent spread of infection.

Antibiotics against *C. difficile* (e.g. metronidazole or oral vancomycin) should be started following diagnosis. The disease is more severe in the elderly and rarely colectomy may be required for toxic megacolon or perforation.

8. Other large bowel disorders

Questions
■ What are the complications of diverticular disease?
■ What is the management of diverticular disease?
■ What are the clinical features of ischaemic colitis?

Lower GI bleeding can result from a number of causes (Fig. 3.8.1).

Diverticular disease

A diverticulum is an outpouching that occurs in the wall of a hollow organ. The presence of diverticulae in the colon is termed diverticular disease.

Epidemiology

Diverticular disease affects 50% of those >50 years of age in Western countries.

Pathogenesis

Diverticular disease is usually acquired, although there are rare congenital forms (e.g. Meckel's diverticulum). The number of diverticulae within the colon ranges from few to numerous. Diverticulae can occur anywhere within the colon, but in most patients the sigmoid colon is affected and in 50% the disease solely affects this area. Right-sided diverticulae are more common in Asian populations and in those < 40 years.

A diverticulum is formed from herniation of the mucosa and submucosa of the colon through the muscularis layer. They are thought to be caused by high intraluminal pressure at mechanically weak areas of the bowel wall, for example at points where blood vessels penetrate the muscularis layer.

Clinical features

Most patients with diverticular disease are asymptomatic. However left iliac fossa discomfort, flatulence, abdominal distension and altered bowel habit can occur. Examination is usually normal.

Investigations

Double-contrast barium enema and CT colonography show the outpouchings within the bowel wall. CT of the abdomen is useful if there is associated infection (diverticulitis). Colonoscopy allows direct visualization of the diverticular pockets within the lumen and is used to exclude coexisting colorectal cancer.

Management

A high-fibre diet eases the discomfort of constipation and may have a role in prevention of diverticular disease. Osmotic laxatives soften the stool by increasing the amount of water in the large bowel, while bulk-forming laxatives increase faecal mass, stimulating peristalsis. Antispasmodic drugs relax intestinal smooth muscle and reduce painful spasm.

Complications

There are a number of potential complications of diverticular disease (Fig. 3.8.2)

Diverticulitis. Infected or inflamed diverticulae cause abdominal pain, fever and raised ESR and CRP. Abdominal CT can show the area of inflammation, abscess formation or perforation. Management consists of i.v. antibiotics, i.v. fluids and analgesia.

Diverticular haemorrhage. Diverticulae are often close to colonic intramural arteries, increasing the risk of haemorrhage. In profuse rectal bleeding, sigmoidoscopy may be difficult and colonic angiography can be used to identify the source. Most patients improve with supportive management and fluid resuscitation, although some require surgery.

Ischaemic colitis

Ischaemic colitis is mucosal damage to the colon caused by a temporary interruption to its blood supply (Fig. 3.8.3).

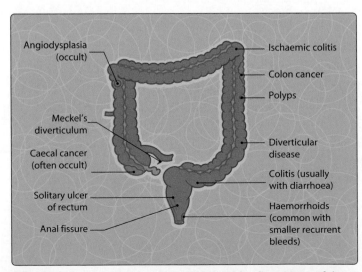

Fig. 3.8.1 Causes of lower gastrointestinal bleeding. Many of these conditions can occur in several locations of the colon.

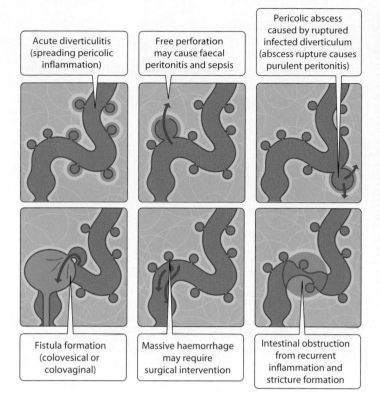

Acute diverticulitis
(spreading pericolic
inflammation)

Free perforation
may cause faecal
peritonitis and sepsis

Pericolic abscess
caused by ruptured
infected diverticulum
(abscess rupture causes
purulent peritonitis)

Fistula formation
(colovesical or
colovaginal)

Massive haemorrhage
may require
surgical intervention

Intestinal obstruction
from recurrent
inflammation and
stricture formation

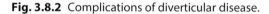

Fig. 3.8.2 Complications of diverticular disease.

Epidemiology

Ischaemic colitis is rare. Patients with cardiovascular disease (particulary atrial fibrillation) and the elderly are more at risk.

Pathogenesis

Vascular occlusion to the colon may be transient (ischaemia) or prolonged (infarction). It usually affects the splenic flexure, which has limited collateral blood supply. The resulting ischaemia causes haemorrhage and ulceration of the colonic mucosa. The blood supply affected may be arterial, venous or smaller vessels. Arterial causes include mesenteric artery thrombosis, cholesterol emboli or aortic dissection. Venous causes include mesenteric venous thrombosis secondary to hypercoagulation states. Small vessels may be affected by vasculitic disorders or diabetes mellitus.

Clinical features

Patients present with a short history of abdominal pain and bloody diarrhoea. Examination may reveal generalized abdominal tenderness, pallor, tachycardia and bloody stool on rectal

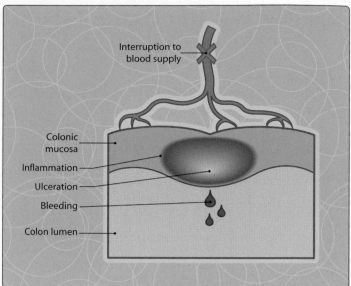

Fig. 3.8.3 Pathogenesis of ischaemic colitis.

examination. Patients with severe disease may show signs of shock or sepsis (tachycardia, hypotension or pyrexia).

Investigations

FBC will show a raised white cell count, and CRP and ESR are elevated. Metabolic acidosis may be present. Abdominal radiograph may exclude other conditions (e.g. toxic megacolon). Flexible sigmoidoscopy shows pale mucosa with petechial haemorrhage, frank bleeding or ulceration and CT angiography will show localized areas of thickened, inflamed colonic wall.

Management

Initial management is with i.v. fluids and broad-spectrum antibiotics. Most patients improve within a few days and the bowel mucosa returns to normal within a few weeks. However, if colonic perforation or peritonitis occurs it is usually within 24 h and may require emergency colectomy. If colonic ischaemia persists, the mucosa ulcerates causing stricture formation as it heals. Stricturoplasty or localized resection may be required. Patients with mesenteric venous thrombosis require long-term anticoagulation with warfarin. Ischaemic colitis rarely recurs.

9. Polyps and colorectal cancer

Questions
- What are the presenting features of colorectal cancer?
- What investigations are performed in suspected colorectal cancer?

Colonic polyps

Colonic polyps are considered premalignant as their incidence mirrors that of colorectal cancer. The average age of patients with polyps is less than those with invasive cancer.

Epidemiology

The incidence of polyps is uncertain as many patients are asymptomatic. However, it is thought that one-third of the population >50 years of age has one or more polyp.

Pathogenesis

A polyp is an elevation of the mucosal surface, although the mechanism of formation is not fully understood. They may be flat (sessile) or stick out into the bowel lumen on a stalk. There are three main histological types:

- adenomatous: most common and have malignant potential; only a minority develop into colorectal cancer (often larger or multiple polyps), but because of this risk they are resected
- hyperplastic: <5 mm in diameter and found incidentally at colonoscopy; as they do not show dysplastic change, they do not need resection
- hamartomatous: develop in children and although there is little chance of malignancy developing they are resected because of their potential to bleed.

Clinical features

Patients are often asymptomatic but may have altered bowel habit or rectal bleeding.

Investigations

Double-contrast barium enema and CT colonography can detect polyps. Colonoscopy allows direct visualization plus biopsy or endoscopic resection of a polyp.

Management

Small colonic polyps can be removed by various endoscopic techniques (e.g. snare or diathermy) but larger polyps may require surgical resection. Polyps should always be sent for histological examination to ensure complete resection and exclude malignant change. Following resection, surveillance colonoscopy is recommended to exclude recurrence.

Colorectal cancer

Epidemiology

Colorectal cancer is the third most common cause of cancer in Europe. Males and individuals >50 years are at increased risk.

Pathogenesis

The cause of colorectal cancer is unknown. The most common area affected is the recto-sigmoid colon. It initially spreads by direct invasion through the bowel wall (Fig. 3.9.1) and may metastasize, often to the liver. Protective factors include a diet high in fruit and vegetables, regular exercise and use of aspirin, hormone replacement therapy and calcium supplements.

Clinical features

Patients present with abdominal discomfort, rectal bleeding, tenesmus (sensation of incomplete evacuation) or a change in bowel habit (Fig. 3.9.2). They may have symptoms of anaemia (e.g. tiredness or breathlessness). Abdominal examination is often normal but a palpable mass or hepatomegaly secondary to metastatic disease may be present.

Investigations

FBC shows iron-deficiency anaemia. Liver function tests are deranged if hepatic metastases are present.

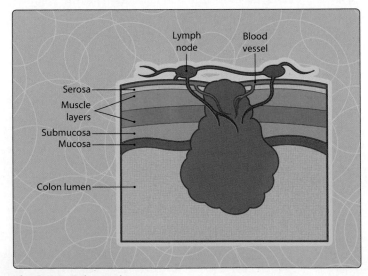

Fig. 3.9.1 Colorectal cancer.

Double-contrast barium enema may show a classic 'apple core' lesion within the lumen and CT colonography can highlight mucosal abnormalities.

Colonoscopy shows a growth protruding from the colonic mucosa and allows biopsy.

Liver ultrasound and chest radiograph may identify metastases and allow staging.

Management

Colorectal cancer is staged according to the TNM system (Table 3.9.1) or Dukes criteria:

Dukes A is limited to the mucosa

Dukes B invades the muscle layer

Dukes C involves lymph nodes

Dukes D indicates distant metastases.

Surgical resection can cure localized colorectal cancer, and patients with Dukes stage A disease have a 5-year survival of 95%. If possible, an end-to-end anastomosis is created but occasionally resection requires formation of a colostomy. Adjuvant chemotherapy is used to minimize the chance of recurrence. If the tumour is not resectable, palliative radiotherapy or chemotherapy may be used to reduce disease bulk and relieve symptoms. Colonoscopic procedures such as local tumour ablation or stent placement may also reduce symptoms.

Hereditary syndromes

Peutz–Jeghers syndrome is an autosomal dominant condition of multiple colonic polyps and mucocutaneous pigmentation.

Familial adenomatous polyposis is inherited in an autosomal dominant fashion and is associated with numerous adenomatous polyps in the colon. In view of the malignant potential, patients are offered prophylactic colectomy.

Gardener's syndrome is a variation of this where patients have extracolonic growths (osteomas, epidermoid cysts and fibromas) in addition to colonic polyps.

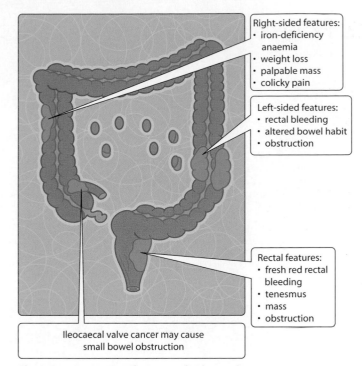

Right-sided features:
• iron-deficiency anaemia
• weight loss
• palpable mass
• colicky pain

Left-sided features:
• rectal bleeding
• altered bowel habit
• obstruction

Rectal features:
• fresh red rectal bleeding
• tenesmus
• mass
• obstruction

Ileocaecal valve cancer may cause small bowel obstruction

Fig. 3.9.2 Presenting features of colorectal cancer.

Non-polyposis coli accounts for approximately 5% of colorectal cancers and is inherited in an autosomal dominant pattern. Affected individuals are at risk of right-sided colorectal cancer at a young age. These patients may also develop extracolonic tumours (e.g. endometrial cancer).

Colorectal screening

Surveillance colonoscopy should be offered to patients in high-risk groups: those with previous history of colorectal cancer, long history of inflammatory bowel disease, any hereditary syndrome linked to increased colon cancer risk or a strong family history.

Table 3.9.1 THE TUMOUR, NODE, METASTASIS (TNM) SYSTEM TO STAGE COLORECTAL CANCER

Stage	Classification			Survival at 5 years (%)
	Tumour	Node (lymph node involvement)	Metastasis	
1	1–2	0	0	~90
2	3, 4	0	0	~60
3	1–4	1,2	0	~30
4	Any	Any	1	~10

Primary tumour: T0, no primary tumour; Tis, carcinoma in situ (has not grown beyond the mucosa); T1, growth into the submucosa; T2, growth into the muscularis propria; T3, growth into the subserosa but not into any neighbouring organs; T4, growth of local tissues or organs. *Node*: N0, no lymph node involvement; N1, 1–3 regional nodes involved; N2, 4 or more regional nodes involved; N3, para-aortic nodes involved. *Metastases*: M0, no distant metastases; M1, distant metastases.

PART V

Disorders of the liver and pancreas

Andrew Fraser

The big picture

The liver

The liver is the largest internal organ in the body and receives 25% of the cardiac output via two different blood supplies: 25% from the hepatic artery (a branch of the coeliac plexus) and 75% from the portal vein. The portal vein is formed from the splenic and superior mesenteric veins, which drain the stomach, spleen, small and large intestines (Fig. 1.1).

The liver is divided into right and left lobes and then further divided into eight functional segments, each of which has its own branch of the hepatic artery, portal vein and bile duct. The functional unit of the liver is the acinus. Blood enters the acinus from the portal tract, containing a branch of the hepatic artery and portal vein (Fig. 1.2 and 1.3). Blood then passes into the endothelial-lined hepatic sinusoids before entering into a branch of the hepatic vein (central vein). In addition to hepatocytes, there are Kupffer cells (specialized macrophages) and stellate cells, which, when stimulated, become contractile and regulate blood flow. A network of bile canaliculi between the plates of hepatocytes join up to form a bile duct in the portal tracts. The ducts combine at a segmental level before eventually becoming the main right and left hepatic ducts, which join at the porta hepatis to form the common hepatic duct. The liver has many important functions and plays a vital role in:

- formation of bile salts, bile acids and bilirubin
- protein production, e.g. albumin
- production of all clotting factors (including vitamin K dependent II, VII, IX and X)
- production of specific transporter proteins, e.g. transferrin and sex hormone-binding protein
- cholesterol synthesis and metabolism of lipoproteins
- glucose homeostasis (glycogenolysis and gluconeogenesis)
- protein and amino acid metabolism
- metabolism, activation or excretion of many drugs.

Liver disorders range from an asymptomatic increase in the amount of fat (hepatic steatosis), resulting in mildly deranged serum liver enzymes, to death of liver cells (massive hepatic necrosis) leading to fulminant hepatic failure. Failure of the liver to maintain function is generally termed hepatic decompensation; classic markers are variceal haemorrhage, portosystemic encephalopathy and ascites.

There has been a marked increase in the reported incidence of liver disease in recent years. This reflects, in part, increased blood testing and so detection, although there does appear to be a genuine rise in some liver diseases. The three most important liver conditions in the developed world are alcohol-related liver disease, non-alcohol-related fatty liver disease and hepatitis C infection.

Liver disease is often detected in 'routine' liver function tests and significant disease may be present before the onset of symptoms or signs. These may be non-specific or reflect the underlying condition rather than the liver dysfunction:

- hepatitis: anorexia, nausea, distaste for cigarettes
- cholestasis: dark urine, pale stools, pruritus
- cholangitis/abscess: pyrexia, rigors
- malignancy: weight loss
- gallstones: right upper quadrant pain.

Although there are patterns of abnormal liver enzymes associated with specific conditions, there is considerable variation and further investigation is often necessary. Ultrasound scanning

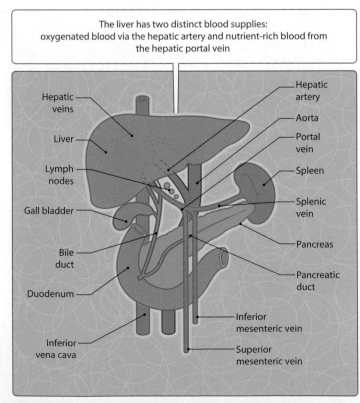

The liver has two distinct blood supplies: oxygenated blood via the hepatic artery and nutrient-rich blood from the hepatic portal vein

Hepatic veins
Liver
Lymph nodes
Gall bladder
Bile duct
Duodenum
Inferior vena cava
Hepatic artery
Aorta
Portal vein
Spleen
Splenic vein
Pancreas
Pancreatic duct
Inferior mesenteric vein
Superior mesenteric vein

Fig. 1.1 Simplified anatomy of the liver, biliary tree and pancreas.

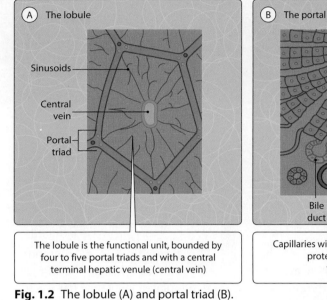

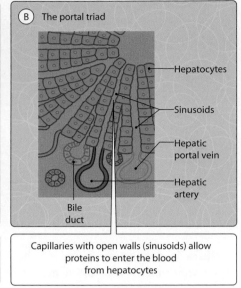

Fig. 1.2 The lobule (A) and portal triad (B).

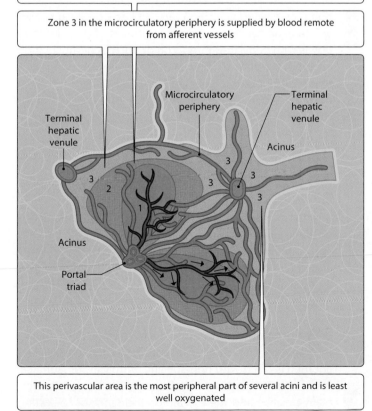

Fig. 1.3 The acinus.

provides information on the shape and structure of the liver along with liver fat content, intrahepatic lesions, biliary dilatation, gallstones and hepatic blood flow. There are limitations to ultrasound as it often underestimates hepatic parenchymal disease and may not detect stones in the bile ducts (choledocholithiasis).

Liver CT or MRI may be useful to identify parenchymal disease or causes of obstruction.

The gallbladder

The gallbladder makes, stores and secretes bile, which consists of water, electrolytes, cholesterol, bile acids and bilirubin. Cholecystokinin is released from the duodenum after a meal, causing the gallbladder to contract and the sphincter of Oddi to relax, with subsequent release of bile into the duodenum. Gallstones are present in up to 20% of the population but most are asymptomatic. They may, however, cause obstruction in the neck of the gallbladder, cystic duct, common bile duct or pancreatic duct and produce pain and obstructive jaundice. Occasionally a gallstone may erode through the gallbladder wall (during an episode of cholecystitis) into the small intestine and cause blockage at the distal ileum (gallstone ileus). Cancer of the gallbladder and bile ducts (cholangiocarcinoma) is uncommon.

The pancreas

The pancreas lies in the retroperitoneum with its head surrounded by the duodenum and tail reaching the spleen. The main pancreatic duct usually meets the common bile duct to drain into the duodenum as a single duct. The pancreas has exocrine and endocrine functions. On appropriate stimulation, the pancreas secretes juices containing digestive enzymes such as amylase, lipase, phospholipase and proteases. The endocrine cells of the pancreas, termed islets of Langerhans, produce insulin, glucagon, somatostatin and pancreatic polypeptide. The pancreas is usually visualized using ultrasound or CT, while endoscopic retrograde cholangiopancreatography (ERCP) can outline the main pancreatic ducts.

High-return facts

1 **Acute liver failure** is defined as failure of the liver to maintain vital functions within 6 months of onset of symptoms in a patient without chronic liver disease. It may present with jaundice and hepatic encephalopathy, proceeding to coma within several days of the onset of symptoms (e.g. paracetamol poisoning) or have a subacute presentation (e.g. autoimmune hepatitis). Acute liver failure should be managed in a specialist unit as it has a high mortality and often requires intensive-care treatment because of multiorgan failure. Liver transplantation is sometimes required.

2 **Chronic liver failure** occurs in individuals who have underlying chronic liver disease. Hepatic decompensation is present when ascites, variceal bleeding or hepatic encephalopathy develops. Ascites is treated with spironolactone or paracentesis. Oesophageal variceal bleeding is managed with vasoconstrictor drugs or endoscopic band ligation. In the event of bleeding not being controlled, a transhepatic portosystemic shunt may be considered. Patients with hepatic encephalopathy usually have an underlying precipitating factor that should be treated, and prognosis depends on the underlying cause. The majority of patients die within 2 years of initial presentation with hepatic decompensation.

3 **Hepatitis A** is an RNA virus usually acquired by the faecal–oral route from contaminated water in areas of high poverty and poor sanitation. It often has a subclinical course but can present as jaundice and an acute hepatitic illness. It is a self-limiting disease with no chronic carrier state. Management is symptomatic and supportive. Active immunization is available with a killed virus or passive immunization with specific immunoglobulin. **Hepatitis E** is a small RNA virus that is spread by the faecal–oral route. There is a high mortality rate in those who acquire the infection during pregnancy although no chronic carrier state exists. Treatment is supportive and there is no available vaccine.

4 **Hepatitis B** is a common DNA virus worldwide, with 350 million having chronic infection. Infection acquired in infancy has a > 90% chance of becoming chronic compared with approximately 5% in adults. Effective immunization is available with a vaccine containing HBVsAg produced by recombinant DNA technology; this can be given at birth to children of infected mothers or to adults at risk of acquiring infection. Chronic infection is associated with high rates of hepatocellular cancer and hepatic decompensation. Treatment of chronic infection is with pegylated interferon or nucleoside/nucleotide analogues. **Hepatitis D** is an incomplete RNA virus that requires the presence of the hepatitis B virus to produce the surface coat for a complete virus. Presence of this virus is associated with an increased incidence of hepatic decompensation.

5 **Hepatitis C** is an RNA virus found worldwide and spread through blood contact. In Western countries, transmission is usually through injecting drug use, while in other areas it is a result of medical intervention with unsterilized equipment. Liver disease is progressive, with approximately 20% having established cirrhosis 20 years after infection. There is no available vaccination. The currently available treatment is with pegylated interferon and ribavirin.

6 **Autoimmune hepatitis** is a form of liver cell inflammation that usually presents in young females. Presentation is often with non-specific symptoms or jaundice. Anti-smooth muscle and anti-nuclear antibodies are normally positive and there is a high incidence of coexisting autoimmune conditions. Treatment is with steroids and azathioprine. Although 50% have cirrhosis at the time of presentation, prognosis is good with treatment. **Primary biliary cirrhosis** is an autoimmune condition of very small bile ducts and usually affects middle-aged females. Anti-mitochondrial antibodies are usually strongly positive. Progression tends to be slow. There is a high incidence of osteoporosis caused by malabsorption of vitamin D in postmenopausal women. Primary biliary cirrhosis was the most common indication for liver transplantation, but better management has reduced the incidence of end-stage liver disease.

7 **Alcohol-related liver disease** covers a wide spectrum of disease from asymptomatic fatty change to end-stage decompensated cirrhosis. Liver changes are reversible with abstinence from alcohol unless cirrhosis has developed. The chance of developing liver disease is related to the amount of alcohol consumed. Patients often require nutritional support in addition to attention to the medical, social and psychological aspects of their disease. The mainstay of treatment is abstinence from alcohol. Survival is dependent on ongoing alcohol use, although there is a high rate of relapse in those who manage to abstain. Patients presenting with acute alcoholic hepatitis may require treatment with oral steroids.

8 **Wilson's disease** is a rare genetic disease of copper metabolism that results in liver and neurological sequelae. Serum copper and the copper-binding protein caeruloplasmin are reduced and copper excretion increases. Prognosis is good if the disease is detected early. **Haemochromatosis** is an autosomal recessive condition with variable penetrance in which a protein that normally regulates iron absorption from the small bowel is defective. Iron continues to be absorbed despite full iron stores and is then deposited in various organs. Venesection is needed to remove iron. There is a high rate of hepatocellular cancer in those with established cirrhosis. α_1-**Antitrypsin deficiency** is an autosomal recessive condition that leads to emphysema and liver disease. Treatment is supportive. **Cystic fibrosis** is the commonest serious inherited disorder in white populations. It is an autosomal recessive condition resulting in multisystem disease; approximately 10% have biliary cirrhosis. The majority of patients with significant liver disease remain stable for many years. Treatment is with ursodeoxycholic acid.

9 **Liver disease in pregnancy** includes cholestasis of pregnancy, which has a familial tendency. Maternal prognosis is good but there is an increased rate of stillbirth at term. Acute fatty liver of pregnancy, the HELLP syndrome (haemolysis, elevated liver enzymes and low platelets) and eclampsia are all related and associated with a high incidence of maternal and fetal death. **Drug-induced liver disease** is common and normally presents within 6 weeks of starting a new drug. Other additional factors such as underlying liver disease or comedication may lead to a clinically detectable reaction. The liver can be damaged by acute toxic effects (e.g. paracetamol overdose) or can suffer progressive damage (e.g. methotrexate). Usually, liver damage subsides with withdrawal of the drug. **Primary sclerosing cholangitis** is an autoimmune condition involving inflammation of the hepatic bile ducts. It is associated with inflammatory bowel disease, particularly ulcerative colitis.

10 **Gallstones** are very common although the majority (80%) are asymptomatic. They more commonly occur in overweight females, pregnancy and those with diabetes mellitus or ileal disease. Gallstones cause complications if they migrate to a position where they obstruct normal function. Acute cholecystitis is managed with antibiotics. Cholecystectomy, the gold standard treatment, is usually performed laparoscopically once the acute episode has settled. **Acute pancreatitis** can be life threatening and is usually caused by alcohol abuse or gallstones. Management is conservative, although occasionally surgery is required. **Chronic pancreatitis** follows repeated episodes of acute pancreatitis and is usually associated with alcohol abuse. It is characterized by severe abdominal pain, features of pancreatic insufficiency and steatorrhoea owing to fat malabsorption. Management involves analgesia and pancreatic enzyme supplements.

11 **Haemangiomata** are abnormal areas of endothelium within the liver that contain blood-filled spaces. **Focal nodular hyperplasia** is an abnormal collection of normal hepatocytes. Neither require treatment. **Hepatic adenoma** is a benign tumour of hepatocytes. Rapidly increasing tumours may be removed because of pressure symptoms or fear of malignant change. **Hepatocellular cancer** is a malignant tumour of hepatocytes that usually occurs upon a background of liver cirrhosis. It is the most common cause of cancer-related deaths worldwide, although it is rare in UK. Prognosis is poor when the tumour becomes symptomatic, with a median survival of < 1 year. Screening programmes may allow detection early when curative treatment is possible. **Cholangiocarcinoma** is an uncommon malignant tumour of bile ducts. Treatment is usually palliative. **Gallbladder tumours** are uncommon and often malignant and prognosis is poor. **Pancreatic cancer** is an adenocarcinoma occurring within the head of the pancreas. It is usually diagnosed by ultrasound or CT. Management is palliative unless an early cancer without tumour invasion of major structures is discovered. The prognosis of pancreatic cancer is dismal.

1. Acute liver failure

Questions
- What is the definition of acute liver failure?
- How does acute liver failure present?

Acute liver failure is defined as the onset of hepatic decompensation with encephalopathy, coagulation disturbance and jaundice (Figs 3.1.1 and 3.1.2) within 6 months of onset of symptoms.

Epidemiology

The cause of acute liver failure varies across the world, with paracetamol poisoning the most common in the UK and viral hepatitis elsewhere. Causes in the UK are:

- drugs (70–80%): paracetamol overdose, NSAIDs, antidepressants, halothane, isoniazid, rifampicin
- cryptogenic (5–10%)
- virus infection (5%): hepatitis virus A–E, herpes simplex
- poisons (<5%): herbal remedies, ecstasy, mushrooms
- miscellaneous (<5%)
  - ischaemic: ischaemic hepatitis, surgical 'shock', acute Budd–Chiari syndrome
  - metabolic: Wilson's disease, fatty liver of pregnancy, Reye's syndrome
  - massive malignant infiltration
  - severe bacterial infection, e.g. leptospirosis.

Patients with fulminant hepatic failure but no identifiable cause are often labelled as having hepatitis non-A–E, as these patients may have infection with a virus yet to be identified.

Pathogenesis

Although the mechanism of liver cell death may vary with different causes, once massive loss of functional liver tissue has occurred similar clinical features develop. These include effects on cerebral functioning, with hepatic encephalopathy and cerebral oedema, coagulation disturbance, metabolic changes (notably hypoglycaemia), infection, renal failure and hypotension.

Clinical features

A careful history should be taken, especially of drug ingestion including herbal remedies, pregnancy, contacts with jaundiced individuals or family history of liver disease.

The patient is often unwell in a non-specific fashion for a short period before signs of acute liver failure develop rapidly, with jaundice, bruising (coagulation disturbance), ascites, tachycardia, hypotension, hyperventilation and signs of encephalopathy (including flapping tremor of the outstretched hands (asterixis),

confusion, drowsiness with inverted sleep pattern, and a sweet smell on the breath of the volatile amine methyl mercaptan (foetor hepaticus)).

Hepatic encephalopathy is defined on a grading scale with four levels.

1. Fluctuant mild confusion, slowing of mentation (thought and affect), sleep disturbance, slurred speech, alternating euphoria and depression
2. Accentuation of grade 1; inappropriate behaviour and drowsiness
3. Marked confusion; the patient sleeps most of the time but is rousable; incoherent speech
4. Coma; unrousable, may or may not respond to noxious stimuli.

The liver is often small by the time jaundice develops and there may be splenomegaly. At this stage, it can be difficult to differentiate acute liver failure from decompensated chronic liver

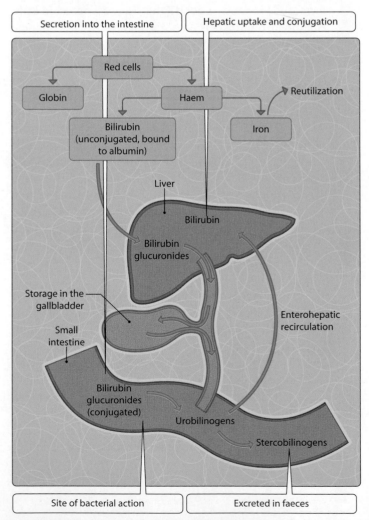

Fig. 3.1.1 Bilirubin metabolism and the liver.

disease, but in the latter, signs of chronic liver disease may be present, for example spider naevi, palmar erythema and leukonychia (pale nails).

Investigations

Prothrombin time or the international normalized ratio (INR) indicates the degree of liver dysfunction, and albumin and liver function tests assess the degree of chronic damage. FBC, fibrin degradation products, immunoglobulins and renal function are also useful. Ultrasound can assess the liver and biliary system. Where necessary, patients should also be screened for paracetamol, alcohol and toxicology.

Serology can identify infection with hepatitis A, B, C and E viruses, and blood, stool and urine cultures will detect other infections.

Management

Treatment is supportive to allow the liver to regenerate or as a bridge to transplantation. Patients with grade 3 and 4 encephalopathy should be managed in a high-dependency or intensive-care unit.

Nasogastric feeding with a diet high in carbohydrate maintains nutrition and prevents hypoglycaemia.

Infection frequently occurs and may be reduced by prophylactic antibiotics and antifungal drugs.

Coagulopathy with prolonged prothrombin time and INR may be treated with vitamin K, while active bleeding may require fresh frozen plasma, clotting factors and platelet transfusion.

Hepatic encephalopathy will require administration of phosphate enemas and lactulose to reduce protein breakdown within the bowel. The use of sedatives should be avoided. Cerebral oedema requires intracerebral pressure monitoring and the use of i.v. mannitol, ultrafiltration, hyperventilation and hypothermia.

Hypotension often requires vasopressor agents (e.g. noradrenaline).

Renal failure may need dialysis or haemofiltration.

A nomogram exists for the use of *N*-acetylcysteine in patients presenting with paracetamol poisoning (see Part VI, Ch. 7). There are well-established criteria for referral for liver transplantation in those with severe paracetamol poisoning (King's criteria).

Liver transplantation needs to be considered in patients in whom there are no contraindications.

Prognosis

The mortality of acute hepatic failure even with good supportive care is approximately 50%. Once grade 3 or 4 hepatic encephalopathy occurs, only 20% survive without transplantation. Liver transplantation survival rates for acute liver failure are less than for chronic liver disease; 1-month survival rates are 60–80%.

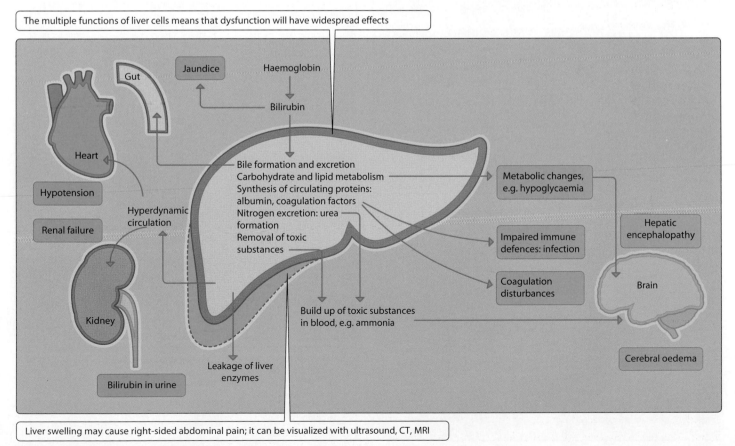

Fig. 3.1.2 Development of clinical features of acute liver failure.

2. Chronic liver failure

Questions
- What are the features of chronic liver failure?
- What is the management of chronic liver failure?

Chronic liver disease leads to loss of synthetic liver function, with reduced serum albumin and reduced production of coagulation factors II, VII, IX and X, leading to prolonged prothrombin time. Liver architecture is progressively disrupted with fibrosis, resulting in regenerative nodules, disturbed intrahepatic circulation and eventually cirrhosis. Figure 3.2.1 shows the physical signs. Causes of chronic liver failure are alcohol excess, chronic viral hepatitis (B or C), non-alcoholic fatty liver disease, immune disease (primary sclerosing cholangitis, autoimmune hepatitis), biliary (primary biliary cirrhosis, cystic fibrosis) and genetic (haemochromatosis, α_1-antitrypsin deficiency, Wilson's disease) disorders.

Portal hypertension occurs when the outflow of the hepatic or portal vein is blocked; this can occur subsequent to pre-, post- or intrahepatic abnormalities (Fig. 3.2.2). In portal hypertension, portal blood will flow into its anastomoses within the systemic system and lead to the formation of varices (Fig. 3.2.3).

Complications of cirrhosis include portal hypertension, portosystemic varices and haemorrhage, ascites, hepatic encephalopathy and hepatorenal syndrome.

Variceal haemorrhage

Approximately 90% of patients with cirrhosis will develop gastro-oesophageal varices over 10 years. Haemorrhage from these varices usually occurs in the distal oesophagus or less commonly in the proximal stomach and has a 25% in-hospital mortality. Patients usually present with both haematemesis and melaena. The immediate priority is resuscitation with fluids, blood and reversal of coagulopathy. Antibiotics are

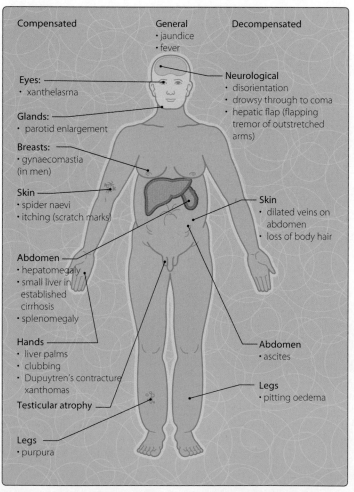

Fig. 3.2.1 Physical signs of chronic liver disease.

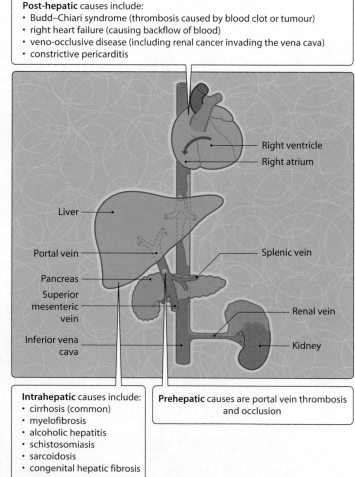

Fig. 3.2.2 Causes of portal hypertension.

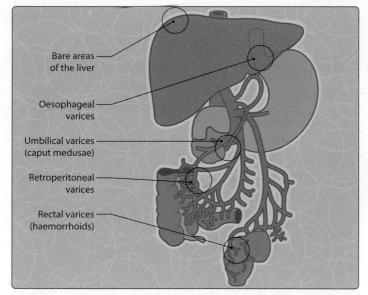

Fig. 3.2.3 Portal hypertension causes enlargement of the veins at the sites of the portosystemic anastomoses. The most important site is the lower oesophagus where oesophageal varices form, which may rupture causing massive blood loss and death.

required for occult infection. Vasoconstrictor therapy with i.v. terlipressin can reduce mortality, and the somatostatin analogue octreotide may also reduce bleeding. Endoscopy with oesophageal band ligation or injection sclerotherapy stops bleeding in 80% and reduces rebleeding. Endoscopic treatment of gastric varices is less effective, and balloon tamponade using a Sengstaken–Blakemore tube may control bleeding. The risk of further bleeding (secondary haemorrhage) can be reduced by:

- non-selective beta-blockers (propranolol or nadolol), which reduce portal pressure
- obliteration of the varices with recurrent courses of endoscopic band ligation
- transjugular intrahepatic portosystemic shunt (TIPSS): insertion of an expandable metal stent between branches of the hepatic and portal veins, resulting in reduction of portal pressure.

In patients with gastro-oesophageal varices, the risk of a first variceal bleed may be reduced (primary prophylaxis) by the use of propranolol or nadolol. Endoscopic band ligation may be used in those intolerant of beta-blockers.

Ascites

Ascites is the accumulation of excess fluid in the peritoneal cavity. Patients present with abdominal distension often with peripheral oedema and occasionally right-sided pleural effusion. Ascites in chronic liver disease can arise from portal hypertension (increases the hydrostatic pressure across capillaries), relative hypoperfusion of the kidneys (activating the renin–angiotensin system and leading to sodium and water retention) and low serum albumin (reduces plasma oncotic pressure).

Generalized abdominal pain, even if mild, suggests spontaneous bacterial peritonitis (SBP). Aspiration of 10–20 ml ascitic fluid should be sent for culture, cytology and protein.

Management
Management includes bed-rest and dietary sodium restriction to 80 mmol/day, while maintaining a high-calorie, high-protein diet. Fluid restriction is used when there is hyponatraemia (sodium < 125 mmol/l) in the absence of renal failure. The aldosterone antagonist spironolactone is the diuretic of choice, furosemide can be added. Paracentesis is used for those with tense ascites, SBP or renal impairment: 8 g i.v. albumin should be given for each litre of ascitic fluid removed.

Broad-spectrum i.v. antibiotic should be given if SBP is suspected; an oral quinolone provides primary prophylaxis.

The use of TIPSS with covered stents should be considered in selected individuals.

Hepatic encephalopathy

Portosystemic encephalopathy is a reversible neuropsychiatric condition ranging from subclinical cognitive changes to coma. It is thought to be caused by increased circulating levels of aromatic amino acids. There may be flapping tremor of the outstretched hands (asterixis), inability to draw a simple object (apraxia) and a sweet smell on breath (foetor hepaticus).

Treatment is of the underlying precipitating factor. Enemas reduce colonic bacterial load and lactulose, an osmotic laxative, reduces colonic pH and limits ammonia absorption.

Hepatorenal syndrome

Hepatorenal syndrome typically occurs in a patient with advanced cirrhosis with jaundice and ascites. There are two forms:

type 1 develops rapidly and if untreated is associated with mortality of > 90% within 1 month

type 2 develops more slowly and presents with ascites unresponsive to diuretic therapy.

Type 1 is treated with i.v. terlipressin and albumin, but recurrence rates are high. Type 2 is managed with paracentesis and avoidance of diuretics, which may exacerbate renal impairment. Malnutrition is common and requires a high-calorie, high-protein diet with oral supplements or nasogastric feeding.

3. Viral hepatitis: overview and hepatitis A and E

Questions
- What is the main population at risk in the UK for each type of hepatitis virus?
- How is hepatitis A transmitted?

Hepatitis A, B, C, D and E are known as hepatotrophic viruses as they primarily present with symptoms and signs of liver disease. All can cause an acute hepatitis, with fever, jaundice and joint pains. All cases should be notified to the relevant public health authorities. Table 3.3.1 summarizes the main differentiating features of these viral infections.

Other viruses can cause an acute hepatitis as part of their clinical spectrum, including Epstein–Barr virus, cytomegalovirus, herpes simplex virus, varicella-zoster virus and flaviviruses (causing yellow fever in Africa and South America and potentially leading to necrotic hepatitis).

Hepatitis E (HEV) is a small RNA virus that is endemic in many developing countries although probably rare in UK. It is transmitted by the faecal–oral route from sewage contamination of drinking water. Infection is associated with travel to the Indian subcontinent although the number of cases identified in the UK has recently increased. Clinical features resemble acute hepatitis A (HAV) infection but it may present with fulminant liver failure especially in pregnancy. There are serological tests available for diagnosis, but treatment is supportive as no drugs have proven to be effective.

Hepatitis A
Epidemiology
A large proportion of the world's population is at risk for HAV. Approximately 90% of young adults in developing countries have antibodies indicating previous infection with HAV, compared with < 20% in developed countries. In endemic areas, the majority of patients become infected in early childhood and are asymptomatic, which means that the diagnosis of acute infection is never made. Those infected as an adult may present with acute hepatitis and jaundice.

Table 3.3.1 DIFFERENTIATING FEATURES OF HEPATITIS VIRUSES

	A	B	C	D	E
Transmission	Faecal–oral	Parenteral, sexual, perinatal	Parenteral, sexual, perinatal	Parenteral	Faecal–oral
Incubation (average days (range))	28 (10–50)	90 (40–160)	60 (15–160)	(20–50)	40
Main population at risk in UK	Travellers to endemic areas; sewage workers; contacts of infected person	Injecting drug users; multiple sexual partners (homo- or heterosexual); infants of carriers; healthcare workers	Recipients of un-screened blood products; injecting drug users	Injecting drug users	Travellers to endemic areas; sporadic
Chronic carriage	None				None
Chronic sequelae	None	Chronic hepatitis; cirrhosis; hepatoma	Chronic hepatitis; cirrhosis; hepatoma	Chronic hepatitis; cirrhosis	None
Diagnosis					
Direct detection	–	+	+	+	–
IgM	+	+	–	+	+
IgG	+	+	+	+	+
Prevention					
Active	Inactivated vaccine	Recombinant vaccine		Hepatitis B immunization	
Passive	Human normal immunoglobulin	Hepatitis B-specific immunoglobulin			
Virus type	Picornavirus (RNA)	Hepadnavirus (DNA)	Pestivirus (RNA)	Defective virus (RNA)	Calicivirus (RNA)

Pathogenesis

HAV is most commonly spread via the faecal–oral route and may occur sporadically or in epidemics (e.g. from contaminated water, shellfish or other foodstuffs). There have been reports of parenteral transmission in injecting drug users and haemophiliacs.

The ingested virus crosses the wall of the alimentary tract and is transported to the liver. The virus is not cytopathic and liver damage occurs through T cell-mediated immune responses. There is a short viraemic phase before the onset of symptoms, which explains the possibility of parenteral transmission. Viral replication occurs within the liver cell, and virus is released into the bile in vesicles. The virus may be shed in high numbers in the faeces for up to a month.

Clinical features

The incubation period between infection and clinical presentation is 10–50 days. There is usually a mild non-specific prodromal illness followed by jaundice. Other symptoms include fever, malaise, anorexia, nausea, vomiting and upper abdominal pain. Patients may present with jaundice associated with joint pains and occasionally a rash. However, in many instances, examination is normal.

Investigations

Investigations give varying results depending on the stage after exposure (Fig. 3.3.1). Anti-HAV IgM antibodies are usually present at the onset of symptoms and decline over 3–6 months

(Fig. 3.3.2). Anti-HAV IgG antibodies reflect immunity from previous exposure (or immunization).

Liver function tests show markedly raised alanine and aspartate aminotransferase (ALT and AST, respectively) in the prodromal phase followed by a rise in bilirubin.

Management

There is no specific therapy for HAV and management is supportive. Fulminant liver failure rarely occurs (< 0.1%). Good sanitation and personal hygiene are the most important forms of prevention.

Active immunization with killed virus provides protection. A single dose provides cover from 2 weeks after the injection for up to 1 year. If a booster is given between 6 and 12 months, protection is extended to 25 years. Human immunoglobulin offers short-term, immediate, passive protection (e.g. for susceptible contacts of an infected individual).

Prognosis

Prognosis is excellent, although approximately 10% relapse before recovery. Rarely there can be a prolonged cholestatic illness or aplastic anaemia. There is no chronic carrier state and chronic liver disease (with enzyme abnormalities) does not occur.

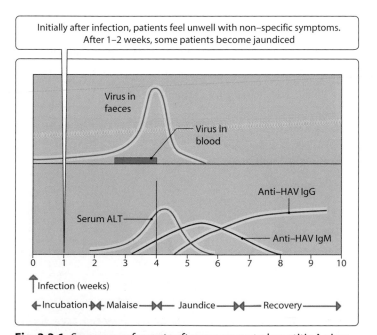

Initially after infection, patients feel unwell with non–specific symptoms. After 1–2 weeks, some patients become jaundiced

Fig. 3.3.1 Sequence of events after exposure to hepatitis A virus (HAV). ALT, alanine aminotransaminase.

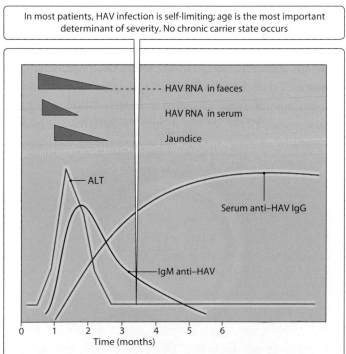

In most patients, HAV infection is self-limiting; age is the most important determinant of severity. No chronic carrier state occurs

Fig. 3.3.2 Virological, serological and clinical events after hepatitis A infection. ALT, alanine aminotransaminase.

5. Hepatitis C

Questions
- How is hepatitis C transmitted?
- How is hepatitis C treated?

Epidemiology
Hepatitis C (HCV) was first recognized in 1989 and is now considered endemic, affecting 175 million individuals across the world. The prevalence of chronic HCV infection ranges from 0.1 to 5% in different countries.

Pathogenesis
HCV is spread through blood contact, with the most important risk factors being:
- current or previous injecting drug use (95% of new cases in the UK)
- previous transfusion of blood or blood products before screening and heat treatment were introduced
- use of unsafe medical practices (in particular poorly sterilized reusable instruments)
- needle-stick injuries.

Vertical or sexual transmission may occur but is rare. Since 1991, all blood donations in the UK have been screened. Blood products, in particular clotting factor concentrates, have undergone heat treatment since the mid-1980s, effectively removing the chance of HCV transmission.

After transmission, the virus infects hepatocytes and virions are produced. This phase is asymptomatic in 90% but in a minority non-specific or typical hepatitis symptoms, including jaundice, occur (Fig. 3.5.1). The immune response results in viral clearance in 20–40% of infected individuals but the majority go on to have persistence of detectable HCV RNA in the blood. Viral clearance in the acute stages is more likely in young females with jaundice. In those who fail to clear the virus, there is ongoing liver inflammation and development of liver fibrosis. The degree of inflammation and fibrosis is variable. Factors influencing progression of liver disease in patients infected with HCV include (Fig. 3.5.2):
- host factors: immunodeficiency, high alcohol consumption, coinfection with hepatitis B or HIV, older age at infection, gender, obesity
- viral factors: viral load at initial innoculum, high level or ongoing viraemia.

Clinical features
Acute infection in the UK is usually through injecting drug use. It is, therefore, difficult to identify the exact time of infection, and the lack of symptoms results in few patients attending for testing. Individuals presenting with a defined infection point (e.g. needlestick injury) should be monitored for 3–6 months as up to 40% will clear the virus without antiviral therapy. There may be a mild non-specific flu-like illness followed by jaundice and some patients present with fever, malaise, anorexia, nausea, vomiting and upper abdominal pain. There may be tender hepatomegaly and joint pains.

Chronic infection is usually discovered following testing in a patient with a known risk factor or as a result of investigation of deranged liver enzymes or liver disease. The patient is usually asymptomatic, although some may have chronic fatigue, arthritis and depression. There may be evidence of previous injecting drug use or tattoos, or joint deformities linked to haemophilia. If there has been progression to cirrhosis, there may be signs of chronic liver disease.

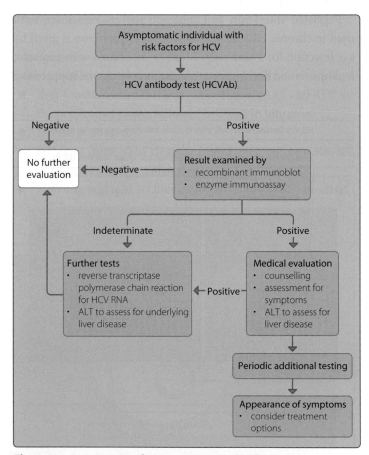

Fig. 3.5.1 Assessment of asymptomatic individuals with risk factors for hepatitis C (HCV) infection: ALT, alanine aminotransferase.

Investigations

Liver function tests often show a small rise in aminotransferases. Antibodies (IgG) to HCV confirm infection. There is no HCV IgM test to confirm acute infection. After acute infection, it may take 6–12 weeks for IgG antibodies to HCV to appear, during which time only tests for HCV RNA may be positive. In those who are immunocompromised, IgG antibodies to HCV may never be detectable.

HCV RNA testing (nucleic acid testing; previously described as PCR) indicates viraemia, ongoing viral replication and, therefore, infectivity. HCV can also be genotyped. There are six genotypes: in the UK, genotype 1 predominates followed by 3 and then 2.

In chronic HCV infection, both IgG antibodies to HCV and HCV RNA remain positive. By comparison, those who clear the virus remain positive for IgG antibodies to HCV but become negative for HCV RNA.

Management

There is no specific treatment for acute HCV infection as up to 40% will clear the virus spontaneously. Those failing to clear the virus spontaneously after 6 months may be offered treatment with pegylated interferon for 12–24 weeks, with successful viral clearance rates of 80–95%.

Those with chronic HCV infection may be offered the combination of pegylated interferon and oral ribavirin. The decision to undertake treatment requires the patient to avoid high-risk behaviour.

Recommended treatment duration is currently 12–48 weeks depending on genotype, viral load, degree of liver damage and initial virological response to therapy. Approximately 20% develop serious side-effects that result in treatment discontinuation.

Treatment was previously restricted to those with moderate or severe disease, but as a result of cost–benefit analyses, the offer of antiviral therapy has now been extended to those with mild disease. Response to treatment is variable (Fig. 3.5.3): the majority suppress the virus so that it is undetectable in blood while on treatment but a minority do not suppress the virus (non-responders). Some responders have detectable virus again 6 months after treatment (relapsers).

Sustained viral clearance is defined as undetectable HCV RNA in blood 6 months after the end of treatment. The clearance rate for genotype 1 is 40–50%, with 70–80% for genotypes 2 and 3. Recurrence rates in those who have achieved sustained viral clearance are <1% per year.

Prognosis

Those with acute HCV infection who clear the virus are thought to have a prognosis similar to uninfected individuals. In those with chronic HCV infection, approximately 20% develop cirrhosis 20 years after infection, depending on coexisting risk factors. Progression is more likely in males, those infected after the age of 40 and those with ongoing alcohol excess. Patients with cirrhosis related to HCV infection have a 2–4% annual risk of developing hepatocellular cancer and should have abdominal ultrasound every 6 months (and perhaps α-fetoprotein) to detect tumours at an early, treatable stage. HCV-related liver disease is now the most common indication for liver transplantation in the Western world.

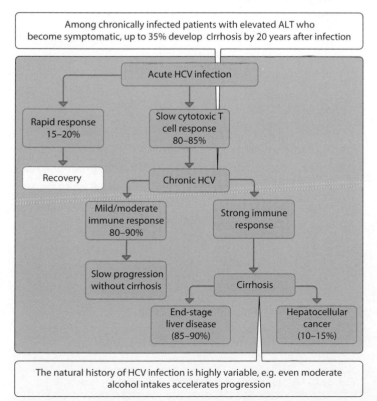

Fig. 3.5.2 Progression of infection with hepatitis C.

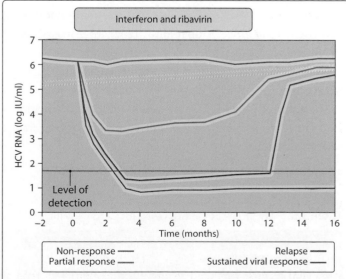

Fig. 3.5.3 Response to antiviral therapy in chronic hepatitis C infection.

6. Autoimmune liver disease

Autoimmune hepatitis

Epidemiology

Autoimmune hepatitis (AIH) usually presents in late childhood or early adulthood, with a female:male ratio of 8:1. The prevalence is estimated to be approximately 15/100 000 in northern European populations.

Pathogenesis

There have been many theories as to the triggers for AIH, but no consistent links have been established. There is an association with different autoantibodies but these do not appear to be of pathological significance (Table 3.6.1). There is mononuclear infiltration of the liver, predominantly T lymphocytes but it may include plasma cells. Inflammation extends from the portal tracts into the liver parenchyma, causing cirrhosis.

Clinical features

Presentation is usually in young females aged 20–50 years; AIH is clinically indistinguishable from acute viral hepatitis in up to 30%. Patients may have a more insidious onset of non-specific symptoms over many months, with up to 50% having cirrhosis at initial diagnosis. Anorexia, joint pains, fatigue, abdominal pain (from liver enlargement) and amenorrhoea often occur. Approximately two-thirds have associated autoimmune disease, particularly Hashimoto's thyroiditis, renal tubular acidosis or rheumatoid arthrititis.

Jaundice, hepatomegaly (which may be tender) and splenomegaly, along with signs of chronic liver disease (e.g. palmar erythema and spider naevi) may be present. Rarely, presentation is with either decompensated cirrhosis or fulminant liver failure with encephalopathy, ascites and variceal bleeding.

Investigations

Liver function tests show raised aminotransferases (ALT and AST) and serum IgG is raised with other immunoglobulins normal.

Anti-nuclear antibodies and anti-smooth muscle antibodies are usually positive (80% and 70%, respectively), but other autoantibodies may be detected.

Liver biopsy may be required.

Management

Prednisolone alone or in combination with azathioprine may induce remission during exacerbations of active and symptomatic disease. Maintenance therapy is with low-dose prednisolone and/ or azathioprine. Immunosuppression can be discontinued after at least 2 years of remission but there is a high rate of relapse.

Prognosis

AIH is characterized by exacerbations and remissions but most patients eventually develop cirrhosis and its complications. Untreated, the 5-year mortality is 50%, but with modern management this falls to approximately 10%. Liver transplantation may be required in advanced disease. The disease may recur in the liver graft, although this is rarely clinically relevant.

Primary biliary cirrhosis

Epidemiology

The prevalence of primary biliary cirrhosis (PBC) is 7.5/100 000 with a 1–6% increase in first-degree relatives. It usually presents in middle age, with a female:male ratio of 9:1.

Pathogenesis

The cause of PBC is unknown. There is chronic granulomatous inflammation causing progressive destruction of the smaller bile ducts, with portal tract infiltration predominantly of lymphocytes and plasma cells. This may progress to fibrosis and eventually cirrhosis (Fig. 3.6.1). While immune activity is a feature of both AIH and PBC, there are distinct differences (Table 3.6.2).

Table 3.6.1 FREQUENCY OF AUTOANTIBODIES IN CHRONIC NON-VIRAL LIVER DISEASE AND HEALTHY PEOPLE

Disease	Anti-nuclear antibody (%)	Anti-smooth muscle antibody (%)	Anti-mitochondrial antibody (%)
Healthy controls	5	1.5	0.01
Autoimmune hepatitis	80	70	15
Primary biliary cirrhosis	25	35	95

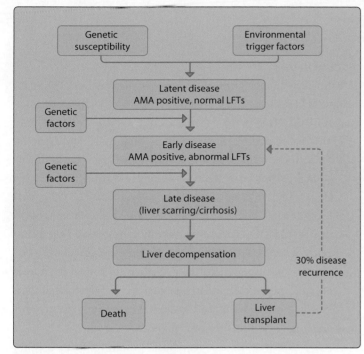

Fig. 3.6.1 Natural history of primary biliary cirrhosis. AMA, anti-mitochondrial antibody; LFTs, liver function tests.

Clinical features

At the time of diagnosis, the majority of patients are asymptomatic, with abnormal liver function tests discovered during 'routine' screening. Generalized pruritus from deposition of bile salts within the skin, sometimes associated with fatigue, occurs before cirrhosis develops. Jaundice is a late feature. Some patients have right upper quadrant pain. There are often associated autoimmune conditions, particularly systemic sclerosis, Sjögren's syndrome, coeliac disease and autoimmune thyroiditis.

Examination may show xanthalasma, palmar erythema and skin pigmentation early in the disease, with features of chronic liver failure found after the development of cirrhosis.

Investigations

Liver function tests show raised alkaline phosphatase and gamma-glutamyl transpeptidase. Serum cholesterol is often raised and serum IgM is elevated.

Anti-mitochondrial antibody is present in high titre in > 95%, with antibodies to the M2 antigen being specific.

Rarely, liver biopsy is necessary to establish the diagnosis.

Management

The synthetic bile salt ursodeoxycholic acid may improve liver biochemistry. Pruritus (itching) is the main symptom requiring treatment. Colestyramine, an anion-binding resin, adsorbs bile salts within the gut and can reduce itching. Alternatives are antihistamines, rifampicin and naltrexone. The fat-soluble vitamins A, D and K may need to be replaced by oral supplements or parenteral injection. Associated osteoporosis is particularly troublesome; calcium and vitamin D intake should be encouraged and a bisphosphonate considered.

Prognosis

Patients with PBC who are asymptomatic and without cirrhosis are expected to live for > 15 years. Prognosis is relatively good for those with cirrhosis, but when bilirubin reaches 100 μmol/l, life expectancy is < 2 years. PBC was previously the most common indication for liver transplantation in the UK, with a 5-year post-transplant survival > 80%. However, in recent years, better management of early disease has led to a reduction in the number of patients with PBC progressing to end-stage liver disease.

Table 3.6.2 DIFFERENCES BETWEEN AUTOIMMUNE HEPATITIS (AIH) AND PRIMARY BILIARY CIRRHOSIS (PBC)

	AIH	PBC
Age	Young adult	Middle age
Gender	Female preponderance	Female preponderance
Liver enzyme increases	Transaminases	Alkaline phosphatase and gamma-glutamyl transpeptidase
Immunoglobulins	IgG ↑	IgM ↑
Autoantibodies	Anti-nuclear, anti-smooth muscle, anti-liver/kidney microsomal	Anti-mitochondrial
Treatment	Steroids, azathioprine	Symptomatic with ursodeoxycholic acid

7. Alcohol-related liver disease

Questions

- What level of alcohol intake is associated with liver disease?
- How should alcohol-related liver disease be managed?

Epidemiology

The quantity of alcohol required to produce alcohol-related liver disease (ALD) varies between individuals. Approximately 20% of heavy drinkers (100 units/week) will develop serious liver disease, with continuous drinking being more dangerous than binge drinking. Males drinking, on average, < 40 g alcohol/day (5 UK units) are highly unlikely to develop serious liver disease unless there is an associated liver disorder, while those drinking 210 g daily (around a standard bottle of spirits) often develop cirrhosis. The amount of alcohol required to cause liver disease is considerably less in females than in males, but ALD does not occur below thresholds of 21 units/week in women and 28 units/week in men. Table 3.7.1 shows the amount of alcohol in an average drink.

There has been a steady rise in the total consumption of alcohol in the UK in recent years, with a subsequent increase in the number of hospital admissions and deaths as a result of ALD. Criteria indicative of alcohol dependence are:

- narrowing of the drinking repertoire (restriction to one type of alcohol, e.g. spirits)
- priority of drinking over other activities
- tolerance of effects of alcohol
- repeated withdrawal symptoms
- relief of withdrawal symptoms with further drinking
- subjective compulsion to drink
- reinstatement of drinking behaviour after abstinence.

Other factors, including concomitant hepatitis C infection, obesity and drug misuse, may increase the likelihood of developing liver disease.

Table 3.7.1 AMOUNT OF ALCOHOL IN AN AVERAGE DRINK

Alcohol type	Alcohol by volume (%)	Amount	Units (UK)
Beer	4	440 ml (1 pint)	2
	9	440 ml (1 pint)	4
Wine	12	125 ml	1.5
Spirits (e.g. rum, vodka, whisky)	37.5	25 ml	1
'Alcopops'	6	330 ml	2

Pathogenesis

Alcohol is metabolized almost exclusively by the liver. The spectrum of liver disease ranges from reversible fatty change to end-stage cirrhosis (Fig. 3.7.1).

Fatty liver disease. Alcohol is converted to acetaldehyde by the mitochondrial enzyme alcohol dehydrogenase; acetaldehyde is converted, in turn, to acetate and then to fatty acids (Fig. 3.7.2). Alcohol is calorie rich, producing 8 kcal/g, and is often consumed in drinks with high sugar content. Fat is deposited in the liver (steatosis) initially around the central veins (zone 3) and later throughout the parenchyma. If alcohol consumption ceases, the liver then returns to normal; if not, inflammation and fatty change occurs (steatohepatitis). Fibrosis, initially around the central veins, may occur, progressing to cirrhosis in some patients.

Alcohol-related cirrhosis. Cirrhosis resulting from alcohol consumption is typically micronodular with steatosis. In some patients, however, there is little evidence of fatty change by the time cirrhosis is present. If alcohol consumption ceases, the cirrhosis may become macronodular with very little inflammatory change.

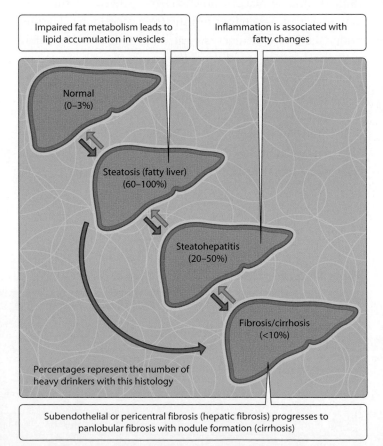

Impaired fat metabolism leads to lipid accumulation in vesicles

Inflammation is associated with fatty changes

Normal (0–3%)

Steatosis (fatty liver) (60–100%)

Steatohepatitis (20–50%)

Fibrosis/cirrhosis (<10%)

Percentages represent the number of heavy drinkers with this histology

Subendothelial or pericentral fibrosis (hepatic fibrosis) progresses to panlobular fibrosis with nodule formation (cirrhosis)

Fig. 3.7.1 Pathological changes in the liver of heavy drinkers.

Acute alcoholic hepatitis. In addition to fatty change, there may be infiltration with polymorphonuclear leukocytes and hepatic necrosis, resulting in hepatomegaly, fever, abdominal pain, jaundice and hepatic decompensation. Acute alcoholic hepatitis may occur on a background of cirrhosis or, in those without underlying cirrhosis, the liver may return to normal with nutritional support and abstinence from alcohol.

Clinical features

There may be a clear history of alcohol excess over many years and the patient may be under the influence of alcohol on presentation. However, patients may also conceal their alcohol intake and it may only become apparent after discussion with friends or relatives. The patient may have stopped drinking prior to presenting with signs of acute alcohol-related hepatitis or end-stage liver disease. Signs of chronic liver disease are common in those with cirrhosis, for example spider naevi, palmar erythema, jaundice, hepatomegaly (which may be tender), splenomegaly and parotitis.

Investigations

FBC may show a raised mean corpuscular volume (MCV) and thrombocytopenia. Liver function tests include raised gamma-glutamyl transpeptidase and AST (usually greater than ALT). There may be slight increases in IgA and IgG.

Increases in the prothrombin time or international normalized ratio (INR) reflect coagulation disturbances and serum albumin is decreased; both indicate reduction in the synthetic function of the liver.

Liver ultrasound may show an enlarged echo-bright fatty liver or an irregular shrunken liver in macronodular cirrhosis.

Other causes of chronic liver disease should be excluded.

Management

Management requires abstinence from alcohol. It may be necessary to manage acute alcohol withdrawal by careful prescription of benzodiazepines (e.g. diazepam), especially in those with cirrhosis. Intravenous thiamine (vitamin B_1) followed by long-term oral administration may prevent Wernicke's encephalopathy (a triad of confusion, ataxia and ophthalmoplegia). Nutrition is often poor and so nasogastric or occasionally i.v. nutrition is required. Liver transplantation may be required in those who have chronic decompensated liver disease despite alcohol abstinence or in those who develop hepatocellular cancer.

Prognosis

Prognosis is dependent on the stage of liver disease at presentation. Those with only fatty liver disease who abstain from alcohol have an excellent prognosis. If a patient presents with decompensated cirrhosis, the 5-year survival is approximately 65% in those who abstain from alcohol. However, this falls to approximately 35% in those who continue to drink, with most deaths occurring in the first year.

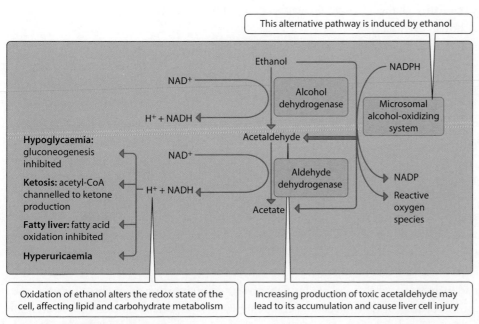

Fig. 3.7.2 Metabolism of alcohol.

8. Genetic disorders affecting the liver

Questions
- Which genetic disorders cause liver disease?
- How are Wilson's disease and haemochromatosis diagnosed?

Wilson's disease

Wilson's disease (hepatolenticular degeneration) is a rare autosomal recessive disorder of copper metabolism, with the genetic defect located on chromosome 13. Prevalence is estimated at 3/100 000, with a carrier frequency of 1:90.

In healthy individuals, copper is absorbed from the upper GI tract and transported to the liver bound to albumin. It is then incorporated into a copper-binding protein (caeruloplasmin), secreted into the blood and excreted into the bile with a smaller quantity excreted in the urine. In Wilson's disease, caeruloplasmin is reduced and copper is deposited in the liver, in a predominantly periportal distribution, as well as in the basal ganglia within the brain and renal tubules.

Young children usually present with liver disease whereas older children and young adults tend to present with neurological complications. Liver damage may range from acute fulminant hepatitis to slow progression to cirrhosis. Wilson's disease is undetectable before 5 years but thereafter may present with:

- signs of chronic liver disease
- neuropsychiatric manifestations, e.g. personality change, psychosis, tremor, dysarthria, rigidity, chorea; eventually resulting in dementia
- renal tubular acidosis
- Kayser–Fleischer rings: brown deposits at the corneal edge.

Investigations show reduced serum copper and caeruloplasmin, with increased 24 h urinary copper excretion. Liver disease may be reversed by the chelating agent penicillamine. Liver transplantation may be required.

Haemochromatosis

Normal dietary intake of iron is 10–20 mg/day but only approximately 1–2 mg is absorbed. In haemochromatosis, failure of iron homeostasis and increased iron absorption occurs even when there is a body iron overload. Total body iron may reach 20–60 g (normally 4–5 g). Other causes of iron overload include:

- secondary iron overload: parenteral iron loading (e.g. repeated blood transfusions), iron-loading anaemia (e.g. thalassaemia, sideroblastic anaemia), chronic liver disease, dietary iron overload (prolonged oral iron therapy)
- complex iron overload: alcoholic liver disease, porphyria cutanea tarda, African iron overload (Bantu siderosis).

Haemochromatosis is a condition in which the total body iron is increased. It is an autosomal recessive change in the gene *HFE*, located on chromosome 6. The rate of homozygosity for the C282Y mutant in Europe is 1:200 to 1:300, but the rate of iron overload and clinical disease is much less. The HFE protein is located in the villi of the upper small intestine and regulates iron absorption. There is increased progression to end-stage liver disease in those who are homozygous for the C282Y mutation and who also drink alcohol to excess or are coinfected with hepatitis C virus.

Iron is deposited in tissues, resulting in damage to the liver, pancreas, endocrine tissues, heart, joints and skin. Patients may present with decompensated liver disease, diabetes mellitus, impotence, heart failure, joint pains or leaden-grey pigmentation owing to iron deposition and excess melanin within the skin.

Investigations show increased serum iron, transferrin saturation and ferritin. Liver biopsy reveals iron deposition and fibrosis, which may have progressed to cirrhosis. There is a high incidence of hepatocellular cancer in those with cirrhosis.

Management is with weekly venesection of 500 ml blood (250 mg iron) until serum iron is normal, which may take 2 years or more. This is continued as required to keep serum ferritin normal. Liver and cardiac diseases are improved by venesection but diabetes and joint pains are usually unchanged. First-degree family members should be investigated by genetic screening.

Deficiency of α_1-antitrypsin

Deficiency in α_1-antitrypsin is an autosomal recessive condition affecting a gene on chromosome 14. The genetic defect alters the configuration of α_1-antitrypsin, a glycoprotein synthesized in the liver and secreted by the hepatocytes, preventing its release. The normal phenotype is PiMM, with variants PiSS and PiMZ associated with slightly reduced levels of circulating protein and PiZZ commonly associated with circulating levels ≤ 10% of normal. In the lungs, α_1-antitrypsin protects against antiproteases; loss of this protection allows destruction of alveolar walls and causes emphysema. Accumulation of α_1-antitrypsin in hepatocytes destroys these cells and ultimately leads to liver disease.

Patients may present with liver disease or chronic airflow obstruction and emphysema (especially smokers). Presentation may be with juvenile liver failure through to cirrhosis at any age. Replacement therapy is becoming available and liver transplantation may be necessary for end-stage liver disease.

Cystic fibrosis

Cystic fibrosis is the most common serious genetic disorder in white populations. It is an autosomal recessive condition with a prevalence of 1:2500 newborns. The defect is located on chromosome 7 and mutations affect the gene for the cystic fibrosis transmembrane conductance regulator, which controls the transport of chloride ions across cell membranes in the chloride channel. Mucus-secreting cells transport chloride into the secreted mucus; sodium ions and water follow passively, keeping the mucus moist. Impaired transport of chloride out of the cytoplasm creates sticky, viscous mucus secretions in the pancreas, lungs and other organs (Fig. 3.8.1). Cystic fibrosis commonly causes pancreatic insufficiency and 20% of patients also develop significant liver disease (Table 3.8.1). Sclerosing cholangitis damages intrahepatic ducts, resulting in portal hypertension and occasionally liver failure. Ursodeoxycholic acid may improve liver biochemistry. Patients may require liver transplantation but in the majority prognosis is determined by respiratory disease.

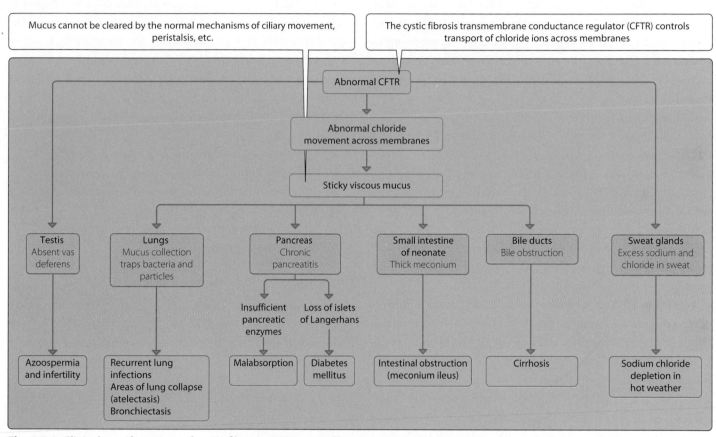

Fig. 3.8.1 Clinical manifestations of cystic fibrosis. CFTR, cystic fibrosis transmembrane conductance regulator.

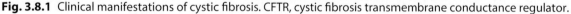

Table 3.8.1 GASTROINTESTINAL AND LIVER EFFECTS OF CYSTIC FIBROSIS

Organ	Disorder	Management
Liver	Fatty change (steatosis); cirrhosis with hepatic decompensation	Ursodeoxycholic acid; liver transplantation
Pancreas	Exocrine insufficiency (85% of newborns); pancreatitis	Pancreatic enzyme supplements and fat-soluble vitamins
Oesophagus	Gastro-oesophageal reflux	Prokinetic drug plus antacid
Small bowel	Meconium ileus; distal intestinal obstruction	Gastrograffin enema or surgery
Colon	Constipation	Dietary advice, laxatives
Rectum	Rectal prolapse	Resolves with pancreatic enzymes

9. Miscellaneous liver disorders

Questions
■ Which liver disorders occur in pregnancy?
■ Which drugs cause liver disease?

Liver disease in pregnancy

In normal pregnancy, there is an increase in the blood supply to the liver, and oesophageal varices may be seen at endoscopy even in the absence of portal hypertension. Liver disease may present for the first time in pregnancy, or pregnancy may influence preexisting liver disease. Jaundice may occur in up to 1:1500 pregnancies, with non-pregnancy-related conditions such as viral hepatitis or gallstones being responsible for the majority.

Cholestasis of pregnancy occurs in 1:200 pregnancies and causes generalized pruritus in the third trimester. There is a familial tendency and it often recurs in subsequent pregnancies or with oral contraceptive pill use. In severe cases, deepening jaundice, dark urine and pale stools develop. It usually resolves within 2–4 weeks after delivery and treatment is with ursodeoxycholic acid. The prognosis for the mother is excellent, although there is an increased risk of premature labour and stillbirth. Elective delivery before the 38th week is often recommended.

Acute fatty liver of pregnancy is a rare and serious condition of uncertain cause. Abnormal fatty acid metabolites produced by the fetus are thought to overcome liver mitochondrial oxidation in the mother. It more commonly occurs during the first pregnancy and in twin pregnancies. It rarely recurs. Fulminant hepatitis may develop in the third trimester, with jaundice, vomiting, abdominal pain and, occasionally, signs of liver failure. Treatment is immediate delivery of the child and, rarely, liver transplantation for the mother.

HELLP syndrome (haemolysis, elevated liver enzymes and low platelets) is associated with hypertension and renal failure, making it difficult to distinguish from eclampsia (Fig. 3.9.1). It is rare and tends to present in older multiparous Caucasian females. It often occurs in the second trimester when the fetus may not be viable. It tends to resolve after delivery of the fetus but there are reports of spontaneous resolution following treatment with plasma expansion, plasmapheresis, steroids, prostacyclin, nifedipine or transplantation.

Eclampsia is a medical emergency associated with seizures in addition to hypertension, proteinuria and oedema. Elevations of aminotransferases are found in those with severe eclampsia. The causes of the liver disease are multifactorial and include fibrin deposition, segmental vasospasm, generalized vasculopathy and microangiopathy. Treatment involves delivery of the child.

Drug-induced liver disease

Drug-induced liver abnormalities are common as the liver is the major site of drug metabolism and is also the first destination of drugs leaving the GI tract. Drug reactions are responsible for 2% of all patients in hospital with jaundice and 25% of patients with acute fulminant liver failure. Most reactions occur within 3 months of starting the drug, but some may occur after long-term treatment (e.g. methotrexate, which can cause progressive fibrosis). A particular drug may cause different forms of liver disease in different individuals or a combination of drugs may interact to cause liver disease; common drug effects include:

■ cholestasis: chlorpromazine, high-dose oestrogens
■ cholestatic hepatitis: NSAIDs, coamoxiclav, statins
■ acute hepatitis: rifampicin, isoniazid, pyrazinamide
■ non-alcoholic steatohepatitis: amiodarone
■ venous outflow obstruction: busulfan, azathioprine
■ fibrosis: methotrexate.

Pathogenesis

Liver damage may be predictable (or toxic) and dose related, or non-predictable (idiosyncratic) and non-dose related. These subdivisions are artificial and a single drug reaction may have components of both. Coexisting liver disease, alcohol ingestion, enzyme inducers and malnutrition may affect the metabolism of drugs and metabolite clearance. Possible mechanisms of drug-

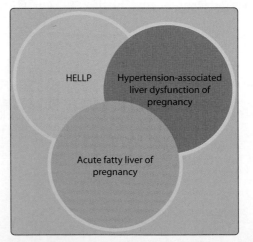

Fig. 3.9.1 Overlap in the acute conditions of acute fatty liver of pregnancy, HELLP and eclampsia.

related liver injury include disruption of calcium homeostasis or bile canalicular transport mechanisms, formation of new compounds that present on liver cell membrane as antigens, induction of apoptosis and mitochondrial dysfunction.

Paracetamol is conjugated in the liver and in overdose toxic metabolites cause liver cell necrosis. The severity of the liver disease is dose related but those who are malnourished or have hepatic enzyme induction, (e.g, from chronic alcohol ingestion or drugs) can have serious liver damage at lower doses of paracetamol. *N*-Acetylcysteine and methionine are specific antidotes to paracetamol poisoning as they enable the replenishment of glutathione, which protects against oxidative stress and is deleted by a metabolite of paracetamol. There is a nomogram for the use of *N*-acetylcysteine based on plasma paracetamol levels and the length of time from drug ingestion (see Part VII, Ch. 4). Recommended plasma levels of *N*-acetylcysteine are lower in those with enzyme induction than those without.

Clinical features

Patients present with any degree of liver disease from mild asymptomatic elevation of liver enzymes to fulminant liver failure. In order to diagnose drug-induced liver disease, a high degree of clinical suspicion is required, along with an accurate drug history and exclusion of other conditions. Presentation varies from non-specific flu-like symptoms with joint pains to acute jaundice and encephalopathy in fulminant liver failure. GI bleeding may occur in those with coagulopathy or portal hypertension. A careful drug history including all drugs taken within the last 3 months must be obtained, as some reactions may present after the course has been completed (e.g. coamoxiclav-induced cholestasic hepatitis and halothane-induced hepatitis). Factors to be considered in the diagnosis of drug-induced liver disease are shown in Fig. 3.9.2.

Investigations

Liver function tests show elevated aminotransferases and bilirubin. FBC (eosinophilia, thrombocytopenia) and coagulation screen (prolonged prothrombin time/international normalized ratio) may be abnormal. If paracetamol poisoning is possible, serum paracetamol should be measured. A liver biopsy may be necessary.

Management

Withdrawal of the toxic agent and supportive therapy is all that is required in the majority.

Prognosis

The outcome is favourable in the majority of inadvertent cases although there are a few fatalities and occasionally the resultant damage is irreversible, for example amiodarone-induced cirrhosis.

Primary sclerosing cholangitis

Primary sclerosing cholangitis is a chronic inflammatory condition affecting both intra- and extrahepatic ducts, resulting in fibrosis and cholestasis. Mean age of diagnosis is approximately 40 years, with 60% being male and 75% having coexisting inflammatory bowel disease, especially ulcerative colitis. The onset may predate the diagnosis of inflammatory bowel disease by many years. Symptoms include chlolestasis with pruritus, and jaundice with dark urine and pale stools. Some patients develop secondary bacterial cholangitis.

Diagnosis is by MR cholangiopancreatography or endoscopic retrograde cholangiopancreatography, with subtle intrahepatic disease requiring liver biopsy. Ursodeoxycholic acid may improve liver biochemistry but does not prevent progression. Stenting of dominant strictures of the common bile duct can assist.

Secondary sclerosing cholangitis is caused by previous bile duct surgery resulting in strictures, bile duct stones causing cholangitis and intrahepatic infusion of 5-fluorodeoxyuridine. In HIV/AIDS, this is probably caused by cytomegalovirus or cryptosporidium infection.

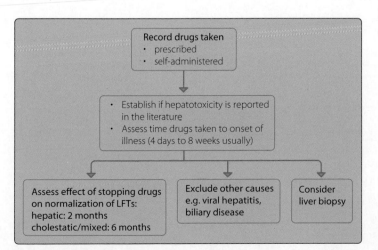

Fig. 3.9.2 Diagnosis of drug-induced liver disease.

10. Disorders of the biliary tree and pancreas

Questions
- What are the complications of gallstones?
- What are the features of acute pancreatitis?
- What is the treatment of chronic pancreatitis?

Gallstones

Gallstones are very common although most (80%) are asymptomatic. The main types are mixed (80%), made up of cholesterol, bile pigments and calcium salts; pigmented (10%), which contain calcium bilirubinate and are more common with haemolytic anaemia; and mainly cholesterol (10%). Risk factors for gallstones include increased cholesterol secretion (old age, female, pregnancy, obesity, rapid weight loss), impaired gallbladder emptying (pregnancy, fasting, total parenteral nutrition, spinal cord injury) or reduced bile salt secretion (pregnancy).

Clinical features

Presentation depends on where the gallstones are (Fig. 3.10.1). Biliary colic causes epigastric pain sometimes radiating to the right shoulder, nausea and vomiting. Symptoms usually settle once the stone has passed. Acute cholecystitis is caused by an impacted stone and is usually associated with bacterial infection. Charcot's triad describes rigors, obstructive jaundice and pain (upper right quadrant, radiating to shoulder) caused by stones in the common bile duct.

Investigations

In biliary obstruction liver function tests show raised aminotransferases, bilirubin and alkaline phosphatase. Amylase is raised if pancreatitis is present. Ultrasound can demonstrate gallstones, thickened gallbladder, intra- and extrahepatic biliary tree dilatation and collections. Endoscopic retrograde cholangiopancreatography (ERCP) allows visualization of the common bile and pancreatic ducts plus retrieval of stones.

Management

Biliary colic and acute cholecystitis are usually managed with fluids, analgesia and i.v. antibiotics (e.g. cephalosporin and metronidazole). More serious complications usually necessitate ERCP to drain the biliary tree. Dye is injected into the biliary tree and identified stones extracted. Cholecystectomy is the gold standard for symptomatic gallstone disease; this is usually performed laparoscopically once the acute episode has settled or if conservative measures or ERCP fails in the acute setting.

Acute pancreatitis

In the UK, the incidence of acute pancreatitis requiring hospital admission is 15–40/100 000 population; most (80%) is caused by alcohol or gallstone disease. Other causes include drugs (e.g. steroids, thiazides, valproate, azathioprine), abdominal trauma, post-ERCP, viral infection (mumps, coxsackie B), hyperlipidaemia, hypercalcaemia, hypothermia and malignancy (periampullary or pancreatic cancer). Although the causes are diverse, a common

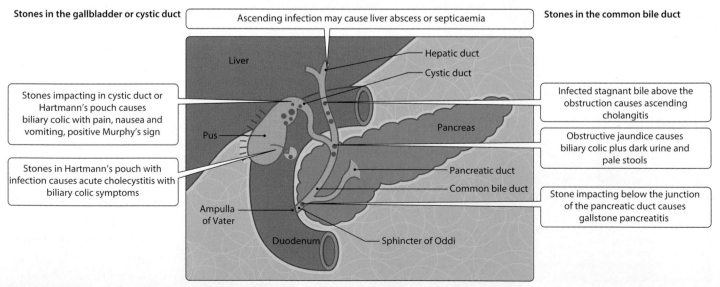

Fig. 3.10.1 Presentation of gallstones.

pathway is usually present in which an increase in intracellular calcium and activation of pancreatic enzymes result in autodigestion of the pancreas, with cell necrosis and inflammation.

Clinical features

Most patients present with upper abdominal pain radiating to the back and nausea and vomiting. Obstructive jaundice (jaundice, dark urine and pale stools) may be present if gallstones are the cause. Severe life-threatening pancreatitis occurs in approximately 20%. Examination may reveal only epigastric tenderness, but in severe disease there may be associated pyrexia, hypotension, tachycardia and hypoxia with ileus and jaundice. In haemorrhagic pancreatitis, bruising in the flanks (Grey–Turner's sign) or in the periumbilical region (Cullen's sign) may be found. Patients may have a history of long-standing alcohol abuse and have signs of chronic liver disease.

Investigations

The **Glasgow Severity Score** (see the box) incorporates the main parameters. Serum amylase is usually elevated >3 times the upper limit of normal.

Erect chest radiograph will exclude perforation or pneumonia mimicking pancreatitis. A plain abdominal radiograph may reveal the calcification of chronic pancreatitis or an isolated dilated jejunal loop (sentinel loop) associated with inflammation in the body and tail of the pancreas. CT of the abdomen allows assessment of the degree of necrosis, formation of abscesses or pseudocysts and involvement of surrounding areas.

Management

Treatment is according to cause and severity. Pancreatitis from obstruction of the ampulla of Vater should be managed with ERCP and sphincterotomy. Severe acute pancreatitis requires oxygen, i.v. fluids and occasionally inotropic support.

Nasogastric suction is often necessary for functional gastric outlet obstruction, although nutritional support may be given by nasojejunal or i.v. feeding. Transient secondary diabetes mellitus is treated with insulin. Late complications such as pancreatic pseudocyst or abscess may need drainage. Prognosis is dependent on the severity of the episode, with a mortality of < 2% in those with a mild episode rising to approximately 15% in those with severe acute pancreatitis.

Chronic pancreatitis

Chronic pancreatitis occurs in approximately 13/100 000; the most common cause in developed countries is alcohol abuse (60–80%). Rarer causes include gallstones and stenosis of the ampulla of Vater (obstructive), malnutrition, hereditary conditions (e.g. cystic fibrosis, α_1-antitrypsin deficiency) and pancreas divisum (found in 7–10% of the normal population).

Pathogenesis

Inappropriate activation of pancreatic enzymes including trypsinogen results in protein precipitation, which may progress to formation of plugs or stones. Blockage of pancreatic ducts increases pressure and causes further damage. Chronic alcohol intake is believed to increase trypsinogen relative to its inhibitor.

Clinical features

Severe epigastric pain (exacerbated by alcohol and relieved by sitting forward) radiating to the back is the most common presentation. In advanced disease, loss of pancreatic exocrine function may result in anorexia, malabsorption, diarrhoea and weight loss. Steatorrhoea owing to fat malabsorption may amount to fat loss of 30 mmol/24 h. Loss of endocrine function manifests as secondary diabetes mellitus.

Investigations

Serum amylase is often normal. Plain abdominal radiograph may reveal calcification and CT may demonstrate pancreatic calcification, atrophy, features of portal hypertension or a pseudocyst. MRCP or ERCP is used to outline the anatomy of the gland. Faecal elastase is reduced in moderate-to-severe disease. The fluorescein dilaurate test relies on pancreatic esterase to release fluorescein, which is then absorbed and excreted in the urine.

Management

The mainstay of management is analgesia, the avoidance of alcohol and the treatment of complications. Opioids, NSAIDs and tricyclic antidepressants may be required. Occasionally, coeliac axis nerve block may be tried. Steatorrhoea is treated by pancreatic enzyme supplements, a proton pump inhibitor and low-fat diet. Secondary diabetes mellitus usually requires insulin.

 USING THE GLASGOW SCORE FOR ASSESSING SEVERITY OF ACUTE PANCREATITIS

Three or more of the following factors indicate severe acute pancreatitis (CRP > 20 mg/l is also associated with poor prognosis):

- age > 55 years
- white cell count ↑, > 15 ×10⁹/l
- plasma glucose ↑, > 10 mmol/l
- plasma lactate dehydrogenase ↑
- plasma AST ↑
- urea ↑, > 16 mmol/l
- Ca²⁺ ↓, < 2 mmol/l (most significant prognostic factor for death)
- albumin ↓, < 32 g/l
- arterial O₂ partial pressure ↓ (Pao₂ < 8 kPa).

11. Tumours of liver, pancreas and biliary tree

Questions
- What is the prognosis of hepatocellular cancer?
- What are the presenting features of pancreatic cancer?

Liver

The liver is a common site for metastatic spread of cancer, particularly from the stomach, colon, oesophagus, breast and lung. Primary liver tumours are less common and may arise from the different cellular components of the liver.

Haemangiomata

Haemangiomata are the most common benign tumours of the liver and are frequently found coincidentally during ultrasound or CT. They appear bright on ultrasound owing to blood content and are occasionally calcified. Haemangiomata may be multiple but the vast majority are asymptomatic and do not require further investigation or treatment.

Hepatic adenoma

Hepatic adenomas are collections of hepatocytes without portal tracts or central veins. They are usually found coincidentally but may present with right upper quadrant pain from rapid expansion or, rarely, with bleeding. There is an association with use of oral contraceptives. Adenomas should be monitored to ensure there is no progression as there have been reports of malignant change. Larger lesions can grow and haemorrhage during pregnancy and may require resection.

Focal nodular hyperplasia

Focal nodular hyperplasia is a collection of benign hepatocytes with a central scar and often a central feeding artery. The finding of the central scar distinguishes this from hepatic adenoma. They may be multiple and do not require further intervention unless expanding rapidly. Although it is more common in young females there is no connection with the oral contraceptive.

Hepatocellular cancer

Hepatocellular cancer is a primary malignant tumour of hepatocytes. It often occurs on a background of liver cirrhosis caused by hepatitis B or C virus, haemochromatosis and alcohol consumption. It is one of the most common malignant tumours in the world although relatively uncommon in the UK (Fig. 3.11.1). The incidence is rising because of the increased prevalence of cirrhosis in alcohol-related liver disease and hepatitis C infection. Anabolic steroids and aflatoxin (fungal contamination of food) are rare associations.

Clinical features include weight loss, anorexia, fever, right upper abdominal discomfort and ascites, usually in those with chronic liver disease. Serum alpha-fetoprotein is raised in 60% and ultrasound shows filling defects in the liver in 90%. Screening with 6-monthly liver ultrasound and alpha-fetoprotein is suggested for patients with cirrhosis.

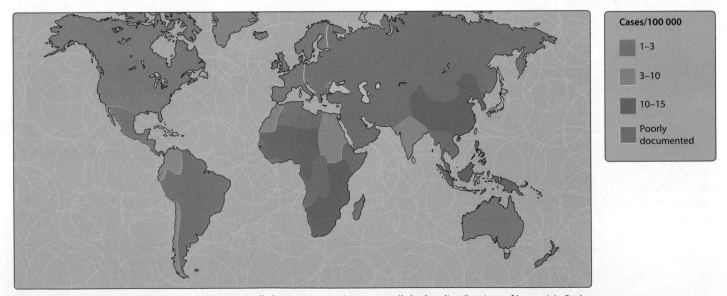

Cases/100 000
- 1–3
- 3–10
- 10–15
- Poorly documented

Fig. 3.11.1 Worldwide distribution of hepatocellular cancer; it almost parallels the distribution of hepatitis B virus.

Table 3.11.1 COMPARISON OF HEPATOCELLULAR CANCER AND CHOLANGIOCARCINOMA

	Hepatocellular carcinoma	Cholangiocarcinoma
Symptoms	Non-specific; weight loss; pain	Jaundice
Associations	Cirrhosis; hepatitis B and C virus; alcohol excess	Rarely primary sclerosing cholangitis
Site	Intrahepatic	Extrahepatic or at porta hepatis
Tumour markers	Alpha-fetoprotein	None in widespread use
Treatment	Resection; liver transplantation; radiofrequency ablation; chemoembolization	Resection; palliative stenting; photodynamic therapy

Small tumours in patients with compensated cirrhosis may be resectable. Liver transplantation may be indicated. Chemoembolization or radiofrequency ablation may be used as palliation. Median survival in symptomatic disease without resection or transplantation is approximately 6 months.

Biliary tree

Gallbladder tumours are uncommon. They usually present with jaundice or an upper abdominal mass, or are found incidentally following removal of a gallbladder. Prognosis is poor.

Cholangiocarcinoma

Cholangiocarcinoma is a rare cancer of the biliary tree. It is associated with choledochal cyst, primary sclerosing cholangitis and chronic parasitic infection of the biliary tree. It presents with obstructive jaundice and pruritus and is confirmed by spiral CT and MR cholangiopancreatography. Cholangiocarcinoma of the common bile duct may occasionally be resectable. Jaundice may be relieved with stenting of the biliary tree. Table 3.11.1 compares hepatocellular cancer and cholangiocarcinoma.

Pancreas

The incidence of pancreatic cancer (adenocarcinomas) is approximately 10/100 000 population, of whom approximately 60% are males. Pancreatic cancer is twice as common in smokers, and there is an increased risk in patients with chronic pancreatitis.

Clinical presentation

Patients present with anorexia, weight loss and abdominal pain (Fig. 3.11.2). Pancreatic tumours often present late because 75% occur in the head of the pancreas and will have an effect only when big enough to compress the bile duct, causing painless obstructive jaundice. Cancers at or near the ampulla of Vater present with jaundice earlier as they impact upon the bile duct. Jaundice often causes intractable pruritus.

Physical examination often only has signs of weight loss, although there may be jaundice and a palpable gallbladder. Courvoisier's law states that a palpable gallbladder in the presence of painless jaundice is unlikely to be caused by gallstones.

Investigations

Transabdominal ultrasound may demonstrate a tumour but as the pancreas is retroperitoneal it is often obscured by bowel gas. Abdominal CT may reveal the cancer and allow assessment of its stage. Endoscopic ultrasound can give additional information on the potential for surgery and enable biopsy.

Management

Only 10% of pancreatic tumours are suitable for resection. Surgical resection is a major procedure and involves a Whipple's resection (a pylorus-preserving proximal pancreatico-duodenectomy). Endoscopic retrograde cholangiopancreatography and stenting of the biliary obstruction may provide symptom relief. Chemotherapy is becoming available. The 5-year survival for pancreatic cancer is approximately 2%, with less than 10% alive at 1 year.

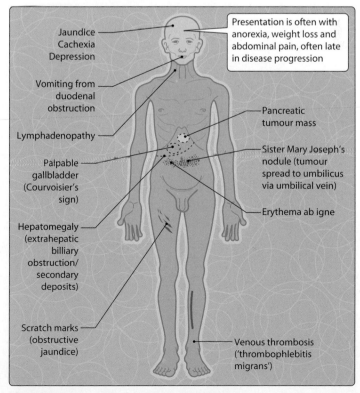

Fig. 3.11.2 Features of pancreatic cancer.

PART VI

Renal disorders

VI

Sian Finlay and Carol Brunton

The big picture

The kidney is an organ with multiple functions:

- regulatory: intravascular fluid volume, electrolytes, acid–base balance
- endocrine: regulating blood flow (renin), vascular tone (prostaglandins), red blood cells (erythropoietin), calcium and bone (1,25-dihydroxycholecalciferol)
- metabolic: vitamin D, proteins, gluconeogenesis, conjugation of drugs.

The blood flow to the kidneys is approximately 20% of the cardiac output. Each kidney has approximately 1 million nephrons (Figs 1.1 and 1.2). The glomerular flow rate (GFR) is approximately 120 ml/min. The kidney, therefore, 'filters' approximately 135–180 litres every day. Since about 2 litres of urine is passed daily, a massive amount of tubular reabsorption occurs.

Renal medicine covers disorders involving glomeruli, tubules, interstitium and renal vasculature. Renal disease can be primary or a complication of systemic illness. All age groups are affected, although those with diabetes mellitus, vascular disease and aged over 65 years are at higher risk (Fig. 1.3).

Established renal failure is irreversible and ultimately requires regular dialysis or transplantation. Renal replacement therapy (RRT) accounts for 1–2% of the UK NHS expenditure.

There are many diseases of the kidney that can be successfully treated and do not lead to renal failure. Some conditions are self-limiting while others progress so slowly that they do not have an impact on lifespan. When kidneys begin to fail, sometimes careful control of blood pressure, diet and intervention to prevent complications can enable individuals to survive in good health for many years.

Acute renal failure

Acute renal failure occurs in 2–5% of hospital patients, with an overall mortality of approximately 50%. Mortality on intensive care can be as high as 80%. Acute tubular necrosis (ATN) is the commonest aetiology, followed by pre- and then postrenal causes. In ATN, 90% of patients who survive will recover kidney function, though not always completely.

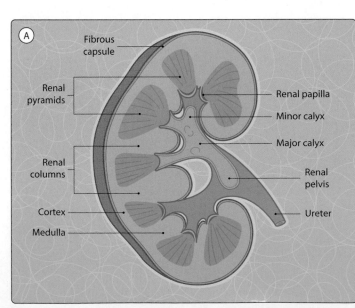

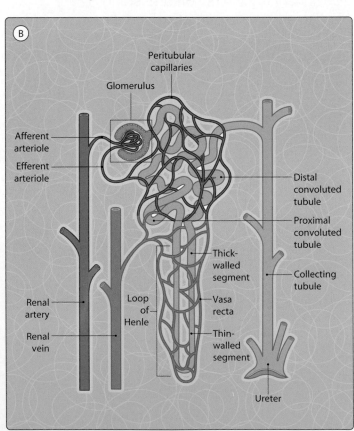

Fig. 1.1 Functional anatomy of the kidney. A, Anatomical relationships; B, A single nephron.

Chronic kidney disease

Chronic kidney disease is a worldwide health problem and a major cause of morbidity and mortality. The ageing population and increasing prevalence of diabetes mellitus and hypertension suggest that it will become even more common in the future. Chronic kidney disease is defined as the presence of structural or functional abnormalities of the kidneys (e.g. microalbuminuria) that persist for at least 3 months, or a sustained fall in GFR to < 60 ml/min per 1.73 m². Early recognition and treatment can delay progression and reduce the risk of cardiovascular complications and premature death.

End-stage renal failure

The number of patients being accepted on to dialysis programmes has increased annually since the mid-1980s, reaching 100–125 patients/1 000 000 population. The median age of patients starting dialysis is also rising; 50% are now > 65 years (Fig. 1.4). The commonest identifiable cause of renal failure is diabetic nephropathy, which now accounts for almost 20% of patients starting RRT. Other important causes are glomerulonephritis, chronic pyelonephritis, and renovascular disease. More than 20% of patients have renal failure of uncertain aetiology.

The prevalence of patients requiring RRT has also increased over recent years and is now > 600/1 000 000 population. By the end of 2002, 46% of these patients had a functioning renal transplant, 39% were on haemodialysis and 15% were on peritoneal dialysis. All patients on RRT have a higher relative risk of death, which is most pronounced in the young; those on dialysis aged 20–24 years have a 121-fold higher risk of death compared with a similar aged person in the general population. Recent UK data indicate that the overall 5-year survival of patients on RRT is 43%, falling to only 14% in those > 65 years at the start of RRT. Heart disease is the most common cause of death in patients with renal disease.

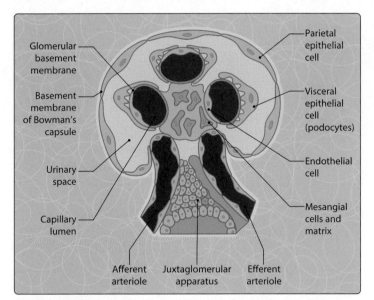

Fig. 1.2 The structure of a glomerulus.

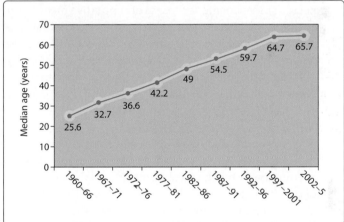

Fig. 1.4 Median age of patients starting renal replacement therapy, 1960–2005.

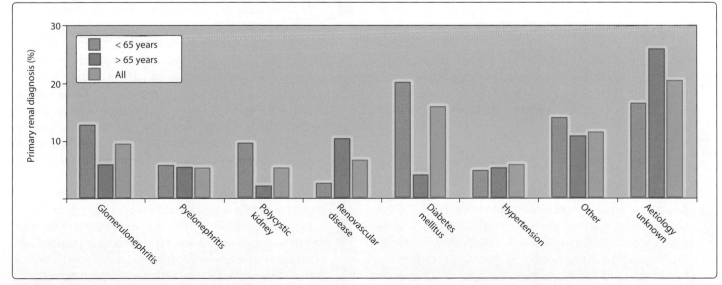

Fig. 1.3 Primary renal diagnoses at varying ages.

High-return facts

1 **Acute renal failure** is a rapid deterioration in kidney function over hours or days that results in accumulation of nitrogenous waste and fluid. The causes of acute renal failure are classified as prerenal (reduced perfusion of the kidneys), postrenal (obstruction) and intrinsic (glomerulonephritis, acute interstitial nephritis, acute tubular necrosis). Management consists of supportive measures to optimize fluid balance and renal perfusion, withdrawal of nephrotoxic drugs and treatment of the underlying cause where possible. Indications for dialysis are refractory hyperkalaemia or metabolic acidosis, fluid overload that is resistant to diuretics, uraemic pericarditis and uraemic coma. The overall mortality is approximately 50%.

2 **Chronic kidney disease** is often asymptomatic until it becomes very advanced. It is defined as the presence of structural or functional abnormalities of the kidneys that persist for at least 3 months or a sustained fall in glomerular filtration rate to <60 ml/min per $1.73\,m^2$. The commonest causes are diabetes mellitus, glomerulonephritis, hypertension and vascular disease. Management is aimed at slowing progression to end-stage renal failure and treating any complications that arise (renal anaemia, renal osteodystrophy). Renal replacement therapy is commenced when symptoms of uraemia, refractory fluid overload, hyperkalaemia or acidosis develop. The options include haemodialysis, peritoneal dialysis and renal transplantation. Transplantation is the treatment of choice (although performed in a minority of individuals) since it improves quality of life and mortality compared with dialysis. Conservative management may be appropriate in some elderly patients.

3 **Glomerulonephritis** describes a group of disorders in which there is immune-mediated injury to the glomeruli. It may be idiopathic or occur in association with a systemic disease or infection. The main types are IgA nephropathy, minimal change disease, focal segmental glomerulosclerosis, membranous nephropathy, mesangiocapillary glomerulonephritis, post-streptococcal glomerulonephritis and rapidly progressive glomerulonephritis.

Some types of glomerulonephritis respond to specific treatment, such as steroids or immunosuppression. Others do not respond to such therapy, and the goal of treatment is to control symptoms and delay progression to end-stage renal failure.

4 **Nephrotic syndrome** is defined by the combination of proteinuria (in excess of 3.5 g in 24 h), hypoalbuminaemia and oedema. It may occur as a result of primary kidney disease (e.g. certain types of glomerulonephritis) or be secondary to systemic diseases (e.g. diabetes mellitus and amyloidosis). In children it is usually caused by minimal change disease and responds to steroids. The prognosis of nephrotic syndrome is largely dependent on the underlying cause. **Tubulointerstitial disease** is an important cause of both acute and chronic renal failure and is often secondary to drugs. Causes include acute and chronic interstitial nephritis, analgesic nephropathy, Balkan nephropathy and urate nephropathy. Treatment involves withdrawal of any implicated drug. Acute interstitial nephritis may respond to high-dose steroids.

5 **Renovascular disease** is commonly caused by atherosclerotic renal artery stenosis or fibromuscular dysplasia. It can be diagnosed using digital subtraction angiography or MRI of the renal arteries. Treatment involves control of hypertension and aggressive management of cardiovascular risk factors. Some patients benefit from angioplasty and stenting of the renal arteries. **Renal tubular acidosis** (RTA) is caused by a failure of the kidneys to regulate acid–base balance within the body by excreting hydrogen ions and reabsorbing bicarbonate in response to acidaemia. There are three main types of RTA but all result in metabolic acidosis. Type 1 (distal) results from an inability to secrete hydrogen ions into the distal tubule. Type 2 (proximal) results from an inability to reabsorb bicarbonate in the proximal tubule. Type 4 is caused by either aldosterone deficiency or resistance. Types 1 and 2 are treated with potassium replacement and alkali therapy. Type 4 is treated with dietary potassium restriction or fludrocortisone.

6 **Inherited renal diseases** include adult polycystic kidney disease, Alport's syndrome, nephronophthisis and medullary cystic disease. Some may progress to end-stage renal failure. Diagnosis in one individual should prompt screening within the family for other cases. Management consists of blood pressure control and treating complications of renal failure. **Systemic disease** can affect the kidneys. Diabetic nephropathy is the commonest cause of end-stage renal failure in Western society. It is managed with ACE inhibitors and tight glycaemic control. Multisystem diseases such as systemic lupus erythematosus (SLE) and vasculitis often involve the kidneys and usually respond to immunosuppression. Multiple myeloma and amyloidosis can also cause renal failure. Haemolytic uraemic syndrome caused by the enteric pathogen *Escherichia coli* 0157H is the commonest cause of acute renal failure in children.

7 **Urinary tract infection** is far more common in females than males, and most episodes are short lived and uncomplicated. Vesicoureteric reflux can cause recurrent infections in childhood and lead to long-term kidney damage. Asymptomatic bacteruria in pregnant women should always be treated, since there is a risk of progression to pyelonephritis. **Urinary stones** are common and often recur. Approximately 80% of stones are composed of calcium (usually oxalate or phosphate) and the remainder of urate, cystine or struvite: knowing the composition can help in preventing recurrence. Stones may be diagnosed using plain radiographs or intravenous pyelography. Management consists of a high-fluid, low-salt diet, alkalinization of the urine and sometimes specific drug treatments. Stones that do not pass spontaneously may require lithotripsy or surgical intervention.

8 **Obstruction of the urinary tract** can occur anywhere from the renal calyces to the urethral meatus. Anatomical abnormalities are the commonest cause in infancy, while prostatic enlargement and malignancy predominate in older patients. Ultrasound is the investigation of choice and also identifies the level of obstruction. A normal urine output does not exclude partial obstruction. Prompt relief of obstruction with a urinary catheter, nephrostomy or ureteric stent is vital, as the probability of recovering kidney function diminishes with time. Relief of obstruction may be followed by a large diuresis requiring fluid and electrolyte replacement. **Tumours** of the urinary tract can arise within the kidney or from the urothelium lining the renal pelvis, ureters and bladder. The most common types in adults are renal cell cancer and transitional cell cancer. Patients present with painless haematuria, loin pain or an abdominal mass. Prognosis depends on the stage of tumour at presentation. Wilm's tumour (nephroblastoma) occurs in children and with treatment has a 5-year survival of 90%.

1. Acute renal failure

Questions
- What are the causes of acute renal failure?
- How should acute renal failure be managed?

Acute renal failure (ARF) is deterioration in renal function over hours or days, resulting in accumulation of nitrogenous waste and fluid. It has a high mortality and should be treated as a medical emergency. It can also be referred to as acute kidney injury.

Epidemiology

ARF occurs in 2–5% of hospital patients. Acute tubular necrosis (ATN) is the most common cause, followed by prerenal and then postrenal causes.

Pathogenesis

The causes of ARF can be classified as prerenal, postrenal or intrinsic (Fig. 3.1.1)

Prerenal failure occurs through a reduction in renal blood flow, leading to underperfusion of otherwise normal kidneys. This is usually a result of a fall in systemic blood pressure, dehydration, blood loss, septicaemia or reduced cardiac output. Prolonged prerenal failure may progress to intrinsic renal failure. Acute vascular syndromes (renal vein thrombosis, renal artery dissection, or atheroembolic disease) are rarer causes of underperfusion.

Postrenal failure is caused by obstruction of the urinary tract, leading to increased intratubular pressure and a fall in glomerular filtration rate (GFR).

Intrinsic renal failure refers to injury within the kidney itself. The commonest cause is ATN (usually as a result of prolonged hypotension or nephrotoxins). Intrinsic renal failure can also be caused by acute interstitial nephritis, acute glomerulonephritis and intratubular obstruction. In intratubular obstruction, the tubules can be blocked by crystals (urate nephropathy) or protein (myoglobin in rhabdomyolysis and casts in multiple myeloma).

Clinical features

Clinical signs and sequelae reflect the functional area that is deranged (Table 3.1.1). The context in which ARF occurs often provides a major clue to its cause. There may be a history of exposure to i.v. contrast or nephrotoxic drugs, recent myocardial infarction, blood loss, dehydration, crush injury or systemic infection. Patients may describe symptoms of an underlying vasculitis (malaise, joint pains, rash, haemoptysis) or those of bladder outlet obstruction (hesitancy, nocturia, poor urinary flow). Septic patients may have fever, sweats and rigors. In rhabdomyolysis, there may be muscle pain and swelling. Acute interstitial nephritis (AIN) often presents with fever and a rash. As renal failure advances, patients may also report symptoms of uraemia or fluid overload. Breathlessness can occur from pulmonary oedema or metabolic acidosis. Reduced urine output (oliguria) is common but not universal.

There may be signs of hypovolaemia (hypotension, reduced skin turgor, dry mucous membranes) or fluid overload (gallop rhythm, raised jugular venous pressure, pulmonary oedema). Respiratory rate may be elevated as patients attempt to compensate for metabolic acidosis. A pericardial rub is audible in uraemic pericarditis. There may be signs of an underlying vasculitis or systemic disease. Infected patients may have a fever and peripheral vasodilatation, and a rash may be visible in AIN or atheroembolic disease.

Investigations

Serum urea and creatinine are elevated and serum potassium is frequently high. ECG may show features of hyperkalaemia. Urine biochemistry can help to distinguish prerenal from renal failure (Table 3.1.2).

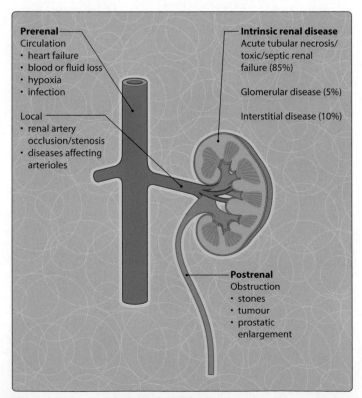

Prerenal
Circulation
- heart failure
- blood or fluid loss
- hypoxia
- infection

Local
- renal artery occlusion/stenosis
- diseases affecting arterioles

Intrinsic renal disease
Acute tubular necrosis/ toxic/septic renal failure (85%)

Glomerular disease (5%)

Interstitial disease (10%)

Postrenal
Obstruction
- stones
- tumour
- prostatic enlargement

Fig. 3.1.1 Causes of acute renal failure.

Table 3.1.1 CHANGES IN KIDNEY FUNCTIONS IN RENAL FAILURE

Functional change	Clinical signs/sequelae
Retention of waste products	Uraemic symptoms: anorexia, nausea, pruritis
Retention of sodium chloride and water	Oedema, hypertension
Retention of potassium	Cardiac arrhythmia
Retention of acid	Breathlessness, acidotic 'Kussmaul's respiration'
Retention of phosphate, failure of vitamin D metabolism	Renal bone disease: bone pain
Retention of drugs	Toxicity

Table 3.1.2 DISTINCTION BETWEEN PRERENAL AND RENAL FAILURE ON URINALYSIS

	Prerenal	Renal
Urine specific gravity	> 1.020	< 1.01
Urine osmolality (mOsm/kg)	> 500	< 350
Urine sodium (mmol/l)	< 20	> 40

Chest radiograph may show pulmonary oedema or haemorrhage. Arterial blood gases may show metabolic acidosis.

Creatine kinase is raised in rhabdomyolysis, and white blood cell count and CRP are elevated in sepsis. Eosinophilia may occur in acute interstitial nephritis.

Immunological tests may show the presence of anti-neutrophil antibodies (ANCA) or anti-glomerular basement membrane (GBM) antibodies, and complement may be reduced in glomerulonephritis.

Ultrasound of the renal tract is necessary to exclude obstruction. If the cause of ARF is not apparent, renal biopsy is required.

Management

Patients should be assessed for fluid balance. Hypovolaemia should be corrected aggressively with i.v. fluids or blood transfusion. A central venous catheter is often useful to guide fluid replacement, and accurate charting of fluid intake and output is essential. If hypotension persists after rehydration, inotropic support may be required to achieve an adequate blood pressure.

Hyperkalaemia should be treated promptly, since it can cause life-threatening cardiac arrhythmias and sudden death. Intravenous calcium (gluconate or chloride) stabilizes the myocardium and reduces the risk of arrhythmia. Infusion of insulin and dextrose increases potassium uptake by cells, and temporarily lowers serum levels. Nebulized beta-adrenergic agonists (e.g. salbutamol) also reduce serum potassium. These measures buy time for elimination of potassium from the gut using calcium resonium resin. Correction of metabolic acidosis with bicarbonate supplementation may also have a beneficial effect on hyperkalaemia.

If a patient remains anuric or oliguric despite adequate fluid replacement and adequate blood pressure, they are likely to require dialysis.

An attempt should also be made to correct the underlying cause of ARF where possible. If there is evidence of obstruction, this must be relieved immediately by insertion of a urinary catheter or nephrostomy. Any nephrotoxic drugs suspected of causing interstitial nephritis should be discontinued. AIN may respond to oral steroids. Vasculitis should be treated with immunosuppression (usually cyclophosphamide and prednisolone ± plasma exchange). Intratubular obstruction is treated with i.v. fluids to maintain a high urinary output where possible.

Prognosis

The overall mortality from ARF is 50–80%. The outcome is worse in older patients and those with multi-organ failure. In ATN, 90% of patients who survive will recover some degree of renal function.

2. Chronic kidney disease

Questions
- What are the clinical features of chronic kidney disease?
- What forms of renal replacement therapy are available?

Chronic kidney disease (CKD) is defined as structural or functional renal abnormalities, for example microalbuminuria persisting for >3 months, or a sustained fall in glomerular filtration rate (GFR) to <60 ml/min per 1.73 m².

Epidemiology
The prevalence of CKD in the general population is 5%. The incidence of end-stage renal failure caused by CKD has risen steadily particularly in those >65 years. The commonest causes are diabetes mellitus, glomerulonephritis, hypertension and vascular disease.

Pathogenesis
After renal injury, the kidneys initially compensate by increasing filtration through remaining nephrons (adaptive hyperfiltration). Increased glomerular pressure contributes to progressive renal damage and glomerulosclerosis.

As renal failure progresses, the kidneys lose ability both to excrete phosphate and produce 1,25-dihydroxycholecalciferol (active form of vitamin D); serum phosphate rises while calcium falls. This stimulates increased parathormone (PTH), causing secondary hyperparathyroidism and eventually bone disease (renal osteodystrophy). Anaemia develops because the kidneys stop producing erythropoietin, which stimulates erythropoiesis. Impaired excretion of potassium and hydrogen ions results in hyperkalaemia and metabolic acidosis.

Clinical features
Symptoms (Fig. 3.2.1) often only appear when CKD is advanced.

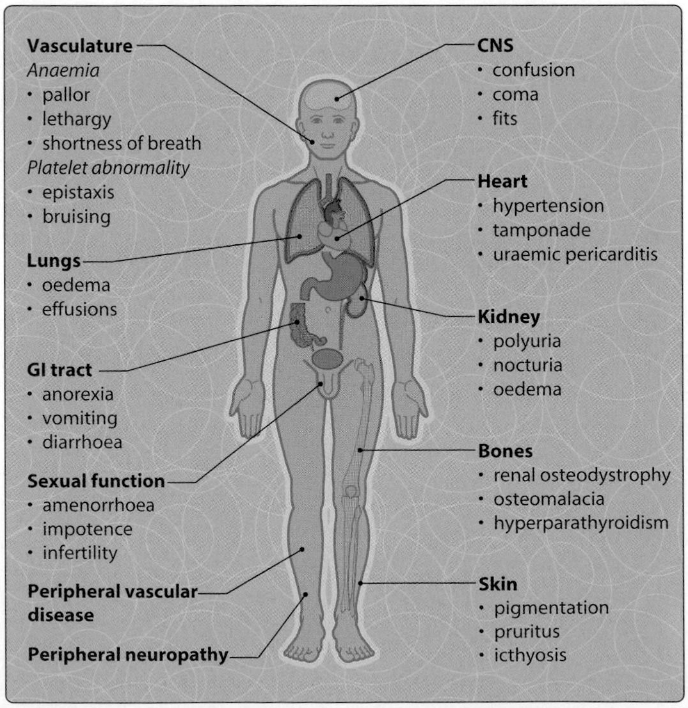

Investigations
Investigations are as for acute renal failure. Serum creatinine is raised as filtration fails (Fig. 3.2.2).

Renal ultrasound scan may show small scarred kidneys, large polycystic kidneys or hydronephrosis of one or both kidneys with loss of cortical thickness.

Management
Once CKD is confirmed, management is directed at slowing progression to end-stage renal failure and treating complications. Blood pressure should be <130/80 mmHg and controlled using ACE inhibitors or angiotensin receptor blockers, unless renovascular disease is present. Good glycaemia control is important in those with diabetes. Risk factors for cardiovascular disease (hypercholesterolaemia and smoking) should also be addressed.

Vasculature
Anaemia
- pallor
- lethargy
- shortness of breath
Platelet abnormality
- epistaxis
- bruising

Lungs
- oedema
- effusions

GI tract
- anorexia
- vomiting
- diarrhoea

Sexual function
- amenorrhoea
- impotence
- infertility

Peripheral vascular disease

Peripheral neuropathy

CNS
- confusion
- coma
- fits

Heart
- hypertension
- tamponade
- uraemic pericarditis

Kidney
- polyuria
- nocturia
- oedema

Bones
- renal osteodystrophy
- osteomalacia
- hyperparathyroidism

Skin
- pigmentation
- pruritus
- icthyosis

Fig. 3.2.1 Clinical features of chronic kidney disease.

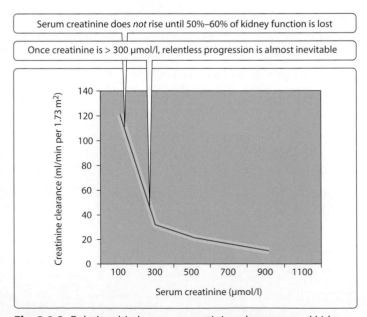

Serum creatinine does *not* rise until 50%–60% of kidney function is lost

Once creatinine is > 300 µmol/l, relentless progression is almost inevitable

Fig. 3.2.2 Relationship between creatinine clearance and kidney function.

Fluid overload. Restrict salt and water intake or give loop diuretics. Failure to respond to diuretics is an indication to start dialysis.

Anaemia. Use s.c. recombinant erythropoetin beta and/or oral or i.v. iron.

Secondary hyperparathyroidism. Reduce dietary phosphate intake and give oral phosphate binders (e.g. calcium acetate or carbonate) to reduce phosphate gut absorption. If calcium is low, activated vitamin D_2 (calcitriol) is given to maintain PTH levels < 300 ng/l. If this fails, surgical parathyroidectomy may be required.

Hyperkalaemia and metabolic acidosis. Reduce dietary potassium and give oral sodium bicarbonate. Persisting acidosis or hyperkalaemia despite these measures is an indication to start renal replacement therapy (RRT).

Renal replacement therapy

RRT should be commenced when a patient with CKD develops symptoms of uraemia, refractory fluid overload, hyperkalaemia or acidosis.

Haemodialysis. Haemodialysis requires either cannulation of a central vein or creation of an arteriovenous fistula (usually in the arm). An alternative is synthetic grafts, which have a higher complication rate but can be used sooner. During dialysis, solutes diffuse across the membrane in either direction down concentration gradients (e.g. urea in blood will diffuse into the dialysate, while bicarbonate in the dialysate will diffuse into the blood) (Fig. 3.2.3). Application of hydrostatic pressure across the membrane allows removal of water from the blood (ultrafiltration). Most patients need to dialyse for 4–5 h three times a week. Survival on haemodialysis at 1, 5 and 10 years is 80%, 40%, and 18%, respectively.

Peritoneal dialysis. Continuous ambulatory peritoneal dialysis (CAPD) requires the permanent placement of a catheter into the abdominal cavity (Fig. 3.2.4). Dialysis fluid is infused and left to dwell while solutes diffuse across the peritoneal membrane, down their concentration gradients. At least three to four exchanges of dialysis solution are required every day. The major complication is peritonitis, which presents with abdominal pain and cloudy dialysate. Treatment is with intraperitoneal (and sometimes systemic) antibiotics, and removal of the catheter if there is recurrent or persistent infection.

Renal transplantation. Transplantation improves quality of life and mortality compared with dialysis and involves the insertion of a single kidney, from a live or cadaveric donor, into the recipient's iliac fossa. Rejection is most likely to occur in the first 3–6 months and immunosuppressive drugs are started immediately (prednisolone, azathioprine, mycophenolate, tacrolimus or ciclosporin). Rejection presents with fever, pain over the graft and rising serum creatinine. If biopsy confirms rejection, high-dose steroids are often effective. Chronic rejection (chronic allograft nephropathy) results in gradual decline in renal function and scarring on biopsy and does not respond to increased immunosuppression.

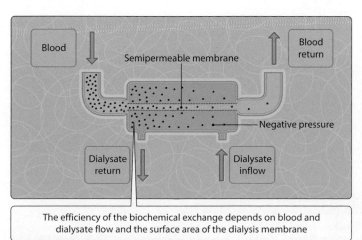

The efficiency of the biochemical exchange depends on blood and dialysate flow and the surface area of the dialysis membrane

Fig. 3.2.3 Principles of haemofiltration.

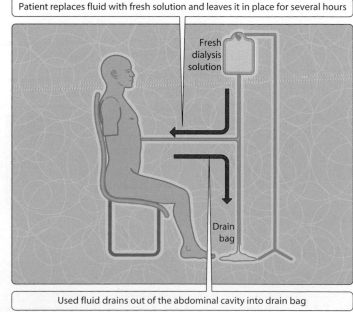

Patient replaces fluid with fresh solution and leaves it in place for several hours

Used fluid drains out of the abdominal cavity into drain bag

Fig. 3.2.4 Peritoneal dialysis.

3. Glomerulonephritis

Questions
- What are the types of glomerulonephritis?
- What is the treatment of IgA nephropathy?

Glomerulonephritis describes disorders with immune-mediated injury to the glomeruli. This can be transient and reversible or lead to progressive renal failure. It is subdivided according to the histological appearance on renal biopsy (Fig. 3.3.1).

Epidemiology

End-stage renal failure is frequently caused by glomerulonephritis. The most common type worldwide is IgA nephropathy, which typically presents in men aged 18–30 years (Fig. 3.3.2). Mesangiocapillary glomerulonephritis also occurs principally in young adults. Membranous nephropathy and rapidly progressive glomerulonephritis (RPGN) are more common in patients aged 40–60 years. Focal and segmental glomerulonephritis (FSGS), minimal change disease and post-streptococcal glomerulonephritis can affect any age, though the latter two are more common in children.

Pathogenesis

Glomerulonephritis may be idiopathic or be secondary to systemic disease or infection. Formation or deposition of immune complexes within the glomeruli is recognized as one pathogenetic mechanism. This results in complement activation and inflammation, which damages the glomeruli. In Goodpasture's disease, circulating antibodies directed against the glomerular basement membrane (anti-GBM) mediate the injury, allowing blood and protein to leak into the urine. Cross-reactivity with alveolar membranes leads to pulmonary haemorrhage.

Clinical features

Patients may be asymptomatic but have microscopic haematuria or proteinuria on urinalysis. Others present with nephrotic syndrome or nephritic syndrome (Fig. 3.3.1).

IgA nephropathy.   Presentation may be with recurrent episodes of frank haematuria with upper respiratory tract infections. Some patients are hypertensive or have symptoms of progressive renal failure. Henoch–Schönlein purpura is a variant of IgA nephropathy that presents with abdominal pain, arthralgia and a purpuric rash on extensor aspects of legs and arms.

Minimal change disease.   This is the most common glomerulonephritis in children and usually presents with periorbital oedema, abdominal swelling and nephrotic syndrome. Urinalysis shows proteinuria but no haematuria. Hypertension and renal impairment are rare.

Focal and segmental glomerulonephritis and membranous glomerulonephritis.   Both usually present as nephrotic

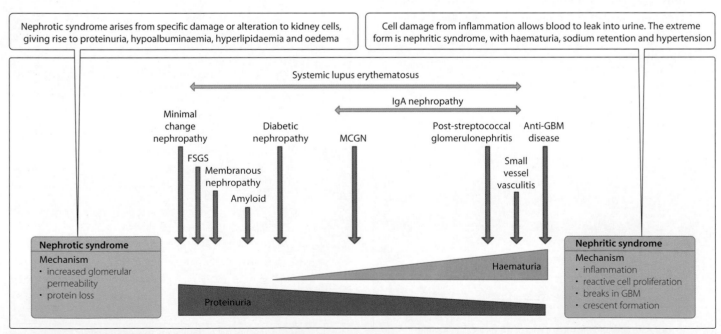

Fig. 3.3.1 Spectrum of glomerular disease. FSGS, focal segmental glomerulosclerosis; GBM, glomerular basement membrane; MCGN, mesangiocapillary glomerulonephritis.

syndrome. Urinalysis shows proteinuria with or without haematuria.

Mesangiocapillary glomerulonephritis. Presentation may be with features of nephritic or nephrotic syndrome.

Post-streptococcal glomerulonephritis. Presentation is as an acute nephritic syndrome several weeks after a streptococcal throat infection. Urinalysis shows microscopic haematuria and proteinuria.

Rapidly progressive glomerulonephritis. Presentation is with systemic symptoms (e.g. general malaise, weight loss, arthralgia, and fever). There may be evidence of vasculitis affecting other organs (respiratory and nasal symptoms, rash, neuropathy). In Goodpasture's disease, lung haemorrhage and haemoptysis occur, almost exclusively in smokers. Urinalysis shows microscopic haematuria and proteinuria. Renal failure often progresses rapidly and patients may present with uraemia, oliguria, and fluid retention.

Investigations

Urine microscopy may show dysmorphic red cells or red cell casts. Depending on the type of glomerulonephritis, there may be nephrotic syndrome (low serum albumin, high cholesterol), renal impairment (raised urea and creatinine) or systemic inflammation (raised CRP, thrombocytosis, eosinophilia). Chest radiograph may show alveolar haemorrhage or pulmonary nodules. Specific associations include:

- post-streptococcal glomerulonephritis: anti-streptolysin O (ASO) titre may be elevated
- mesangiocapillary and post-infectious glomerulonephritis and in systemic lupus erythematosus (SLE; lupus nephritis): serum complement levels (especially C3) are often reduced

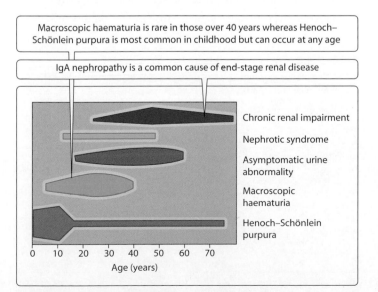

Fig. 3.3.2 Features of IgA nephropathies with age.

- Goodpasture's disease: anti-GBM antibodies
- Wegener's granulomatosis: cytoplasmic anti-neutrophil antibodies (cANCA).

Renal biopsy is the gold-standard method for diagnosing and classifying glomerulonephritis.

Management

Some types respond to specific treatments (e.g. immunosuppression) but others do not and the goal is to control symptoms and slow progression. Oedema is managed with diuretics and restriction of fluid intake. ACE inhibitors or angiotensin II receptor blockers are used to control hypertension and reduce proteinuria. Lipid-lowering agents and anticoagulation are beneficial in nephrotic syndrome.

IgA nephropathy. Hypertension or proteinuria should be treated. In patients with heavy proteinuria and rapidly deteriorating renal function, immunosuppressive drugs (e.g. prednisolone, cyclophosphamide, azathioprine) may slow progression. Despite treatment, 20% of patients develop end-stage renal failure at 20 years.

Minimal change disease. Prednisolone resolves proteinuria in >90%. Approximately 50% of patients relapse and some become steroid dependent. Other immunosuppressants (e.g. cyclophosphamide or ciclosporin) can be tried. Renal function does not usually decline.

Focal and segmental glomerulonephritis. Approximately 10–20% of patients respond to steroids. The remainder are treated with diuretics and ACE inhibitors. End-stage renal failure within 10 years of diagnosis occurs in 80%.

Membranous nephropathy. Spontaneous remission occurs in 15–30%, while 20–30% progress to end-stage renal failure within 20 years. The remainder have persistent nephrotic syndrome with stable or slowly deteriorating renal function. Management is with ACE inhibitors, diuretics and statins; immunosuppresssion using steroids and chlorambucil or cyclophosphamide can be tried.

Mesangiocapillary glomerulonephritis. End-stage renal failure develops within 10 years in 50%.

Post-streptococcal glomerulonephritis. Treatment is supportive with antibiotics for persisting infection; 1% of adults may develop chronic kidney disease.

Rapidly progressive glomerulonephritis. Without treatment, RPGN progresses to end-stage renal failure in weeks to months. Immunosuppression with high-dose steroids and cyclophosphamide improves the prognosis. Plasma exchange may remove circulating anti-GBM antibodies in Goodpasture's disease. Recovery of function depends on the extent of renal damage when treatment commences.

4. Nephrotic syndrome and tubulointerstitial disease

Questions
- What is the pathogenesis of nephrotic syndrome?
- What drugs cause tubulointerstitial disease?

Nephrotic syndrome

Nephrotic syndrome is proteinuria ($\geq$3.5 g in 24 h; Table 3.4.1), hypoalbuminaemia and oedema. Hypercholesterolaemia and an increased thrombotic tendency are other features. Nephrotic syndrome can be primary or secondary to systemic diseases (Table 3.4.2). Prognosis depends on the underlying cause.

Epidemiology

Nephrotic syndrome is 15 times more common in children than in adults, with an annual incidence of 2–7/100 000 children. The peak incidence is between 2 and 6 years.

Pathogenesis

Changes in permeability in glomerular capillaries result in increased loss of protein in urine and hypoalbuminaemia (Fig. 3.4.1).

Clinical features

The main symptom is oedema, which may be periorbital or dependent. Accumulation of fluid elsewhere can lead to pleural effusions or ascites. Some patients have frothy urine. Less commonly, presentation is with thrombotic complications such as deep venous thrombosis of the calf veins. Hypertension is rare.

Investigations

Urinalysis shows heavy proteinuria. Serum albumin is low (<30 g/l) and cholesterol is high.

Renal function is often normal if nephrotic syndrome is caused by minimal change disease, but it may be impaired if secondary to other types of glomerulonephritis or systemic disease.

Renal biopsy is helpful in adults but seldom necessary in children, where nephrotic syndrome can be assumed to be caused by minimal change disease.

Management

Management targets specific features (Table 3.4.3). Daily weight measurements are useful in monitoring response to treatment. ACE inhibitors reduce proteinuria. Hyperlipidaemia usually resolves with resolution of the nephrotic syndrome but if persistent it may be treated with a statin.

Prednisolone is the treatment of choice in minimal change disease and leads to complete resolution of proteinuria in over 90% of patients. Approximately 50% of patients will relapse, and some have frequent relapses or become steroid dependent. These patients may respond to immunosuppressants such as cyclophosphamide or ciclosporin.

Tubulointerstitial disease

In tubulointerstitial disease the predominant histology is interstitial inflammation and tubular damage. It is an important cause of acute and chronic renal failure and is often secondary to drugs.

Analgesic interstitial nephropathy. Chronic tubulointerstitial nephritis and papillary necrosis are caused by long-term ingestion of analgesics, especially phenacetin.

Urate nephropathy. Deposition of urate crystals in the tubules and collecting ducts can cause acute tubular inflammation and intrarenal obstruction (crystal nephropathy), while chronic hyperuricaemia may cause interstitial fibrosis.

Table 3.4.1 QUANTIFYING PROTEINURIA

24 h urinary protein (g)	Protein/creatinine ratio	Status
<0.03	<2.5 (men); <3.5 (women)	Normal
0.03–0.3	3.5–15	Microalbuminuria
0.3–0.5	15–50	Detectable on dipstick
0.5–2.5	50–250	
>2.0	>250	Glomerular disease likely
$\geq$ 3.5	>400	Nephrotic range

Table 3.4.2 CAUSES OF NEPHROTIC SYNDROME

Cause	Examples
Glomerular disease	Minimal change, membranous and mesangiocapillary glomerulonephritis; focal segmental glomerulosclerosis
Drug/toxin induced	Gold; other heavy metals; penicillamine
Extrarenal causes	Infection (e.g. infective endocarditis, malaria, hepatitis B) Malignancy (e.g. lymphoma, leukaemia, myeloma, lung cancer) Multisystem disorders (e.g. systemic lupus erythematosus, Henoch–Schönlein purpura, rheumatoid arthritis, diabetes mellitus) Injecting drug abuse

Balkan nephropathy. A progressive interstitial nephritis of unknown cause endemic in rural areas of the Danube basin.

Epidemiology

Interstitial nephritis can develop in response to drugs:

- NSAIDs
- antibiotics: penicillins, aminoglycosides, vancomycin, rifampicin, sulphonamides
- diuretics: furosemide
- anticonvulsants: phenytoin, valproate
- others: allopurinol, cimetidine, ranitidine.

Crystal nephropathy occurs in patients with massive overproduction of urate caused by lymphoproliferative disorders or rapid tumour lysis after chemotherapy. Chronic urate nephropathy typically occurs in middle-aged males with gout.

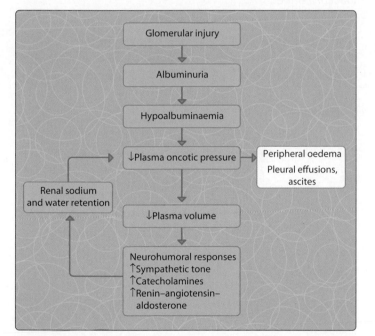

Fig. 3.4.1 Pathogenesis of oedema in nephrotic syndrome.

Pathogenesis

Acute interstitial nephritis (AIN) is a hypersensitivity reaction to a drug. There is an intense cellular infiltrate (often containing eosinophils) in the interstitium and tubules. In chronic interstitial nephritis, there is progressive interstitial fibrosis and tubular atrophy. Impaired ability to concentrate urine causes polyuria. Ischaemic injury to the papillae can lead to papillary necrosis. Damaged papillae may slough off and cause urinary tract obstruction. There is an increased incidence of urothelial tumours in both analgesic and Balkan nephropathy. Crystal nephropathy occurs when urate crystals accumulate in the tubules causing obstruction.

Clinical features

Detailed drug history is vital. AIN may be associated with features of a hypersensitivity reaction such as rash, fever and arthralgia. Papillary necrosis may present as loin pain, haematuria and renal colic. Chronic interstitial nephritis may be asymptomatic until advanced renal failure develops. There may be a history of gout and gouty tophi may be visible in urate nephropathy.

Investigations

Serum urea and creatinine are elevated. In urate nephropathy, serum urate level is elevated. Eosinophilia is common in AIN. Sterile pyuria may occur in analgesic nephropathy. Renal biopsy confirms interstitial inflammation or scarring. In analgesic nephropathy, clubbed calyces and papillary necrosis may be seen on intravenous pyelogram or CT.

Management

Implicated drugs should be discontinued. AIN may respond to high-dose steroids, but there is no specific treatment for chronic disease. Urate nephropathy is treated with a high fluid intake, alkalinization of the urine and allopurinol.

Table 3.4.3 FEATURES OF NEPHROTIC SYNDROME AND THEIR MANAGEMENT

Feature	Pathogenesis	Outcome	Management
Hypoalbuminaemia	Urinary loss exceeds liver synthesis	Reduced oncotic pressure; oedema	Diuretics; low-sodium diet
Sodium retention	Low intravascular volume; secondary hyperaldosteronism	Oedema	Diuretics; low-sodium diet
Hypercholesterolaemia	Low oncotic pressure causes increased synthesis in liver	Possibly atherosclerosis	Lipid-lowering drugs (e.g. statins)
Hypercoagulability	Loss of inhibitors (e.g. antithrombin III, protein C, protein S) and increased synthesis of clotting factors	Venous thromboembolism	Anticoagulation
Infection	Urinary loss of gammaglobulin	Pneumococcal infection	Consider vaccination

5. Renovascular disease and renal tubular acidosis

Questions
- What are the causes of renovascular hypertension?
- What are the types of renal tubular acidosis?

Renovascular disease

Renovascular disease (renal artery stenosis) is an important cause of progressive renal failure. It is potentially treatable if recognized before irreversible ischaemic injury occurs. The commonest causes in adults are atherosclerotic renal artery stenosis and fibromuscular dysplasia (FMD).

Epidemiology

Atherosclerotic renal artery stenosis (Fig. 3.5.1) occurs mainly in males > 45 years, who often have evidence of vascular disease elsewhere (coronary, cerebral or peripheral). Smoking is an important risk factor. FMD occurs principally in young females and is much less common than atherosclerosis.

Pathogenesis

Atherosclerosis is a systemic disease characterized by the development of cholesterol plaques within arteries. It typically affects the proximal part of the renal artery and may be unilateral or bilateral. The rate of progression is highly variable.

FMD is caused by fibrodysplasia or collagen deposition within the artery wall. The cause is not known. It progresses more slowly than atherosclerosis and rarely leads to arterial occlusion.

As the artery narrows, the kidney responds to ischaemia by activating the renin–angiotensin–aldosterone system. This promotes salt and water retention and hypertension. Treating hypertension may reduce intraglomerular pressure below normal (caused by the stenosis), and the kidney will then try to maintain perfusion by constricting the efferent arteriole (a process mediated by angiotensin II). Introduction of an ACE inhibitor (blocks angiotensin II formation) will prevent this autoregulation and can cause a sharp deterioration in renal function (Fig. 3.5.2).

Clinical features

Patients may have signs and symptoms of vascular disease elsewhere (angina, transient ischaemic attacks or intermittent claudication). Hypertension is common and may be difficult to control. Some patients have recurrent 'flash' pulmonary oedema.

Investigations

Urinalysis is often normal. Serum creatinine is often elevated and may rise sharply after introduction of an ACE inhibitor.

Renal ultrasound may demonstrate asymmetrical kidney size. Magnetic resonance angiography of the renal arteries or digital

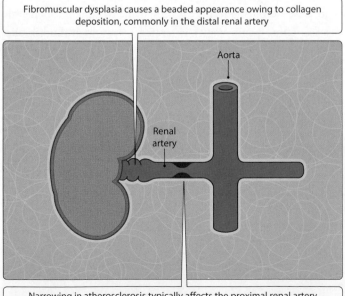

Fibromuscular dysplasia causes a beaded appearance owing to collagen deposition, commonly in the distal renal artery

Aorta

Renal artery

Narrowing in atherosclerosis typically affects the proximal renal artery

Fig. 3.5.1 Appearances of renovascular disease seen at angiography.

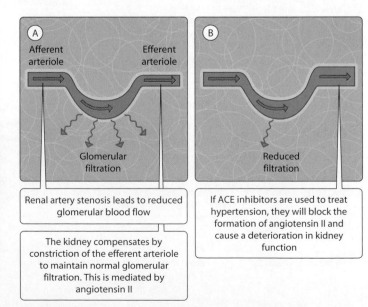

A

Afferent arteriole

Efferent arteriole

Glomerular filtration

Renal artery stenosis leads to reduced glomerular blood flow

The kidney compensates by constriction of the efferent arteriole to maintain normal glomerular filtration. This is mediated by angiotensin II

B

Reduced filtration

If ACE inhibitors are used to treat hypertension, they will block the formation of angiotensin II and cause a deterioration in kidney function

Fig. 3.5.2 Use of ACE inhibitors in renovascular disease.

Table 3.5.1 METABOLIC DEFECTS IN RENAL TUBULAR ACIDOSIS

	Type 1 (distal)	Type 2 (proximal)	Type 4
Basic defect	Distal acidification ↓	Proximal bicarbonate reabsorption ↓	Aldosterone deficiency
Urine pH during acidaemia	> 5.3	< 5.3 (can be variable)	Usually < 5.3
Plasma bicarbonate untreated (mEq/l)	May be < 10	Usually 14–20	Usually > 15
Plasma potassium	Low	Low	Raised
Non-electrolyte complications	Nephrocalcinosis; renal stones	Rickets and osteomalacia	None

subtraction arteriography confirms the location and severity of the stenosis (Fig. 3.5.1).

Management

Patients with atherosclerosis require aggressive management of cardiovascular risk factors (aspirin, statins, smoking cessation). Hypertension should be treated, but may be difficult to control and frequently needs numerous antihypertensive drugs. Percutaneous angioplasty and stent placement should be considered in patients with refractory hypertension, recurrent 'flash' pulmonary oedema or progressive renal failure.

Atheroembolic renal disease is a complication of angioplasty or aortic manipulation but can also occur spontaneously. It is caused by a shower of cholesterol emboli lodging in the kidney and is characterized by an abrupt decline in renal function. Extrarenal emboli may cause digital gangrene, livedo reticularis and eosinophilia. Treatment is supportive.

Renal tubular acidosis

The kidneys play an important role in regulating acid–base balance within the body by excreting hydrogen ions and reabsorbing bicarbonate in response to acidaemia. Renal tubular acidosis (RTA) describes conditions in which this regulatory process fails, resulting in the development of metabolic acidosis. There are three major types of RTA: type 1 (distal), type 2 (proximal) and type 4 (Table 3.5.1).

Epidemiology

Types 1 and 2 RTA can present at any age but are uncommon in adults. Type 4 RTA is rare.

Clinical features

Type 1 RTA presents with failure to thrive in early childhood, or later with symptoms of renal stone disease. Muscle weakness can occur as a result of hypokalaemia. Type 2 presents with polyuria and polydipsia. Bone pain may occur as a result of osteomalacia or rickets. Examination is not usually very helpful although there may be evidence of rickets, muscle weakness or hyperventilation.

Investigations

Patients with RTA have a metabolic acidosis with a normal anion gap. Serum potassium is usually low in types 1 and 2 RTA, but elevated in type 4 RTA.

Type 1 RTA. Inability to excrete an acid load results in urinary pH remaining > 5.5 despite the presence of metabolic acidosis. There may also be evidence of renal stone disease and hypercalciuria.

Type 2 RTA. The filtered bicarbonate load exceeds the limited reabsorptive capacity in the proximal tubules. Diagnosis requries identification of alkaline urine (pH 7.5) after a bicarbonate infusion.

Type 4 RTA. This is characterized by hyperkalaemia and mild metabolic acidosis. Urinary pH is usually appropriately low (< 5.3) in the presence of acidosis.

Management

Type 1 and 2 are treated with potassium replacement and alkali therapy. Type 4 is treated with dietary potassium restriction or fludrocortisone.

6. Inherited kidney disease and secondary kidney dysfunction

Questions
- How does polycystic kidney disease present?
- How does diabetic nephropathy progress?

Inherited kidney diseases

Epidemiology

Adult polycystic kidney disease (APKD) affects 1/1000 of the population (Fig. 3.6.1). Although spontaneous mutations can occur, it is usually autosomal dominant with defects on chromosomes 16 or 4. Approximately 30% of patients also have hepatic cysts, although liver function is rarely compromised. Intracranial berry aneurysms occur in 10–20% of patients and may lead to subarachnoid haemorrhage.

Infantile polycystic kidney disease is much rarer and may cause renal insufficiency in utero, resulting in oligohydramnios and pulmonary hypoplasia. Liver involvement is common and may lead to hepatic failure.

Alport's syndrome is a rare condition comprising hereditary nephritis, progressive renal failure and high-frequency nerve deafness. It mainly affects young males.

Nephronophthisis is a chronic tubulointerstitial nephritis causing impaired concentrating ability and sodium conservation and resulting in polyuria and polydipsia. It presents in childhood and leads to progressive renal failure.

Medullary cystic disease is a variant of nephronophthisis, presenting with nephrogenic diabetes insipidus in young adults.

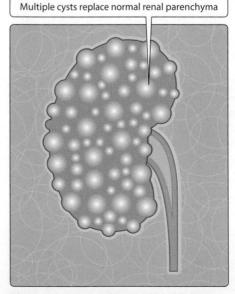

Multiple cysts replace normal renal parenchyma

Fig. 3.6.1 Adult polycystic kidney disease.

Clinical features

APKD is frequently diagnosed through screening in affected families. Patients may have loin pain, haematuria from bleeding into a cyst or symptoms of progressive renal failure.

Infantile polycystic kidney disease may be detected during antenatal screening. In the neonatal period, there may be symptoms of liver and renal failure, or respiratory distress as a result of pulmonary hypoplasia. Occasionally the condition does not present until later in childhood, when abdominal masses and hypertension are detected.

Nephronophthisis presents with polyuria, polydipsia, growth retardation and progressive renal failure. Extrarenal manifestations include retinitis pigmentosa, cerebellar ataxia and liver fibrosis.

Investigations

APKD is diagnosed by the identification of multiple renal cysts on ultrasound, although cysts may not be detectable until about 20 years of age. Ultrasound will also identify liver and renal cysts in infantile polycystic kidney disease.

In Alport's syndrome, patients have haematuria on urinalysis. Renal biopsy confirms the diagnosis.

Renal biopsy is usually not necessary in nephronophthisis, since the diagnosis can be made from polyuria, normal urinalysis and normal ultrasound in a patient with extrarenal manifestations and positive family history.

Management

Management is based on control of hypertension and treatment of renal failure.

Diseases having secondary kidney dysfunction

Diabetes mellitus

Diabetes mellitus is the commonest cause of end-stage renal failure in Western society. Diabetic nephropathy typically develops 10–15 years following the diagnosis of diabetes; the incidence being highest in patients with poor glycaemic control and microalbuminuria. Renal biopsy shows glomerular basement membrane thickening and nodular glomerulosclerosis (Kimmelstiel–Wilson lesions). Microalbuminuria is followed by overt proteinuria and a fall in glomerular filtration rate (GFR; Fig. 3.6.2). Diabetic nephropathy is managed with ACE inhibitors or angiotensin II receptor blockers to control hypertension and limit proteinuria. Tight glycaemic control slows disease progression.

Systemic vasculitis

Systemic vasculitides are multisystem disorders caused by inflammation of blood vessels (Table 3.6.1). Glomerulonephritis often occurs in Wegener's granulomatosis, polyarteritis nodosa or Churg–Strauss syndrome. Renal involvement may result in crescentic glomerulonephritis. Wegener's granulomatosis is also characterized by necrotizing granulomatous lesions in the upper airway and lungs. It is usually treated with immunosuppression (steroids, cyclophosphamide) and sometimes plasma exchange.

Connective tissue disorders

Systemic lupus erythematosus most commonly affects females aged 20–30 years and can be associated with any type of glomerulonephritis. It usually responds to oral immunosuppression.

Amyloidosis

Amyloidosis may occur in association with myeloma or secondary to chronic inflammation or infection (e.g. rheumatoid arthritis, bronchiectasis). It is caused by the production of an abnormal degradation-resistant protein (amyloid), which can be deposited in the kidneys, heart, liver, spleen, and throughout the body. Management involves chemotherapy as well as treatment of any underlying condition.

Myeloma

Myeloma mainly affects those > 70 years of age. It can cause renal failure through cast nephropathy, light chain deposition, hypercalcaemia or amyloidosis. Myeloma is treated with chemotherapy or bone marrow transplantation and bisphosphonates are used to correct hypercalcaemia.

Haemolytic uraemic syndrome

Haemolytic uraemic syndrome (HUS) is the commonest cause of acute renal failure in children. It typically develops after enteric infection with the 0157H strain of *Escherichia coli*, although it may also occur after *Shigella dysenteriae* infection and certain drugs. HUS is characterized by a triad of microangiopathic haemolytic anaemia, thrombocytopenia and acute renal failure. There is usually a history of bloody diarrhoea or purpuric rash. Thrombotic thrombocytopenic purpura (TTP) is a variant in which neurological symptoms dominate. HUS may resolve with supportive management or require plasma exchange.

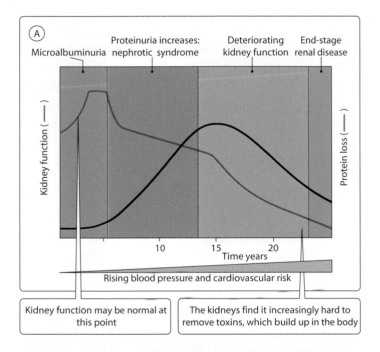

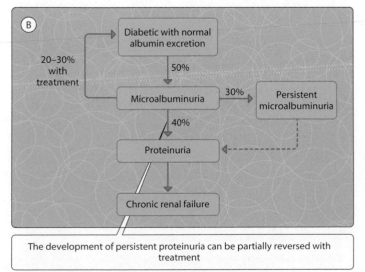

Fig. 3.6.2 Progression of diabetic nephropathy. A, loss of kidney function (GFR); B, proportion of diabetic patients affected.

Table 3.6.1 SYSTEMIC VASCULITIS ACCORDING TO BLOOD VESSEL SIZE

Vessel	ANCA positive	ANCA negative
Small	Wegener's granulomatosis	Goodpasture's syndrome
	Microscopic polyangiitis	Henoch–Schönlein purpura
		Cryoglobulinaemia
Medium	Churg–Strauss syndrome	Polyarteritis nodosa
		Kawasaki disease
Large		Giant cell arteritis
		Takayasu arteritis

ANCA, anti-neutrophil cytoplasmic antibodies.

7. Urinary tract infection and stones

Questions
- What are the common organisms that cause urinary infection?
- What predisposing factors cause urinary stones?

Urinary tract infection

Urinary tract infection (UTI) is more common in females than males. Most episodes are short lived and uncomplicated, but ascending infection can lead to acute pyelonephritis. Recurrent infections in childhood can lead to long-term kidney damage. Table 3.7.1 gives the common infecting organisms.

Epidemiology

About 50% of women experience at least one UTI during their lifetime. The incidence increases during pregnancy, when 2–6% will have asymptomatic bacteriuria.

Pathogenesis

Most urinary tract infections result from organisms entering the urinary tract via the urethra and ascending to the bladder (causing cystitis) or kidneys (causing pyelonephritis).

Vesicoureteric reflux occurs in children and results from incompetence of the valve mechanism that prevents urine refluxing into the ureters during bladder contraction (Fig. 3.7.1). It can lead to chronic pyelonephritis, renal scarring and, eventually, end-stage renal failure from reflux nephropathy.

Clinical features

Symptoms include urinary frequency, urgency, suprapubic discomfort, pain on micturition (dysuria) and frank haematuria. If pyelonephritis develops, there may be renal angle pain, fever and rigors. Uncomplicated UTIs can be asymptomatic. In children or older adults, there may be few localizing symptoms, and the patient may present unwell with fever, malaise, vomiting or meningism.

Investigations

Urinalysis may be positive for leukocytes (pyuria), nitrite, blood or protein. Presence of leukocytes without bacteriuria is termed sterile pyuria and may occur in papillary necrosis, interstitial cystitis, bladder tumour, tuberculosis, stones or partially treated UTI.

Bacteriuria is considered significant if a mid-stream specimen contains more than 10^5 colony-forming units (CFU) of the same organism per millilitre. Recurrent UTI in women or children (or any UTI in males) requires investigation for a predisposing cause.

In reflux nephropathy, intravenous urography may show irregular renal outlines and clubbed calyces, and a micturating cystogram will demonstrate vesicoureteric reflux of contrast. Cystoscopy may be required to investigate cystitis in the absence of bacteriuria, or if there is frank haematuria in an older patient (to exclude malignancy). Urodynamic studies assess bladder emptying and urethral flow.

Management

Patients should maintain a high fluid intake. Uncomplicated UTI usually resolves spontaneously or responds to oral antibiotics. Asymptomatic bacteriuria in pregnant women should always

Table 3.7.1 ORGANISMS CAUSING URINARY TRACT INFECTION

Organism	Frequency (%)
Esherichia coli and coliforms	68
Proteus mirabilis	12
Klebsiella aerogenes	4
Enterococcus faecalis	6
Staphylococcus saprophyticus, *S. epidermidis*	10

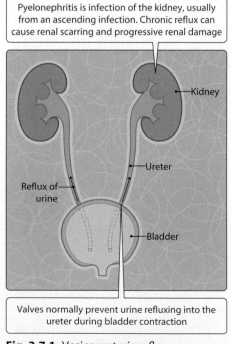

Pyelonephritis is infection of the kidney, usually from an ascending infection. Chronic reflux can cause renal scarring and progressive renal damage

Kidney

Ureter

Reflux of urine

Bladder

Valves normally prevent urine refluxing into the ureter during bladder contraction

Fig. 3.7.1 Vesicoureteric reflux.

be treated since there is a risk of progression to pyelonephritis. In contrast, asymptomatic bacteruria in a patient with a urinary catheter does not usually require treatment. Pyelonephritis requires i.v. antibiotics. Urine should be recultured 5–7 days after completion of antibiotics to ensure that infection has resolved. Strategies to prevent recurrent UTI include double-voiding of urine and voiding after sexual intercourse. Low-dose prophylactic antibiotics may be helpful.

Urinary stones

Nephrolithiasis describes formation of stones within the urinary tract. Most stones (80%) are composed of calcium (usually oxalate or phosphate). The remainder consist of urate, cystine or struvite (magnesium ammonium phosphate).

Epidemiology

Nephrolithiasis is common. Approximately 12% of people have a renal stone in their lifetime, with the peak incidence being between ages 20 and 50 years. Males are more commonly affected than females (3:1), with the exception of struvite stones (staghorn calculi), which are associated with urinary tract infections and have a female preponderance. Recurrence of stones is common. Predisposing factors for kidney stones include:

- environmental and dietary: high temperature; low fluid intake and low urine volume; high-protein, high-sodium, low-calcium diet
- urine excretion: high sodium, oxalate or urate; low citrate
- acquired causes: hypercalcaemia of any cause; ileal disease or resection
- inherited causes: cystinuria, medullary sponge kidney, renal tubular acidosis type 1.

Pathogenesis

Stones develop when the urine becomes supersaturated with a stone-forming substance (e.g. calcium, urate or oxalate). Crystals develop and aggregate to form stones. Increased urinary excretion of calcium, urate or oxalate, or reduced excretion of citrate (an inhibitor of stone formation) increases the risk of nephrolithiasis. Stones may remain within the kidney or pass into the ureter and move distally.

Clinical features

Renal stones may be asymptomatic, especially if they remain within the kidney. Stones that pass into the ureter typically give severe colicky loin pain which often radiates to the groin, and associated nausea and vomiting. Patients typically cannot lie still and usually require strong analgesia. Stones within the bladder or urethra may cause haematuria, frequency and pain on micturition.

Investigations

Urine pH should be measured and urinalysis shows microscopic haematuria. Urate stones form in acidic urine, while alkaline conditions favour formation of struvite stones. Analysis of a passed stone and measurement of 24 h urinary excretion of calcium, urate, cystine and oxalate may be useful. Serum urate and calcium should also be measured. As 80% of stones are radioopaque, they can be identified on an abdominal radiograph. CT or MRI scan may be needed to identify non-radioopaque stones. An intravenous pyelogram may identify filling defects within the urinary tract.

Management

High fluid intake should be encouraged and parenteral opioids may be required for pain. If stones do not pass spontaneously, they may need to be fragmented using lithotripsy, or removed endoscopically (Fig. 3.7.2).

Calcium stones. A low-sodium diet will reduce calcium excretion in the proximal tubules (via the sodium/calcium cotransporter). Drug treatment depends on the metabolic abnormality that is identified:

- hypercalciuria: thiazide diuretics; alkalinization of the urine, using potassium citrate or bicarbonate, may also be effective
- hyperoxaluria: colestyramine or calcium carbonate are used to bind oxalate in the gut and reduce absorption
- hypocitraturia: alkalinization enhances citrate excretion.

Urate stones. Treatment is with alkalinization of the urine and allopurinol (xanthine oxidase inhibitor).

Cystine stones. Treatment is with alkalinization of the urine. Penicillamine, captopril or tiopronin can also be tried.

Struvite stones. Often require surgical intervention.

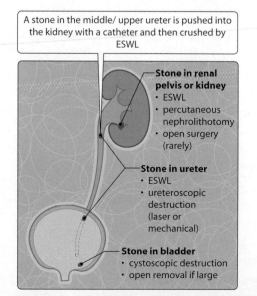

A stone in the middle/ upper ureter is pushed into the kidney with a catheter and then crushed by ESWL

Stone in renal pelvis or kidney
- ESWL
- percutaneous nephrolithotomy
- open surgery (rarely)

Stone in ureter
- ESWL
- ureteroscopic destruction (laser or mechanical)

Stone in bladder
- cystoscopic destruction
- open removal if large

Fig. 3.7.2 Surgical options for urinary stones. ESWL, extracorporeal shock wave lithotrophy.

8. Urinary tract obstruction and tumours

Questions
- What are the causes of urinary tract obstruction?
- How common are urinary tract tumours?

Urinary tract obstruction

Obstruction of the urinary tract can occur anywhere from the renal calyces to the urethral meatus and can be:

- within the lumen: stone, blood clot, sloughed papilla, tumour of renal pelvis or ureter, bladder tumour
- within the tract wall: pelviureteric neuromuscular dysfunction, ureteric or urethral stricture, congenital megaureter, neuropathic bladder
- pressure from outside: prostatic obstruction, phimosis, retroperitoneal fibrosis, aberrant vessels/bands across ureter, tumours (e.g. colon or cervical cancer).

Urinary tract obstruction must be excluded in unexplained kidney failure. Anatomical abnormalities are the commonest cause in childhood, while prostatic enlargement and malignancy within the pelvis or retroperitoneum predominate in older patients. Obstruction is often reversible if identified early.

Epidemiology

Urinary tract obstruction occurs most often in the very young and old. It is frequently seen in men >60 years with prostatic enlargement.

Pathogenesis

Obstruction of the urinary tract at any level can result in increased hydrostatic pressure, which is transmitted back to the renal tubules. The increased tubular pressure leads to a fall in the glomerular filtration rate and, if the obstruction is prolonged, reduction in renal blood flow and loss of nephrons.

Clinical features

Clinical features depend on the site, degree and speed of onset of obstruction (Fig. 3.8.1). Total anuria is suggestive of complete bilateral obstruction (or complete obstruction of a single functioning kidney). Normal urine output does not exclude partial obstruction, and polyuria can occur as a result of impaired concentrating ability in renal tubules. If obstruction develops over a long period of time, it can be asymptomatic. Rectal examination in males may reveal an enlarged or abnormal prostate gland.

Investigations

Ultrasound of the renal tract can usually identify the level of the obstruction. It cannot distinguish between an obstructed urinary system and a low-pressure chronically dilated system, for example an ileal conduit or after previous long-standing obstruction. Radionuclide renogram may show delayed drainage of isotope if functional obstruction is present.

Management

Rapid relief of the obstruction is important because the probability of recovering renal function diminishes with time. Insertion of a urethral or suprapubic catheter may be sufficient in lower urinary tract obstruction. More proximal obstruction requires external drainage of urine via a nephrostomy. Relief of obstruction may be followed by a large diuresis, resulting in loss of sodium and water, necessitating fluid and electrolyte replacement. Subsequent management depends on the underlying cause; surgery is often required, but retroperitoneal fibrosis may respond to medical management alone.

Urinary tract tumours

Tumours of the urinary tract arise within the kidney or the urothelium lining the renal pelvis, ureters and bladder (Fig. 3.8.2). Renal cell cancer (RCC) is the commonest renal tumour

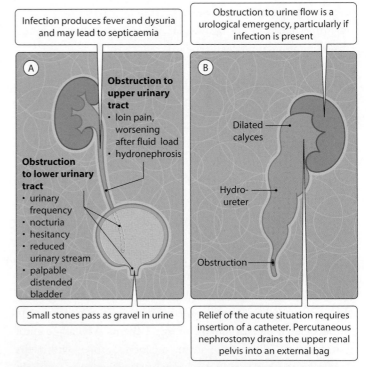

Fig. 3.8.1 Urinary tract obstruction. A, Symptoms depend on level of obstruction; B, hydronephrotic kidney.

in adults (85%), while Wilm's tumour (nephroblastoma) is most frequent in children. Tumours of the urothelium are usually transitional cell cancer (TCC) and the bladder is the usual site.

Epidemiology

Approximately 2–3% of malignant tumours in adults occur in the kidney. RCC is twice as common in males as females, and the peak incidence is 50–70 years. Wilm's tumour accounts for 6% of childhood cancers. TCC has a male preponderance of 4:1, and the incidence increases with age.

Pathogenesis

RCC arises from tubular epithelium as large cells with clear cytoplasm; it may be solitary or multiple. It spreads locally into the renal vein and surrounding tissues, or distally to bone, liver and lungs (cannon-ball metastases). TCC arises from the epithelium of the urinary tract; 90% occur in the bladder. Spread is locally within the pelvis or distally to liver and lungs.

Clinical features

RCC presents with frank haematuria (Fig. 3.8.3), loin pain or an abdominal mass. Other symptoms include pyrexia, malaise and weight loss. Invasion of the left renal vein can lead to left-sided varicocele.

TCC typically presents as painless haematuria, though pain may occur if there is clot retention. Bladder irritation can result in symptoms of urinary tract infection in the absence of positive cultures.

Wilm's tumour usually presents as an enlarging abdominal mass in an infant. Haematuria is uncommon.

Investigations

FBC may show secondary polycythaemia (caused by abnormal production of erythropoietin). Urinalysis may show haematuria and urine cytology can identify malignant cells.

RCC is often detected by ultrasonography. TCC is often detected by an intravenous pyelogram, which identifies filling defects or obstruction within the urinary tract.

Cystoscopy or ureteroscopy is required for biopsy.

Hypercalcaemia may be present if bony metastases are present.

Management

Renal cell cancer. Radical or partial nephrectomy is the treatment of choice for localized disease. Metastatic disease may respond to alpha interferon or hormonal therapy (progesterone). The overall 5-year survival is 40–45%.

Wilm's tumour. Combined use of surgery, radiotherapy and chemotherapy results in a 5-year survival of almost 90%.

Transitional cell cancer. Tumours of the renal pelvis and ureters are treated by nephroureterectomy. Bladder lesions are treated with cystodiathermy, transurethral resection or cystectomy, depending on the stage. Systemic or local (intravesical) chemotherapy may be used as an adjuvant to surgery. Immunotherapy with local instillation of BCG vaccine to stimulate the immune system to attack malignant cells is sometimes used. Since bladder cancer has a high rate of recurrence, surveillance cystoscopies should be performed. The 5-year survival for bladder cancer is about 85% if the disease is superficial but 5% if there is metastatic disease at diagnosis.

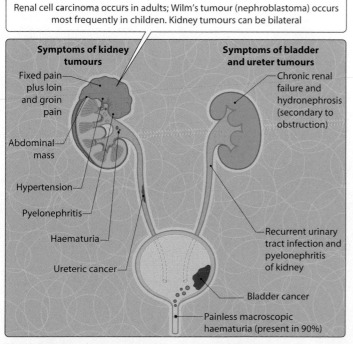

Fig. 3.8.2 Renal tract tumours and clinical features.

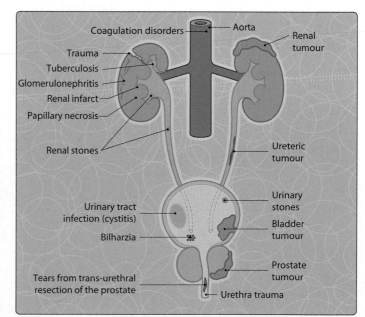

Fig. 3.8.3 Sites and other causes of haematuria.

PART VII

Electrolyte disturbance and poisoning

Graeme Currie and Graham Douglas

The big picture

Normally the volume and composition of both the extracellular and intracellular fluid compartments within the body remain remarkably constant. In health, total body water makes up 50–60% of lean body weight in men and 45–50% in women. In a normal 75 kg man, total body water is approximately 42 litres of which:

- 28 litres (67%) is intracellular fluid
- 9.4 litres (22%) is interstitial fluid bathing the cells
- 4.6 litres (9%) is plasma.

Small amounts of water are also contained in bone, dense connective tissue and secretions, for example within the GI tract and in CSF.

Intracellular and extracellular (interstitial) fluids are separated by cell membranes while interstitial fluid and plasma are separated by the capillary wall (Fig. 1.1). Osmotic pressure is the main determinant of the distribution of water among the three major compartments. The concentrations of major electrolytes in these fluids differ and each compartment has a constituent that is primary to that compartment and, therefore, determines its osmotic pressure:

- potassium salts in the intracellular fluid
- sodium salts in the interstitial fluid
- protein in plasma.

The capillary wall is relatively impermeable to plasma proteins, and cell membranes are impermeable to sodium and potassium ions because the sodium/potassium ATPase pump restricts sodium to extracellular fluid and potassium to intracellular fluid. Sodium stores are the main determinant of extracellular fluid volume. Therefore 1 litre of water given i.v. as 5% dextrose is distributed equally into all compartments whereas the same amount of 0.9% saline remains largely in the extracellular compartment. Intravenous colloid protein increases the oncotic pressure in the vascular compartment and is the treatment of choice for hypovolaemia.

Plasma osmolality

Antidiuretic hormone (ADH) plays a central role in water excretion (Fig. 1.2). At a plasma osmolality of < 275 mOsm/kg, which represents a plasma sodium concentration of < 136 mmol/l, there is no circulating ADH. As plasma osmolality rises above this threshold, secretion of ADH and, therefore, water excretion increases progressively. Ingestion of a water load leads to reduction in plasma osmolality and diminished release of ADH. Water

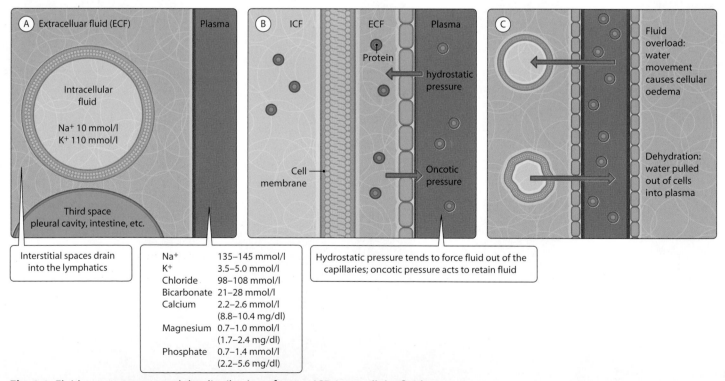

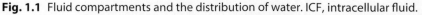

Fig. 1.1 Fluid compartments and the distribution of water. ICF, intracellular fluid.

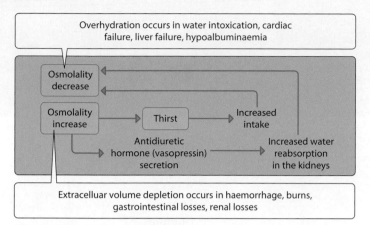

Fig. 1.2 Regulation of water balance.

reabsorption in the renal collecting ducts allows excess water to be excreted in dilute urine. In contrast, water lost through sweating and diarrhoea causes a rise in both plasma osmolality and ADH secretion, enhanced water reabsorption and excretion of a smaller volume of more concentrated urine.

Oedema

Peripheral oedema is caused by expansion of extracellular volume by at least 2 litres (15%). The ankles are usually swollen but in bed-bound patients, oedema may accumulate in the sacral area. Extracellular volume expansion is caused by sodium retention, which occurs in numerous disease states.

Heart failure. Reduction in cardiac output and, therefore, circulating volume and arterial filling leads to activation of the renin–angiotensin–aldosterone system, with release of ADH and increased activity of renal sympathetic nerves. This results in increased peripheral and renal arteriolar resistance and water and sodium retention, causing oedema.

Liver cirrhosis. Peripheral vasodilatation, possibly caused by nitric oxide release, results in reduced effective arterial filling. This leads to effects similar to heart failure. In addition, reduced hepatic synthetic function causes hypoalbuminaemia.

Nephrotic syndrome. Hypoalbuminaemia is a result of heavy proteinuria. Despite this, oncotic pressure remains unchanged and the increase in interstitial fluid results from accumulation of sodium in the extracellular compartment. In addition, reduction in effective circulating volume and fall in cardiac output and arterial filling lead to effects similar to those in heart failure and liver cirrhosis.

Sodium retention. Renal disease with reduced glomerular filtration rate (GFR) decreases the ability of the kidney to excrete sodium. This can occur in acute end-stage renal failure. Numerous drugs also cause renal sodium retention particularly:

- oestrogens: have a weak aldosterone-like effect, the cause of weight gain in the premenstrual phase
- mineralocorticoids and liquorice: aldosterone-like actions
- NSAIDs: cause sodium retention in the presence of activation of the renin–angiotensin–aldosterone system.

Other causes of oedema:

- transient oedema may occur after starting insulin for type 1 diabetes and refeeding after malnutrition
- calcium channel blockers (e.g. nifedipine) can relax precapillary arterioles
- increase in capillary permeability to proteins, for example in ovarian hyperstimulation and in use of interleukin-2 in cancer chemotherapy.

Decreased extracellular volume

Deficiency of sodium and water causes shrinkage of both the interstitial space and the blood volume (hypovolaemia). Salt and water may be lost from the kidneys, GI tract or from the skin. Common causes include:

- **septicaemia**, causing vasodilatation of both arterioles and veins leading to a fall initially in diastolic blood pressure; increased capillary permeability to plasma protein also leads to loss of fluid from the plasma to the interstitium
- **diuretics** used in heart failure may lead to rapid reduction in plasma volume
- **haemorrhage**, either external, as in haematemesis or melaena, or concealed as in leaking aortic aneurysm
- **other GI losses** in either severe vomiting or prolonged diarrhoea or as concealed fluid loss (e.g. in ileus).

Symptoms are variable and include thirst, muscle cramps, nausea and vomiting, and postural dizziness. Severe depletion of circulating volume causes hypotension and impairs cerebral perfusion, causing confusion and eventually coma. Loss of interstitial fluid leads to loss of skin elasticity (turgor), which can be tested by pinching skin over the anterior triangle of the neck or on the forehead. One of the earliest and most reliable signs of volume depletion is postural hypotension, with a > 20 mmHg systolic fall in blood pressure as the subject stands up.

High-return facts

1 **Sodium** is the major extracellular cation and has an essential role in fluid and electrolyte balance and in the generation of action potentials. Hyponatraemia is commonly caused by diuretics or extracellular fluid overload. Symptoms of hyponatraemia include headache, confusion, seizures and coma. Serum sodium should be corrected slowly to avoid permanent neurological damage. Hypernatraemia is less common and usually caused by excess water loss or excess sodium intake. **SIADH**, the syndrome of inappropriate ADH secretion, can be caused by both malignant and non-malignant disorders. **Potassium** is the most abundant intracellular cation and has a role in membrane potentials in nervous and muscle tissue. Hyperkalaemia is caused by increased release from cells or decreased excretion. Severe hyperkalaemia, with muscle weakness and cardiac arrythmias, is a medical emergency and treatment consists of i.v. insulin in 50% dextrose and i.v. calcium chloride or gluconate. Dialysis may be required in life-threatening or severe refractory cases. Hypokalaemia usually results from decreased oral intake, increased cellular uptake or increased loss (e.g. diuretics). Serum potassium < 2.5 mmol/l can cause muscle weakness, muscle cramps, paraesthesia and cardiac arrhythmias. Treatment is with oral or i.v. potassium replacement.

2 Serum **calcium** measurements are affected by serum albumin concentration and should be 'corrected' if albumin is abnormal. Common causes of hypercalcaemia are malignancy (with or without bony metastases) and primary hyperparathyroidism. Clinical features include anxiety, depression, lethargy, abdominal pain, constipation, bone pain, renal stones, cardiac arrhythmias, confusion and coma. Hypocalcaemia may result from disrupted homeostasis, small bowel malabsorption, hypoparathyroidism or high phosphate levels. Symptoms result from neuromuscular irritability. In symptomatic severe hypocalcaemia, i.v. calcium gluconate should be given. **Phosphate** has a crucial role in nucleic acids, signalling molecules and energy and bone metabolism. Hypophosphataemia causes weakness,

encephalopathy, seizures, respiratory depression and heart failure. Hyperphosphataemia usually occurs in chronic renal failure. Low serum **magnesium** is more common than hypermagnesaemia. It is usually asymptomatic but should be suspected in patients with chronic diarrhoea, chronic alcohol abuse, hypocalcaemia, hypokalaemia or arrythmias.

3 **Acid–base balance** aims to maintain arterial pH in the range 7.38–7.42. This tight regulation is achieved by various buffers, most notably the carbonic acid/bicarbonate buffer. There are four major acid–base disorders. Respiratory acidosis is caused by alveolar hypoventilation, leading to an increase in Pco_2. Chronic elevation of Pco_2 leads to renal retention of bicarbonate and normalization of pH, 'compensated respiratory acidosis'. Respiratory alkalosis is caused by hyperventilation, thus reducing Pco_2. This may occur after a brainstem stroke, in acute asthma, in severe pulmonary thromboembolism and with acute panic attacks. Metabolic acidosis is caused by loss of bicarbonate and is found in acute renal failure, diabetic ketoacidosis and disorders causing lactic acidosis, including septic shock and cardiac arrest. Metabolic alkalosis is caused by loss of hydrogen ions through vomiting or nasogastric suction, or retention of bicarbonate as in excess diuretic therapy.

4 Effects of **benzodiazepine** overdose can be severe in the elderly and patients with liver impairment. Symptoms include drowsiness, slurred speech, ataxia and mild hypotension. Alcohol or other sedatives/hypnotics can accentuate the problem, leading to coma, respiratory depression and cardiovascular collapse. Flumazenil, a benzodiazepine antagonist, can be given to reverse the effects of benzodiazepine. Acute **alcohol** intoxication can lead to ataxia, stupor and coma. In severe intoxication, hospital observation with airway maintenance, i.v. fluids, vitamin replacement and dextrose may be required. **Paracetamol** overdose causes liver damage, which can be more severe in those with alcohol excess or poor nutrition. Hepatic necrosis, encephalopathy, acute renal failure and lactic acidosis are features of severe overdose. The specific antidote to paracetamol is i.v. *N*-acetylcysteine or, less commonly, oral methionine.

5 **Aspirin** (acetylsalicylic acid) overdose causes tachypnoea, sweating, epigastric pain and vomiting, tinnitus, blurred vision, agitation, seizures and coma. Gastric lavage with activated charcoal can be beneficial within 1–2 h of the overdose. Features of severe **opioid** overdose include pinpoint pupils, respiratory depression, hypotension, coma and rarely adult respiratory distress syndrome. Naloxone, a pure opioid antagonist, can be administered in i.v. boluses until a response occurs. Overdose with **tricyclic antidepressants** causes dry mouth, blurred vision, urinary retention, confusion, drowsiness and sinus tachycardia.

Severe poisoning can result in seizures, metabolic acidosis, cardiac arrhythmias, respiratory depression and coma. Both **methanol** and **ethylene glycol** (both in antifreeze) cause metabolic acidosis with clinical features similar to ethanol poisoning. Treatment involves i.v. ethanol and possibly haemodialysis. **Organophosphate** poisoning causes anxiety, headache, diarrhoea, vomiting, muscle weakness, sweating, rhinorrhoea, twitching and bronchospasm. Severe toxicity results in cardiac arrhythmias, pulmonary oedema, respiratory failure, coma and death. **Carbon monoxide** poisoning causes tissue hypoxia, with headache, malaise, confusion, irritability, convulsions and coma. Oxygen saturation is often normal as most blood gas machines cannot differentiate oxyhaemoglobin from carboxyhaemoglobin. Management is with high-flow O_2, occasionally hyperbaric O_2.

1. Sodium and potassium

Questions
- What are the main causes of hyponatraemia?
- How do you diagnose and manage SIADH?
- What are the causes and management of hypokalaemia?
- What are the causes and management of hyperkalaemia?

■ SODIUM

Hyponatraemia

Hyponatraemia (sodium <135 mmol/l) is frequently found in individuals taking diuretics or with extracellular fluid overload states (e.g. heart failure) (Fig. 3.1.1 and Table 3.1.1). Spuriously low sodium (pseudohyponatraemia) can also occur with hyperlipidaemia or hyperglycaemia.

Clinical features

Low plasma sodium can produce lethargy and nausea; neurological impairment, such as headache, confusion, seizures and coma, occurs if it falls to <120 mmol/l. It may be asymptomatic if long standing. Patients should be assessed for dehydration or fluid overloaded.

Investigations

U&Es, plasma and urine osmolality and urinary sodium concentration should be measured.

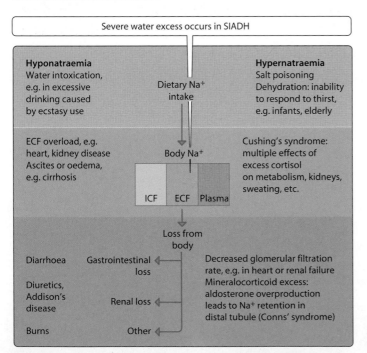

Fig. 3.1.1 Sodium in the body. ECF, extracellular fluid; ICF, intracellular fluid; SIADH, syndrome of inappropriate antidiuretic hormone secretion.

Management

Serum sodium should be increased by 10–12 mmol/l per day at most as too rapid a correction can lead to permanent neurological damage (central pontine myelinolysis). Treatment is either by water restriction (in hypervolaemic hyponatraemia) or sodium and water replacement (in hypovolaemic hyponatraemia). Only in the presence of severe neurological disturbance (e.g. coma or prolonged seizures) should hypertonic (3%) saline be given.

Syndrome of inappropriate antidiuretic hormone secretion

The syndrome of inappropriate antidiuretic hormone (ADH) secretion (SIADH) (Table 3.1.2) is diagnosed in a normovolaemic patient when serum sodium is <130 mmol/l, serum osmolality <275 mosmol/kg, urine sodium >20 mmol/l and urine osmolality exceeds plasma osmolality in the absence of diuretic use, renal dysfunction, hypothyroidism and adrenal insufficiency. Patients should be restricted to 1–1.5 l/day of fluid. Demeclocycline, which reduces the responsiveness of the collecting tubule to ADH, can be useful in refractory cases.

Hypernatraemia

Hypernatraemia (sodium >142 mmol/l) is less common since a rise in plasma osmolality triggers ADH release and thirst. It is usually caused by excess water loss (more common) or excess sodium intake (less common and usually iatrogenic). A long history of thirst and polyuria may indicate diabetes insipidus. Some drugs, including lithium, amphotericin and tetracycline, can cause nephrogenic diabetes insipidus.

Clinical features

Clinical features are non-specific and include nausea, vomiting, lethargy, irritability, confusion, seizures and coma. It is important to assess the fluid volume status, for example skin turgor, and identify pulmonary oedema, peripheral oedema and abnormal jugular venous pressure.

Table 3.1.1 CAUSES OF HYPONATRAEMIA

Hydration state	Causes
Hypovolaemic	Kidney or gastrointestinal loss; diuretics
Normovolaemic	SIADH, adrenal insufficiency hypothyroidism
Hypervolaemic	Heart, liver or kidney failure; primary polydipsia

SIADH, syndrome of inappropriate antidiuretic hormone secretion.

Table 3.1.2 CAUSES OF THE SYNDROME OF INAPPROPRIATE ANTIDIURETIC HORMONE SECRETION (SIADH)

	Examples
Neurological disorders	Head trauma, stroke, subarachnoid haemorrhage, meningitis/encephalitis, Guillain–Barré syndrome, cerebral vasculitis
Malignancy	Small cell lung cancer, pancreatic cancer, lymphoma
Pulmonary disease	Pneumonia, tuberculosis
Drugs	Antipsychotic drugs (e.g. thioridazine, haloperidol, amitryptyline), chlorpropramide, opioids

Management

In diabetes insipidus, desmopressin (an analogue of ADH) should be administered. Hypernatraemia should usually be corrected slowly (over 48 h) at a rate of approximately 10 mmol/l per day to avoid cerebral oedema. In hypovolaemia or normovolaemia, water is given orally, but i.v. 5% dextrose or 0.9% or 0.45% saline can be given where oral intake is difficult. In hypervolaemic hypernatraemic patients, any sodium-containing fluid should be discontinued.

■ POTASSIUM

Hypokalaemia

Hypokalaemia (potassium < 3.5 mmol/l) is common and caused by decreased oral intake, increased cellular uptake or increased loss. Decreased oral intake is rare and is compensated for by the normal kidney, which reduces potassium excretion. Increased cellular uptake can occur in alkalosis, insulin administration, theophylline and β_2-agonist use and in hypothermia. Increased losses can occur in GI (diarrhoea, vomiting, laxative abuse) and urinary (diuretics, primary hyperaldosteronism) tract disturbances, in magnesium depletion, in excessive sweating, or during dialysis and plasmapheresis.

Clinical features

Symptoms are not usually apparent unless plasma concentrations fall to < 2.5 mmol/l. Below this, muscle weakness, muscle cramps, paraesthesia and cardiac arrhythmias occur. (Fig. 3.1.2).

Management

Treatment is with oral or i.v. potassium (≤ 20 mmol/h) replacement. A potassium-sparing diuretic (e.g. spironolactone or amiloride) can be substituted if diuretics are thought to be responsible. Hypomagnesaemia frequently coexists.

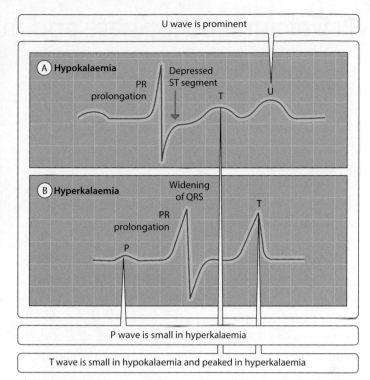

Fig. 3.1.2 ECG features of deranged potassium levels: A, hypokalaemia; B, hyperkalaemia.

Hyperkalaemia

Hyperkalaemia (potassium > 5 mmol/l) is usually caused by increased cell release or decreased excretion.

Clinical features

Clinical features occur at high levels (> 6.5 mmol/l) and relate to muscular weakness and cardiac arrhythmias (Fig. 3.1.2). Serum potassium should be measured in all patients with renal failure and cardiac rhythm abnormalities.

Management

Treatment varies depending upon onset, severity, cause and whether or not ECG changes are present. If plasma potassium is > 6.5 mmol/l, urgent treatment is required:

- stop any supplements or medication (e.g. ACE inhibitors, spironolactone) that may be contributing
- give 10 ml i.v. 10% calcium chloride or gluconate to stabilize the myocardium even if no ECG changes
- soluble insulin (10 units) in 50 ml 50% dextrose over 30 min will reduce serum levels for several hours
- calcium-exchange resins (Resonium) can be given orally in less urgent situations
- dialysis may be required in life-threatening or severe refractory cases.

2. Calcium, phosphate and magnesium

Questions
- What are the causes and management of hypercalcaemia?
- What are the causes of hypomagnesaemia?

■ CALCIUM

More than 90% of the calcium in the body is in bone, where it is combined with phosphate. Calcium also plays a major role in signal-transduction mechanisms regulating cellular activities; consequently, calcium in extracellular fluid and plasma must be controlled precisely (Fig. 3.2.1). Calcium exists in the body as the physiologically important ionized form (50%), a protein-bound form (40%) and a smaller proportion associated with anions (10%). Serum albumin concentration can, therefore, alter the total measured calcium and should be measured; values are subsequently 'corrected' for an abnormally high or low albumin.

Hypercalcaemia

Common causes of hypercalcaemia are malignancy with or without bony metastases (lymphoma, myeloma, breast, lung, thyroid, prostate, kidney) and primary hyperparathyroidism. Other causes are

- tertiary hyperparathyroidism caused by small bowel malabsorption or chronic renal disease
- hyperthyroidism
- drugs (e.g. thiazide diuretics, lithium)
- Paget's disease when immobilized
- sarcoidosis
- Addison's disease
- milk–alkali syndrome
- familial hypocalciuric hypercalcaemia.

Clinical features

Hypercalcaemia can be asymptomatic or present with anxiety, depression, lethargy, abdominal pain, constipation, bony pain, renal stones, hypertension, cardiac arrhythmias, confusion and coma.

Investigations

Investigations may include renal function, measurements of serum parathormone, plasma electrophoresis, urinalysis for Bence–Jones protein, chest radiograph and isotope bone scan.

Management

In malignancy, treatment involves fluid administration, usually with 0.9% saline. If this fails to reduce levels to normal, a bisphosphonate (e.g. pamidronate), which inhibits osteoclast activity, should be given. In refractory cases where malignancy is responsible, oral steroids may be helpful. Surgery is often necessary in patients with primary hyperparathyroidism.

Hypocalcaemia

Hypocalcaemia is less common than hypercalcaemia and may result from disrupted homeostasis, small bowel malabsorption, parathormone insensitivity or high phosphate levels. Causes include:

- hyperphosphataemia: renal failure, phosphate treatment, tumour lysis
- vitamin D deficiency: osteomalacia, rickets, vitamin D resistance
- malabsorption: cystic fibrosis, coeliac disease
- iatrogenic hypoparathyroidism following thyroid or parathyroid surgery
- congenital deficiency: Di George syndrome
- parathyroid resistance (pseudohypoparathyroidism)
- hypomagnesaemia
- hypoparathyroidism
- pancreatitis.

Clinical features

Symptoms result from neuromuscular irritability and include perioral paraesthesia, hyperreflexia, carpopedal spasm, tetany, seizures and prolonged QT interval on ECG. Specific clinical signs are Chvostek's sign (tapping of the facial nerve over the zygomatic arch causes twitching of the facial muscles) and Trousseau's sign (carpopedal spasm when a blood pressure cuff is inflated around limb).

Management

If the calcium level is very low and symptoms are present, 10 ml 10% i.v. calcium gluconate should be given. In more chronic situations, oral supplementation is required.

■ PHOSPHATE

Phosphate has a crucial role in the body, for example in nucleic acids, signalling molecules, energy metabolism and bone. Approximately 80% of the body's phosphate is in bone.

Hyperphosphataemia

Hyperphosphataemia usually occurs as a result of reduced excretion in chronic renal failure. It is usually asymptomatic but can cause calcium phosphate precipitation, resulting in itching, hyperparathyroidism and periarticular calcification. Treatment

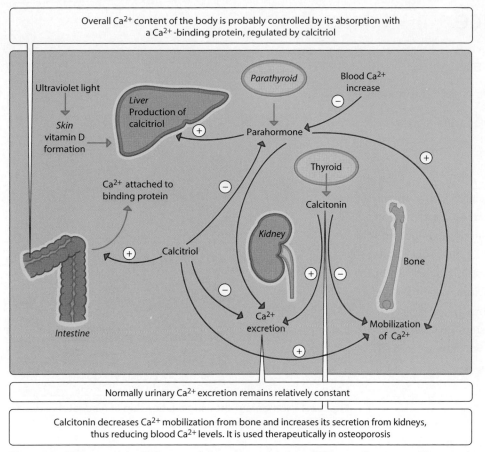

Overall Ca²⁺ content of the body is probably controlled by its absorption with a Ca²⁺-binding protein, regulated by calcitriol

Normally urinary Ca²⁺ excretion remains relatively constant

Calcitonin decreases Ca²⁺ mobilization from bone and increases its secretion from kidneys, thus reducing blood Ca²⁺ levels. It is used therapeutically in osteoporosis

Fig. 3.2.1 Maintenance of plasma calcium concentrations. PTH, parathormone; GI, gastrointestinal tract.

is usually not required, although in hyperphosphataemia caused by chronic renal disease, oral phosphate binders are used.

Hypophosphataemia

Hypophosphataemia may result from reduced absorption, excessive renal losses or redistribution within the body. The most common causes are chronic alcoholism and the ingestion of antacids (Table 3.2.1). Symptoms include weakness, encephalopathy, seizures, respiratory depression (often from diaphragmatic weakness) and heart failure. Management is with oral phosphate supplements or i.v. phosphate in more severely symptomatic individuals.

■ MAGNESIUM

Hypermagnesaemia

Hypermagnesaemia (magnesium >1.1 mmol/l) is uncommon. Symptoms include nausea, flushing, headache and cardiac arrhythmias. The most common cause is ingestion of magnesium-containing salts (e.g. antacids) in the presence of impaired renal function. Any magnesium-containing salts should be stopped; severe toxicity may require dialysis.

Table 3.2.1 CAUSES OF HYPOPHOSPHATAEMIA

Process	Cause
Reduced absorption/intake	Starvation, prolonged vomiting, chronic alcoholism, vitamin D deficiency, antacid ingestion (binds phosphate)
Excess renal loss	Diuretics, renal tubular dysfunction, hyperparathyroidism, familial hypophosphataemic rickets
Redistribution	Diabetic ketoacidosis, refeeding syndrome, respiratory alkalosis, post-parathyroidectomy

Hypomagnesaemia

Hypomagnesaemia (magnesium <0.7 mmol/l) is more common than hypermagnesaemia and tends to occur together with hypocalcaemia and hypokalaemia. It is usually asymptomatic but muscle weakness, tetany, seizures and cardiac arrythmias can occur. Hypomagnesaemia should be suspected in patients with chronic diarrhoea, chronic alcohol abuse, hypocalcaemia, hypokalaemia or arrythmias. Management is with oral replacement in mild cases or intravenous therapy in more severe depletion states or when arrythmias are present.

3. Acid–base balance

Questions
- What are the causes of respiratory alkalosis and respiratory acidosis?
- What are the causes of metabolic alkalosis and metabolic acidosis?

The pH of arterial plasma is tightly regulated and normally maintained between 7.38 and 7.42 (hydrogen ion concentration, 36–44 nmol/l). The normal adult diet contains 70–100 mmol acid and cellular metabolism also creates CO_2 and other acids. However a variety of buffers including intracellular proteins (e.g. haemoglobin) and tissue factors (e.g. calcium carbonate and phosphate in bone) act to prevent large swings in arterial pH.

The carbonic acid/bicarbonate buffer system involves the reaction of hydrogen ions with bicarbonate, which is in relatively high concentration in extracellular fluid (21–28 mmol/l) to form carbonic acid:

$$H^+ + HCO_3^- \rightleftarrows H_2CO_3$$

This is then dissociated by the enzyme carbonic anhydrase:

$$H_2CO_3 \rightleftarrows CO_2 + H_2O$$

These reactions are under constant physiological control via two mechanisms. First, changes in arterial pH affect ventilatory drive to the lungs, which can rapidly compensate for acid–base disturbance. In response to acid accumulation, ventilation is increased, which reduces the arterial partial pressure of CO_2 (Pa_{CO_2}). Conversely, alkalosis leads to reduced ventilation and accumulation of CO_2. Second, when acid accumulates owing to chronic respiratory or metabolic causes, the kidney responds by excreting more acid and retaining bicarbonate. The relationship between arterial pH, bicarbonate and carbonic acid is governed by the Henderson–Hasselbalch equation:

$$pH = 6.1 + \log[HCO_3^-]/[H_2CO_3]$$

Acid–base disorders can be classified based on the abnormal pH (acidosis or alkalosis) and further on the secondary changes in respiration or metabolism depending on the primary abnormality. There is a close interrelationship between the four forms: respiratory and metabolic acidosis and respiratory and metabolic alkalosis (Fig. 3.3.1). Different disorders can lead to the same imbalance but by different mechanisms (Table 3.3.1).

Respiratory acidosis is caused by alveolar hypoventilation leading to a rise in Pa_{CO_2} (Table 3.3.2). This occurs in severe exacerbations of chronic obstructive pulmonary disease (COPD),

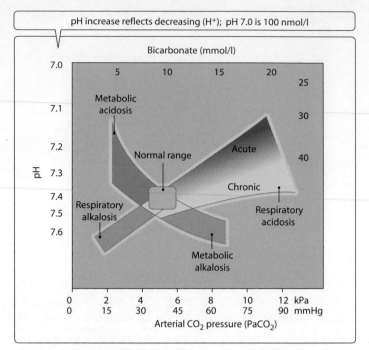

Fig. 3.3.1 Nomogram showing relationship of respiratory arterial pH, Pa_{CO_2} and bicarbonate.

Table 3.3.1 CAUSES OF ACID–BASE DISORDERS

Type	Causes
Metabolic acidosis	
Normal anion gap	Diarrhoea, renal tubular acidosis, Addison's disease, pancreatic fistula
Increased anion gap	Lactic acidosis, renal failure, ketoacidosis, drugs (salicylates, methanol)
Metabolic alkalosis	Vomiting, burns, diuretics
Respiratory acidosis	
Ventilatory failure	
CNS causes	Opioids, sleep apnoea
Chest wall pathology	Kyphoscoliosis, Guillain–Barré syndrome, myasthenia, obesity
Lung pathology	Chronic obstructive pulmonary disease, severe asthma, occasionally severe pulmonary oedema
Respiratory alkalosis	
Decrease in CO_2 production	Hypothermia, hypothyroidism
Increased alveolar ventilation	Primary CNS activation (tumours, infections, trauma); secondary stimulation (lung pathology, anaemia, hypoxia)
Iatrogenic	Mechanical hyperventilation

Table 3.3.2 VARIOUS TYPES OF ACID–BASE DISTURBANCE AND TYPICAL EFFECTS UPON PH, CO_2 AND HCO_3^-

	Decompensated (or partially compensated) respiratory acidosis	Compensated respiratory acidosis	Respiratory alkalosis	Metabolic alkalosis	Metabolic acidosis	Mixed metabolic and respiratory acidosis
pH	↓	↔	↑	↑	↓	↓
Pa_{CO_2}	↑	↑	↓	↑(respiratory compensation)	↔ or ↓	↑
HCO_3^-	↔ or ↑	↑	↔	↑	↓	↓

Pa_{CO_2}, arterial partial pressure of CO_2.
Normal values: pH, 7.35–7.45; P_{CO_2}, 4.6–6 kPa; HCO_3^-, 21–28 mmol/l.

severe pneumonia and severe acute asthma. Elevation in Pa_{CO_2} for more than 2–3 days, as can occur in COPD, neuromuscular disorders and thoracic skeletal deformities, leads to renal retention of bicarbonate and normalization of pH. This pattern of low Pa_{O_2}, high Pa_{CO_2} and rise in bicarbonate with normal pH is known as compensated respiratory acidosis.

Respiratory alkalosis is a result of hyperventilation, leading to reduction in Pa_{CO_2} and raised pH. This can occur at high altitude, following stroke, in the early stages of acute asthma, in severe pulmonary thromboembolism and in hyperventilation.

Metabolic acidosis is caused by loss of bicarbonate, leading to a fall in arterial pH. This stimulates arterial chemoreceptors and results in alveolar hyperventilation and a fall in Pa_{CO_2}. This occurs in metabolic disorders associated with production of organic acids (e.g. acute renal failure, diabetic ketoacidosis) and in shock and after a cardiac arrest, which produces lactic acidosis. Loss of bicarbonate, as can occur in severe diarrhoea, Addison's disease and renal tubular acidosis, can also result in metabolic acidosis.

The anion gap can be useful in determining the cause of metabolic acidosis. The main cations present in plasma are sodium and potassium while the main anions are chloride, bicarbonate and negative charges on albumin, sulphate, phosphate, lactate and other organic acids. The anion gap is therefore:

$$[NA^+ + K^+] - [HCO_3^- + Cl^-]$$

Since there are more unmeasured anions than cations, the anion gap is normally 10–18 mmol/l.

Metabolic alkalosis is caused by either loss of hydrogen ions, as occurs in severe vomiting or nasogastric suction, or retention of bicarbonate, as occurs in high-dose diuretic therapy and excessive alkali ingestion (e.g. milk-alkali syndrome). The increase in arterial pH leads to alveolar hypoventilation and a rise in Pa_{CO_2}.

Any acid–base disturbance results in correction of arterial pH by activating the opposite control system: that is, a primary respiratory problem will be compensated by metabolic pathways via the kidney and a primary metabolic problem will be compensated by ventilatory drive via the lungs.

4. Poisoning I

Questions
- What are the general principles in the management of any overdose?
- What is the management of benzodiazepine overdose?
- What is the management of paracetamol overdose?

Approximately 15% of all medical emergencies are from overdose; alcohol use occurs in over 50% of these. Regardless of the drug taken, similar general principles apply. A period of observation and supportive care is often all that is required, although in some cases (e.g. paracetamol poisoning) a specific antidote is available. On presentation, immediate attention should be taken to secure the airway, assist breathing and optimize cardiovascular status using fluids, inotropes or antiarrhythmic agents. Hypoglycaemia and intracranial abnormalities should be excluded in all who are unconscious or who have prolonged seizures. Seizures should be treated with anticonvulsants (e.g. diazepam) and hypothermia (often associated with alcohol excess) should be managed with passive or active rewarming. Gastric lavage is carried out less commonly but should still be considered when a potentially harmful dose of toxic drug has been ingested within 1 h of presentation. It should be avoided following ingestion of corrosives or in the presence of oesophageal varices. Elimination of some drugs can be hastened with the use of activated charcoal. The National Poisons Bureau should be contacted in difficult cases. Psychiatric evaluation is essential following recovery. Features suggesting that a serious suicide attempt was contemplated include careful planning, a suicide note, a history of serious overdose, lack of regret and measures taken to avoid discovery.

Figure 3.4.1 gives the clinical features of specific drugs taken in overdose.

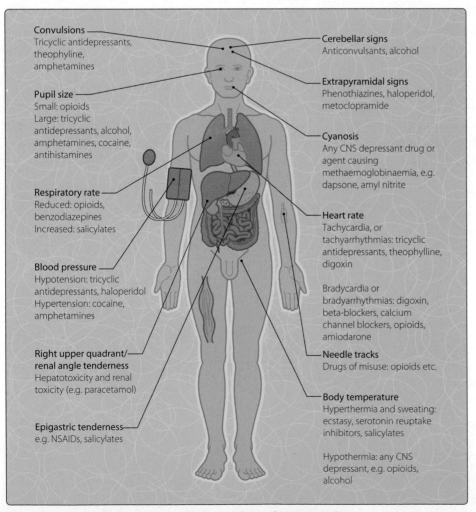

Fig. 3.4.1 Clinical features of specific drugs when taken in overdose.

Benzodiazepines

Benzodiazepine poisoning is common, especially in combination with alcohol and other sedative drugs. Effects can last for days and can be particularly severe in the elderly and patients with liver impairment. Symptoms include drowsiness, slurred speech, ataxia and hypotension. Coma, respiratory depression and cardiovascular collapse are less likely but can occur when combined with alcohol or other sedatives/hypnotics.

Treatment includes initial resuscitation, with management of the airway, breathing and circulation, close observation and supportive management. In severe overdose, the benzodiazepine antagonist flumazenil should be given. Initial dose is 200 μg i.v. with a further 100 μg given every 2–3 min to a maximum of 500 μg. It should not be used as a diagnostic test or in suspected mixed overdose as it can precipitate seizures and cardiac arrhythmia, particularly in patients who are chronic benzodiazepine users.

Alcohol

Acute intoxication with alcohol results in disinhibition, euphoria and incoordination, leading to ataxia, stupor and coma. Complications include acute gastritis, respiratory depression, aspiration pneumonia, hypoglycaemia and accidental injury. Mild to moderate intoxication needs no specific management. In patients with severe intoxication, hospital observation with airway maintenance, i.v. fluids, vitamin replacement and dextrose is sometimes required. Chronic abusers of alcohol should be referred to counselling services.

Paracetamol

Paracetamol is safe when taken in therapeutic doses. The minimum dose believed to cause heptotoxicity is 125 mg/kg or 7.5 g for a 60 kg person. Doses >250 mg/kg produce hepatotoxicity in 60%. Because of its widespread availability, paracetamol accounts for approximately 3% of drug-related overdoses and deaths. Toxicity can be asymptomatic during the initial stages and yet damage to the liver can be occurring, so plasma paracetamol levels should ideally be checked 4 h following ingestion or 4 h after admission (Fig. 3.4.2). The likelihood of liver damage occurring depends on the dose and body weight:

- <150 mg/kg: serious liver damage unlikely
- >250 mg/kg: serious liver damage likely
- >12 g total: potentially fatal.

Paracetamol is conjugated in the liver by glutathione, but if glutathione stores become depleted, toxic metabolites accumulate and cause hepatocellular damage. Risk factors such as alcohol excess or nutritional depletion can, therefore, result in serious liver damage with low levels of ingestion. Toxicity may cause nausea and vomiting during the initial stages. If untreated, features of hepatic necrosis develop, for example right subcostal pain and tenderness, jaundice, vomiting and confusion. Encephalopathy, acute renal failure and lactic acidosis are late features. Investigations should include liver function tests and international normalized ratio (INR).

The specific antidote to paracetamol is i.v. *N*-acetylcysteine and, less commonly, oral methionine. Most patients presenting after a large paracetamol overdose (>150 mg/kg or >12 g) should have treatment commenced. The threshold for commencing *N*-acetylcysteine is lower when additional risk factors are present. Fulminant liver failure has a high mortality and early referral to the local liver unit for advice regarding transplantation may be necessary. If ingestion occurred more than 24 h prior to presentation, plasma paracetamol concentrations are likely to be below the treatment line, although in some instances treatment is required. The regimen for giving *N*-acetylcysteine for paracetamol overdose is as follows:

- 150 mg/kg in 200 ml 5% Dextrose over 15 min
- 50 mg/kg in 500 ml 5% Dextrose over 4 h
- 100 mg/kg in 1000 ml 5% Dextrose over 16 h

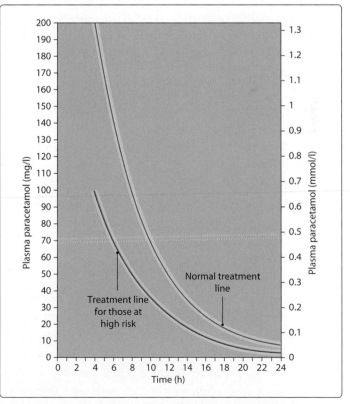

Fig. 3.4.2 Graph used to determine whether specific treatment is required in paracetamol poisoning; high risk includes chronic alcohol abuse, drug-induced hepatic enzyme induction, malnutrition or starvation, individuals with HIV or AIDS. Time is after ingestion (or admission).

5. Poisoning II

Questions

- What drugs have a specific antidote available if taken in overdose?
- What is the management of tricyclic antidepressant overdose?
- What poisons typically cause a metabolic acidosis?
- What are the clinical features and management of carbon monoxide poisoning?

Salicylates

Aspirin (acetylsalicylic acid) is widely taken both as 'over the counter' analgesia and for cardiovascular disease. It is often taken in overdose alone or with other drugs. Clinical features of salicylate toxicity include tachypnoea, sweating, epigastric pain and vomiting, tinnitus, blurred vision and, in extreme cases, agitation, seizures and coma. Complications include GI haemorrhage, acute renal failure and electrolyte abnormalities. Inhibition of platelet function, as well as alteration in vitamin K-dependent clotting factors, results in bruising and bleeding. The severity of poisoning can be assessed by measuring serum salicylate levels; 500–750 mg/l indicates moderate intoxication, while > 750 mg/l indicates severe toxicity.

Serum salicylate < 500 mg/l can be managed with oral or i.v. fluids and correction of any electrolyte abnormalities or dehydration. If ingestion has been within 1–2 h, gastric lavage with activated charcoal can be beneficial. Marked signs and symptoms or serum salicylate > 750 mg/l usually requires forced alkalization of the urine to pH > 7.5 with 1 litre 1.26% sodium bicarbonate solution over 2 h, which will aid clearance. In severe toxicity (> 1000 mg/l) and those with significant metabolic acidosis, haemodialysis may be necessary.

Opioids

Prescribed opioids for pain control may be taken in overdose either deliberately or by accident. Severe opioid overdose most commonly occurs in the drug-abusing population where heroin is taken intravenously or subcutaneously. Clinical features include pinpoint pupils, respiratory depression, hypotension, coma and rarely adult respiratory distress syndrome. Urine toxicology screen can be helpful in difficult cases.

Naloxone is a pure opioid antagonist and can be administered in i.v. boluses of 100–200 μg at 2–3 min intervals until a response occurs. Infusion may be required since naloxone has a shorter half life than most opioids.

Tricyclic antidepressants

Selective serotonin-reuptake inhibitors, which are less toxic in overdose, are now widely prescribed in preference to tricyclic antidepressant and, therefore, overdose is becoming less common. Tricyclic antidepressants (such as amitriptyline and imipramine) prevent reuptake of noradrenaline in nerve endings and exhibit anticholinergic and anti- (and pro-) arrhythmic effects.

Clinical features frequently develop within the first few hours of ingestion and are mainly anticholinergic, for example dry mouth, blurred vision, urinary retention, confusion, drowsiness and sinus tachycardia. Severe poisoning can result in seizures, metabolic acidosis, cardiac arrhythmias, respiratory depression and coma. Management is largely supportive; a single dose of activated charcoal can be given if ingestion has been within an hour of presentation. Following ingestion of larger amounts of tricyclic antidepressants, some patients may require intubation and ventilation, and treatment of arrythmias with 8.4% sodium bicarbonate. Recovery from overdose can be associated with agitation and hallucinations.

Ethylene glycol

Ethylene glycol is found in antifreeze and ingestion causes a metabolic acidosis, through formation of glycolate, and deposition of calcium oxalate crystals (Fig. 3.5.1). Clinical features are similar to ethanol poisoning, although in more severe cases, neurological problems, coma and convulsions develop. Treatment includes inhibition of alcohol dehydrogenase (e.g. with i.v. ethanol, which inhibits the metabolism of ethylene glycol) and vitamins (pyridoxine, thiamine, which stimulate production of less-toxic metabolites). Haemodialysis may also be required in an attempt to remove ethylene glycol and its metabolites.

Methanol

Methanol is also a common constituent of antifreeze and ingestion causes metabolic acidosis. Initial presentation is similar to ethanol intoxication, although blurred vision and reduced visual acuity (and occasionally blindness) develop later. Treatment involves haemodialysis to correct the acidosis and ethanol infusion in an attempt to inhibit methanol metabolism (Fig. 3.5.1).

Organophosphates

Organophosphates are predominantly used as pesticides, and ingestion can be either deliberate or accidental. Organophosphates inhibit acetylcholinesterase, resulting in accumulation of acetylcholine at the neuromuscular junction. Features

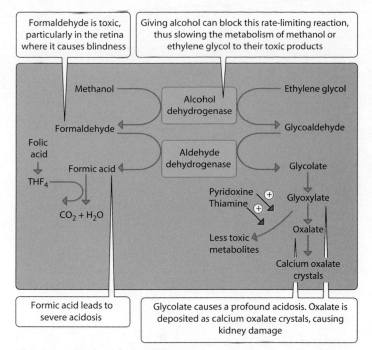

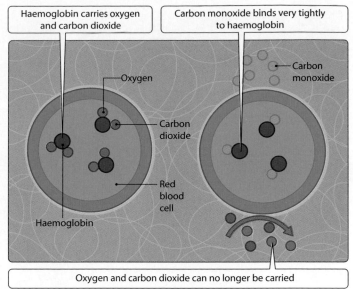

Fig. 3.5.1 Methanol and ethylene glycol themselves are relatively non-toxic, causing mainly CNS sedation. However, their acidic oxidation products are highly toxic.

Fig. 3.5.2 The effects of carbon monoxide inhalation on haemoglobin.

of poisoning include anxiety, headache, diarrhoea, vomiting, muscle weakness, sweating, rhinorrhoea, twitching and bronchospasm. Severe toxicity results in cardiac arrhythmias, pulmonary oedema, respiratory failure, coma and death. Hospital personnel should avoid contamination with protective clothing. Diagnosis requires a high index of suspicion but can be confirmed by measuring red cell cholinesterase activity. Treatment is supportive and involves removal of contaminated clothing and washing. Atropine may be given if severe cholinergic symptoms are present.

Carbon monoxide

Carbon monoxide (CO) poisoning usually occurs from gas leaks from poorly maintained heating systems and domestic gas appliances. CO has greater affinity than O_2 for haemoglobin and, therefore, causes hypoxia to vital organs and tissues (Fig. 3.5.2). Symptoms depend on the degree of exposure but include headache, confusion, irritability, convulsions and coma. A high level of clinical suspicion is often required as mild symptoms are non-specific; symptoms depend on the level of poisoning:

$<30\%$: headaches, dizziness

30–60%: syncope, tachycardia, seizures

$>60\%$: cardiorespiratory failure.

CO levels can be easily checked in most blood gas machines. Oxygen saturation is often normal as most analysers are unable to differentiate oxyhaemoglobin from carboxyhaemoglobin. Management includes delivery of high-flow O_2, but severely affected individuals will also require intubation and mechanical ventilation. Hyperbaric O_2 may be effective in individuals with severe CO poisoning who have been unconscious or who are pregnant.

PART VIII

Diabetes mellitus and other metabolic disorders

Sam Philip

The big picture

The most common metabolic disorder is diabetes mellitus, which is a syndrome of chronic hyperglycaemia caused by relative insulin deficiency and/or resistance. There is a wide range of dysfunctions, reflecting the central role of insulin in energy balance. The estimated number of individuals with diabetes worldwide had risen from 30 million in 1985 to 150 million in 2000 and is expected to rise to almost 350 million by 2025 (Fig. 1.1). Reasons for this increase include an ageing population, rising obesity and sedentary lifestyle. Increasing urbanization, changing dietary patterns and reduction in physical activity also contribute to this growing problem in both developed and developing countries. Although diabetes is usually irreversible, lifestyle interventions (e.g. a healthy diet, increased physical activity and weight reduction where indicated) have been shown to significantly reduce the rate of late complications. Complications include

- macrovascular disease, leading to coronary artery disease, peripheral vascular disease and stroke
- microvascular disease, causing diabetic retinopathy, chronic kidney disease, peripheral neuropathy.

The cost of diabetes mellitus in UK

In addition to the direct costs of the disease, 5–7% of total UK NHS budget, diabetes is associated with

- 10–30% reduction in life expectancy
- 25 times increase in lower limb amputation

- increase in sight loss: the most common cause of blindness in 20–65 year olds
- increased incidence of end-stage kidney disease
- six-fold increase in use of hospital beds and longer hospital stays.

Types of diabetes mellitus

There are two main forms of diabetes mellitus: **type 1** (old term insulin-dependent diabetes (IDDM)) and **type 2** (old term non-insulin-dependent diabetes (NIDDM) or maturity-onset diabetes).

Type 1 diabetes

Type 1 diabetes is caused by autoimmune destruction of pancreatic beta islet cells, mainly by T lymphocytes in response to poorly defined antigens on the beta cells. The process is believed to be initiated by an environmental trigger in genetically susceptible individuals. Although type 1 diabetes typically presents as an acute or subacute illness, it results from chronic autoimmune destruction of beta islets that typically started many years before the disease became evident (Fig. 1.2). Patients become symptomatic after losing more than 90% of their beta cells. Type 1 diabetes is associated with other autoimmune conditions, such as pernicious anaemia and thyroid disease. It is more common in those of northern European ancestry, and in northern Europe its prevalence in children has doubled since 1980 particularly in those under 5 years.

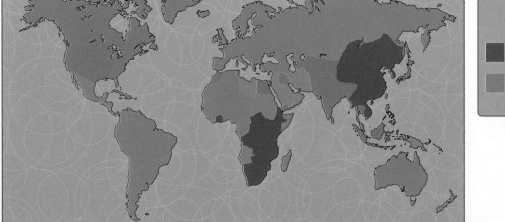

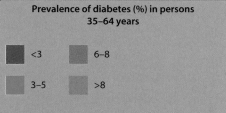

Prevalence of diabetes (%) in persons 35–64 years

- <3
- 3–5
- 6–8
- >8

Fig. 1.1 The worldwide prevalence of diabetes. Number of people with diabetes in 2000: Asia and Australia 83 million; the Americas, 33 million; Europe, 33 million; Middle East, 15 million; Africa, 7 million.

Type 2 diabetes

Type 2 diabetes results from the inability of pancreatic beta islet cells to secrete adequate insulin to meet the increased demand in an insulin-resistant individual (Fig. 1.3). The relative importance of these two key components (insulin resistance and beta islet cell dysfunction) varies from individual to individual. It is common in migrant populations to industrialized countries and is now recognized in children. In Europe and North America, the ratio of type 2 to type 1 diabetes is approximately 7:3.

Diabetes of pregnancy

Diabetes mellitus can also occur during pregnancy (gestational diabetes mellitus). This form resembles type 2 diabetes in several respects. It occurs in 2–5% of all pregnancies and may improve or disappear after delivery. It is fully treatable but requires careful medical supervision throughout the pregnancy. Approximately 20–50% of affected women develop type 2 diabetes later in life.

Other metabolic disorders

Metabolic syndrome has recently been recognized as a group of major risk factors for cardiovascular disease. These include a high fasting blood glucose (usually as a result of type 2 diabetes), hypertension and hyperlipidaemia, which often results in increased waist circumference and obesity. Genetic factors, low birth weight and significant weight gain in adulthood are all factors in the development of the metabolic syndrome.

Obesity, defined as a body mass index (BMI) of >30, is an increasing problem worldwide, with a prevalence in Europe of approximately 20% in adults. It develops in an individual when energy intake exceeds energy expenditure over a long period.

These metabolic disorders are major contributors to total healthcare costs in affluent societies. Direct costs amount to approximately 2–8% of total healthcare costs, including funds diverted for the treatment of obesity. Indirect costs relate to loss of productivity through absenteeism, provision of disability pensions and premature death.

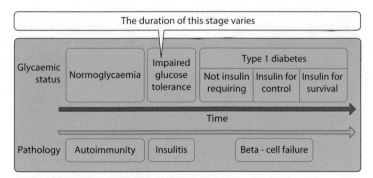

Fig. 1.2 Clinical spectrum of type 1 diabetes. Patients progress along the spectrum at varying speeds.

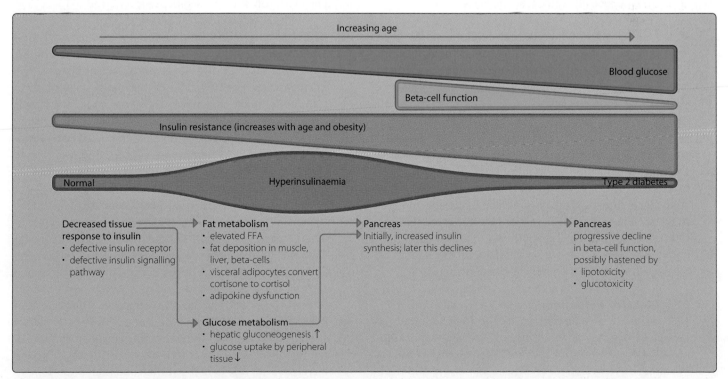

Fig. 1.3 Type 2 diabetes. TG, triglycerides; FFA, fatty acids.

High-return facts

1 **Diabetes mellitus** is caused by a defect in insulin secretion. **Type 1 diabetes** is caused by an absolute deficiency of insulin while type 2 diabetes is characterized by varying degrees of insulin resistance with an inadequate compensatory rise in insulin secretion. Clinical features include polyuria, polydipsia, blurred vision, fungal infections and weight loss. Presentation can be insidious and a minority present initially with complications of diabetes. Type 1 diabetes usually presents subacutely in younger individuals, who may have a personal or family history of other autoimmune conditions. **Type 2 diabetes** tends to occur in middle-aged or elderly obese individuals. Diagnosis of diabetes is confirmed by typical symptoms and either a raised fasting plasma glucose or a raised random blood glucose reading. In the absence of symptoms, two diagnostic tests are needed on separate days. In borderline cases, the glucose tolerance test (OGTT) is used.

2 **Management of diabetes** should aim for tight glucose control to reduce the risk of complications while avoiding the risk of hypoglycaemia. Glycosylated haemoglobin (HbA1c) is used as an index of glycaemic control over the preceding 6–8 weeks (target < 7%). Type 1 diabetes requires treatment with insulin. Different insulin preparations have different speeds of action; these are used to attempt to mimic physiological insulin release. Patients are educated on monitoring and adjusting their glycaemic control and how to deal with changes in circumstance, such as acute illness. Type 2 diabetes requires reduction in weight, which results in improvement in glycaemic control, and drug treatment (usually metformin) if lifestyle changes are not successful. Patients should be examined annually for complications of diabetes.

3 **Diabetic ketoacidosis** is a life-threatening condition. It is characterized by the triad of hyperglycaemia (which may be mild), metabolic acidosis and ketonuria (or elevated serum ketones). Management consists of correcting dehydration, i.v. insulin, identifying and treating precipitating factors, and monitoring and correcting electrolyte abnormalities (mainly hypokalaemia) and blood glucose. **Hyperosmolar non-ketotic coma** (HONK) occurs in type 2 diabetes and presents with altered conscious level and severe hyperglycaemia and elevated serum osmolality without acidosis. Management requires slow correction of dehydration, reduction of hyperglycaemia with i.v. insulin and prevention of thromboembolic complications. **Hypoglycaemia** is the most common side effect of diabetes therapy. Recognition of hypoglycaemia (initial symptoms sweating, tremor and palpitation) is an important protective mechanism and termed hypoglycaemic awareness. If hypoglycaemia is not corrected and blood sugar falls further, neuroglycopenia occurs with confusion, coma and death. Hypoglycaemia is corrected by administering 15–20 g rapidly absorbed glucose (dextrose tablets, gel or solution). In a comatose patient, i.m. glucagon or i.v. 50% glucose is required.

4 The long-term complications of diabetes are classified into macrovascular (ischaemic heart disease, peripheral vascular disease, cerebrovascular disease) and microvascular (retinopathy, nephropathy, neuropathy). **Ischaemic heart disease** is more common in diabetic adults and the risk of fatal myocardial infarction is substantially increased. **Hypertension** is common. **Diabetic retinopathy** is the most common cause of blindness among those of working age in the UK, and diabetic patients should be screened annually. **Diabetic nephropathy** is the most common cause of end-stage kidney disease in the UK. The initial feature of diabetic kidney disease is microalbuminuria, and patients should be screened annually. **Diabetic neuropathy** can involve sensory, motor and autonomic nerves. The most common manifestation is sensory peripheral polyneuropathy, which has a characteristic 'glove and stocking' distribution. **Diabetic foot problems** are common and the feet of the diabetic patient should be checked regularly for any deformities or neurological/vascular compromise. **Erectile dysfunction** increases with age in diabetic men and is an important indicator of increased cardiovascular risk.

5 **Metabolic syndrome** describes a cluster of risk factors for arteriosclerotic cardiovascular disease including elevated fasting glucose, high blood pressure, low levels of high density lipoprotein cholesterol and high triglycerides levels. Insulin resistance is a central component of the metabolic syndrome. Patients with metabolic syndrome are typically overweight and treatment requires lifestyle changes. **Hyperlipidaemia** usually results from a combination of excessive dietary intake and genetic predisposition. Some individuals have inherited abnormalities of lipid metabolism or secondary hyperlipidaemia. Treatment includes a diet low in saturated fats (meat and dairy products) and high in fibre, sometimes with drugs such as statins, fibrates, ezetimibe or anion-exchange resins.

6 **Obesity** is defined as a body mass index (BMI) of > 30. The prevalence of obesity has risen dramatically and now in most countries exceeds 15%. Most obesity is caused by increased consumption of high-energy foods and lack of physical activity. It is associated with an increased risk of cardiovascular disease, diabetes, hypertension, hyperlipidaemia, sleep apnoea, breathlessness, gall bladder disease, osteoarthritis, depression, gout, reduced fertility, complications surrounding pregnancy, low back pain and some malignancies such as colorectal cancer. For effective weight loss, energy intake must be reduced and physical activity increased. This can be attempted through a combination of diet and lifestyle changes and, in selected individuals, drugs or surgery.

1. Presentation of diabetes mellitus

Questions
- What is the prevalence of type 1 and type 2 diabetes?
- What are the criteria for the diagnosis of diabetes mellitus?

Diabetes mellitus can be primary or secondary to an underlying cause. Irrespective of aetiology, a defect in insulin secretion exists that is either absolute or relative to requirements in the presence of coexisting insulin resistance. Insulin is produced by the pancreas (Fig. 3.1.1) and has a direct effect on blood glucose (Fig. 3.1.2). As chronic hyperglycaemia damages blood vessels and nerves, uncontrolled diabetes leads to severe complications.

Epidemiology

The prevalence of diabetes in all age groups worldwide was 2.8% in 2000 and rose to 4.4% in 2003. It is more common among males than females. In the UK, the cumulative risk of developing type 1 diabetes by the age of 20 years is 0.3–0.4%. Annual incidence of type 1 varies worldwide. Type 2 diabetes is more common and the prevalence has tripled since the mid-1970s: current estimates are 6% in Europe, 6–8% in the USA, and 20–25% of adults in some Middle East regions. The greatest increase is in developing countries.

Pathogenesis

Blood glucose is tightly regulated, balancing glucose entry from stored glycogen and meals with uptake by peripheral tissues, particularly skeletal muscle and the brain (Fig. 3.1.3). After meals, insulin is secreted into the portal circulation by the beta cells of the pancreatic islets.

Type 1 diabetes is caused by an absolute deficiency of insulin and **type 2** diabetes is characterized by varying degrees of insulin resistance with an inadequate compensatory rise in insulin secretion. Genetic factors influence both insulin sensitivity and beta cell dysfunction. Although genetic susceptibility is common in type 1 diabetes, the concordance rate in monozygotic twins is only 40%. Environmental factors are, therefore, important in the development of type 1 diabetes as well as type 2 diabetes.

Less commonly, diabetes can be associated with pregnancy (**gestational diabetes**), secondary to diseases or drugs that damage the pancreatic islet cells or caused by endocrine disorders that antagonize the effect of insulin (**secondary diabetes**).

- pancreatic damage: chronic pancreatitis, pancreatectomy, pancreatic tumour, cystic fibrosis, haemochromatosis
- endocrine causes: acromegaly, Cushing's syndrome, hyperthyroidism, phaeochromocytoma, glucagonoma
- drugs: glucocorticoids, alpha-interferon, protease inhibitors, thiazides.

Clinical features

Features (Table 3.1.1) result from the osmotic effects of hyperglycaemia or increased catabolism caused by relative or absolute insulin deficiency:

- hyperglycaemia: polyuria, nocturia, enuresis, thirst, polydipsia, blurred vision (refractive changes in lens), genital candidiasis (pruritus vulvae, balanitis)
- increased catabolic state: recent weight loss, muscle weakness, malaise, tiredness, lack of energy.

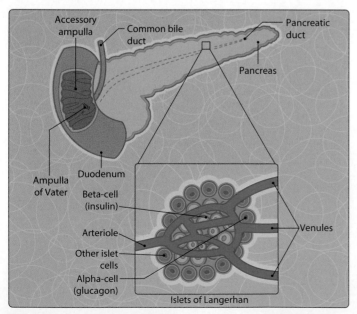

Fig. 3.1.1 Pancreatic structure.

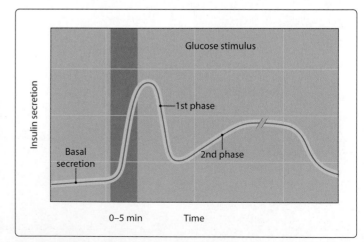

Fig. 3.1.2 The effect of endogenous insulin on blood glucose in a normal individual 5 min after a meal.

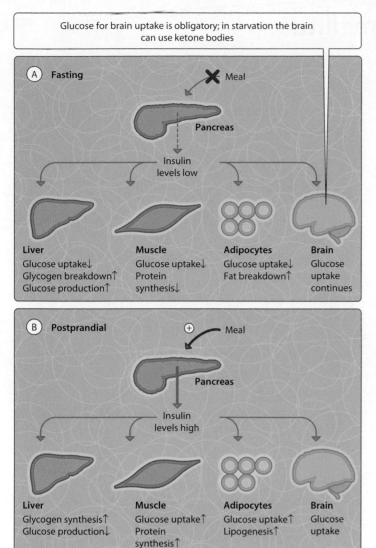

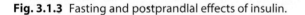

Fig. 3.1.3 Fasting and postprandial effects of insulin.

Investigations

Blood glucose is normally maintained in a very narrow range (3.8–6.6 mmol/l). The diagnosis of diabetes is made on any one of the criteria below performed on two separate occasions:

- symptoms plus a random plasma glucose concentration ≥ 11.1 mmol/l (≥ 2 g/l)
- fasting venous plasma glucose ≥ 7.0 mmol/l (≥ 1.26 g/l)
- oral glucose tolerance test (OGTT): venous plasma glucose ≥ 11.1 mmol/l (≥ 2 g/l) 2 h after glucose bolus.

Impaired fasting glucose tolerance is defined as:

- fasting venous plasma glucose 6–7 mmol/l (1.08–1.26 g/l)
- OGTT venous plasma glucose 7.8–11.1 mmol/l (1.4–2.0 g/l) at 2 h after a glucose load

Among those with impaired glucose tolerance, 5–10% develop overt diabetes every year and are at risk of cardiovascular disease. Patients with impaired glucose tolerance and impaired fasting glucose should be rescreened annually.

Gestational diabetes

Gestational diabetes is more common in the obese, those of black or Hispanic race and those with a family history of type 2 diabetes. All women should be assessed at their first antenatal visit and between 24 and 28 weeks of pregnancy. The diagnostic criteria for gestational diabetes are fasting glucose > 5.5 mmol/l or venous plasma glucose > 9.0 mmol/l 2 h after a 75 g oral glucose dose in the OGTT. Babies born to women with diabetes have a four-fold increase in perinatal death and a three-fold increase in major malformation.

Table 3.1.1 PRESENTATION OF TYPE 1 AND 2 DIABETES

	Type 1	Type 2
Age of onset	Usually < 30 years	Usually > 30 years
Weight	Any body weight	Usually overweight
Family history	Possible	Possible
Duration of symptoms	Variable (from absent to a number of years)	Short period (6–8 weeks)
Osmotic symptoms	Mild to marked	None to marked
Increased catabolic state	Mild to marked	None to marked
Ketoacidosis	Can be a presenting feature	Rare but may be precipitated by intercurrent illness
Clinical insulin dependence	Insulin dependent at diagnosis	Usually takes many years
Autoantibodies (glutamic acid decarboxylase, islet cell)	Present in 70–90%	Absent

2. Management of diabetes mellitus

Questions
- What is the management of type 1 diabetes?
- What lifestyle changes are important in the management of type 2 diabetes?

Good glucose control reduces the risk of long-term complications, albeit with a slightly increased risk of hypoglycaemia. Patients can self-monitor their blood glucose, and recent control can be assessed using measurement of glycosylated haemoglobin (HbA1c; glucose bound to haemoglobin). As red cells live for 8–12 weeks, HbA1c indicates how high blood glucose has been, on average, over the preceding 6–8 weeks. HbA1c of <7% while avoiding significant hypoglycaemia correlates with pre-prandial plasma glucose of 5.0–7.2 mmol/l and a peak postprandial capillary plasma glucose of <10.0 mmol/l.

The management is summarized by the four 'Es'.

Enquiry:
- records: previous investigations
- history: family history, other medical conditions, smoking, vascular risk factors, contraception and sexual history, occupation, driving
- hyperglycaemic symptoms
- glycaemic control: knowledge of self-management (frequency and timing of testing depends on current diabetes therapy, exercise and intercurrent illness)
- medication: dosage, compliance, side-effects, injection technique and rotating injection sites for insulin
- hypoglycaemia: frequency and severity (losing consciousness or requiring third party assistance), awareness
- chronic complications: foot (neuropathic pain, ulcers or claudication), chest pain, erectile dysfunction, visual symptoms.

Evaluation:
- HbA1c: near-patient testing kits
- nephropathy: annual screen for serum creatinine, estimated glomerular filtration rate (GFR) and urine microalbumin
- lipid profile: annual check
- other laboratory measures: urinalysis for ketones, protein, sediment, microalbumin, thyroid-stimulating hormone (in all type 2 and in type 1 if indicated).

Examination:
- every visit: weight and height (in relation to diet and exercise; calculate body mass index), blood pressure, insulin injection sites (if relevant)
- annually or if symptomatic: annual screening for diabetic retinopathy (fundus photography or fundoscopy); peripheral pulses, neuropathy, foot deformities, foot ulcer; and skin, acanthosis nigricans, lipohypertrophy or atrophy.

Encouragement:
- individual glycaemic goals: possibly a higher HbA1c in those with poor awareness of hypoglycaemia, limited life expectancy or significant comorbidity
- weight loss targets if overweight
- vascular risk reduction: smoking, blood pressure and lipids.

Formal specialist dietetic advice can help individuals and self-management education is important.

Pharmacological treatment

Insulin

Insulin derived from extracts of animal pancreases has been almost completely replaced by biosynthetic insulin produced by recombinant DNA technology. Insulin delivery is usually subcutaneous. The speed of action of insulin depends on its type, its lipid solubility and route of delivery. Insulin is available as 100 U/ml (U-100) and preparations can be broadly classified into short acting, intermediate acting and long acting. A 500 U/ml (U-500) preparation is available for severe insulin resistance.

Physiological insulin release consists of a constant background secretion coupled with prandial surge in insulin release in response to a rise in blood sugar following carbohydrate intake (Fig. 3.2.1).

The most commonly used delivery system is the insulin pen device, although a variety of other devices are available such as disposable syringes and pumps. The aim of insulin therapy is to mimic physiological insulin release and meet the demand for rise in blood sugar at meal times. Two commonly used regimens are basal bolus or twice daily premixed insulin (Fig. 3.2.1B,C).

Oral hypoglycaemic drugs

Numerous oral agents are available for type 2 diabetes:
- sulfonylureas: stimulate insulin secretion from pancreatic beta cells
- biguanides: decrease hepatic glucose production, and glucose absorption, increase skeletal muscle glucose uptake
- thiazolidinediones: stimulates the peroxisome proliferative-insulin-activated receptors (PPAR-γ), which have insulin-sensitizing effects on skeletal muscle and adipose tissue and inhibit hepatic gluconeogenesis
- meglitinides: stimulate pancreatic insulin secretion; more rapid and shorter duration of action than sulphonylureas

- α-glucosidase inhibitors: blocks this enzyme on the GI brush border, slowing the breakdown of dietary oligosaccharides and disaccharides.

Type 1 diabetes

Patients with type 1 diabetes are dependent on insulin. Patients should be educated on home blood glucose monitoring, checking urine (or blood) for ketones, insulin administration, insulin dose titration and management of hypoglycaemia. Information is provided on how to deal with acute illness (sick day rules), exercise, driving and medical insurance. All patients should attend a structured education programme to learn how to adjust their insulin therapy according to varying carbohydrate intake and physical activity.

Type 2 diabetes

Losing small amounts of weight (up to 10 kg or 10% of body weight) results in improvements in glycaemic control and a significant reduction (30–40%) in mortality linked to diabetes. Lifestyle changes are difficult to implement and sustain but yield substantial improvements in glycaemic control, blood pressure reduction and general well-being.

Metformin should be considered although lifestyle changes are generally advised as the first treatment option. Treatment should be intensified if patients do not meet glycaemic targets, moving from lifestyle changes through oral drugs and on to insulin.

Gestational diabetes

Gestational diabetes can develop during the second or third trimester of pregnancy; hormones produced by the placenta oppose the action of insulin, making the mother insulin resistant. Treatment depends on the severity of hyperglycaemia and may include dietary modification, metformin and insulin. Most patients discontinue treatment after delivery, although there is a 20–50% increased risk of developing type 2 diabetes within 5–10 years.

Newer therapies

Several new classes of compound that may avoid weight-gain problems will soon become available: glucagon-like peptide 1 analogues and agonists (potentiate insulin secretion, suppress glucagons and may promote beta islet neogenesis), dipeptidyl peptidase 4 (DPP-4) inhibitors (metabolize glucagon-like peptide 1 and gastric inhibitory peptide) and amylin analogues (slow gastric emptying, suppress the release of glucagons and increase satiety).

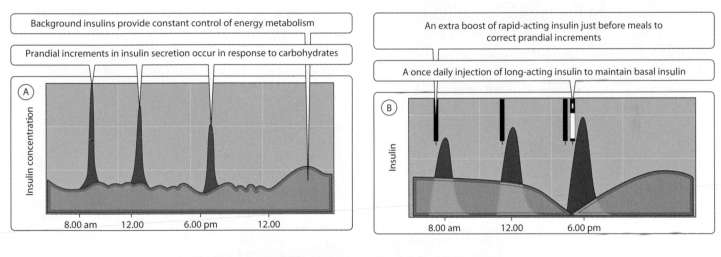

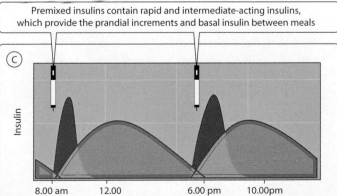

Fig. 3.2.1 Changes in insulin in blood. A, Physiological insulin release; B, under a basal bolus regimen; C, under a twice daily premixed insulin regimen.

3. Common diabetic emergencies

Questions
- What is diabetic ketoacidosis and how is it managed?
- What are the symptoms of hypoglycaemia?

Diabetic ketoacidosis

Diabetic ketoacidosis (DKA) is a life-threatening condition requiring immediate treatment. It usually occurs in previously undiagnosed diabetes or in those who have an interruption of insulin therapy or have an intercurrent illness (Fig. 3.3.1). It presents with severe osmotic symptoms (Fig. 3.3.2), nausea and vomiting and increased respiratory rate. Severe acidosis can result in an altered mood, depressed consciousness and coma.

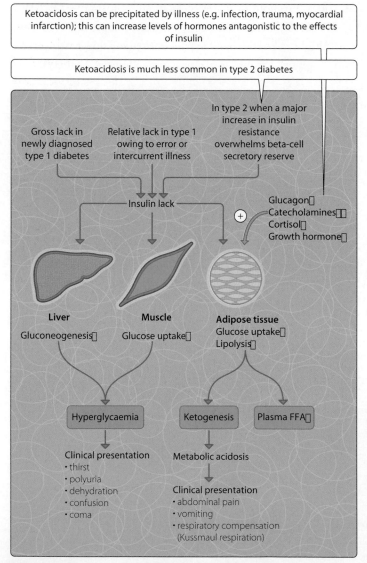

Fig. 3.3.1 Development of diabetic ketoacidosis. FFA, fatty acids.

Clinical features
Clinical features include:
- symptoms: nausea, vomiting, abdominal pain, tiredness, weight loss
- signs: hyperventilation (Kussmaul's breathing as a result of metabolic acidosis), dehydration, ketotic (fruity) breath
- clinical assessment: pulse, blood pressure, respiratory rate, temperature, level of consciousness, precipitating cause.

Common laboratory abnormalities include neutrophilia, hyponatraemia, decreased serum bicarbonate, metabolic acidosis, elevated serum and urinary ketones and raised urea; blood glucose is usually raised but may be normal and serum amylase may be elevated. The diagnosis is confirmed by the presence of hyperglycaemia (which may be mild), metabolic acidosis and ketonuria (or elevated serum ketones).

Management
The main aims of treatment are:
- identifying and treating precipitating factors
- monitoring and correcting electrolyte abnormalities (mainly hypokalaemia), blood glucose and fluid balance.
- correcting dehydration
- delivering insulin.

Airway, breathing and circulation should be assessed and resuscitative measures should be instituted if necessary. Dehydration

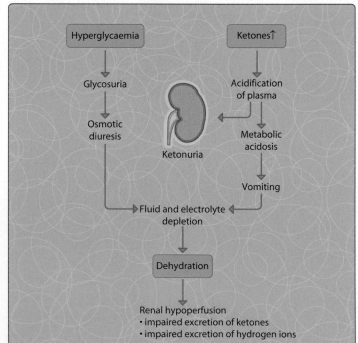

Fig. 3.3.2 Dehydration during ketoacidosis.

should be corrected by replacing the estimated fluid deficit (usually 4–6 litres) using isotonic saline. If there is no suspicion of impaired cardiac function, the first litre should be infused rapidly and subsequent fluid resuscitation should aim at correcting circulating volume. Once the circulating volume is restored, extravascular fluid deficits should be corrected with normal saline at a rate of 150–500 ml/h. Fluid intake and output should be meticulously monitored. In patients with heart failure, severe renal impairment and septic shock, fluid resuscitation should be guided by central venous pressure monitoring.

The aim of giving insulin is to switch off the breakdown of fat into ketones and promote the utilization of glucose, thus correcting hyperglycaemia. Intravenous insulin delivered by a syringe driver should be started at a rate of 6 U/h. When the blood sugar falls to <14 mmol/l, 10% dextrose should be started and insulin infusion rate reduced to 3 U/h to prevent hypoglycaemia and to provide adequate substrate for switching off ketogenesis. Rapid decline in blood sugar and aggressive fluid resuscitation carries a risk of cerebral oedema. Intravenous bicarbonate should only be considered in severe acidosis as it increases the risk of cerebral oedema.

If infection is suspected as a cause of the ketoacidosis, antibiotics should be considered following appropriate cultures. Once food and fluid intake has stabilized, ketonaemia cleared and acidosis corrected, patients should recommence their usual s.c. insulin.

Hyperosmolar non-ketotis

Whenever a patient presents with an altered mental state and severe hyperglycaemia (usually 30–60 mmol/l) hyperosmolar non-ketosis (HONK) should be suspected. It is confirmed by an elevated serum osmolarity (>350 mOsm/kg), with minimal or absent ketonaemia or ketonuria. Prolonged and marked osmotic diuresis causes fluid and electrolyte disturbance. The marked rise in serum osmolality results in dehydration of the brain and the altered mental state. HONK occurs in type 2 diabetes where insulin levels are enough to suppress breakdown of fat but not sufficient to control hyperglycaemia; excessive ketone production and acidosis are not found. In the initial stages, there may be no symptoms, and the severity of metabolic derangement (hyperglycaemia, hyperosmolarity and dehydration) is more severe than with diabetic ketoacidosis.

Treatment consists of correction of dehydration, slow reduction in hyperglycaemia, identification of precipitating factors (e.g. myocardial infarction) and prevention of thromboembolism.

Hypoglycaemia

The major risk of tight glycaemic control is hypoglycaemia. It occurs when a patient has had an excessive amount of insulin either as a result of exogenous insulin administration or drug-

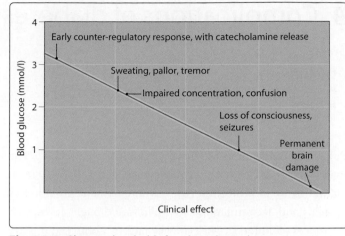

Fig. 3.3.3 Glucose thresholds for physiological responses to hypoglycaemia. Hypoglycaemia unawareness occurs when the thresholds for warning symptoms shifts to values below those for normal brain function.

induced endogenous insulin release relative to the amount of carbohydrate ingested. The human brain is dependent upon glucose as a fuel. Hence a variety of protective responses in the form of counter-regulatory hormone release (e.g. glucagon, cortisol and epinephrine) occurs when the blood glucose falls to <3.2 mmol/l. These cause the initial symptoms of increased sweating, tremor and palpitation (Fig. 3.3.3). Recognition of these symptoms is an important protective mechanism and termed 'hypoglycaemic awareness'. The glucose level at which symptoms develop varies from individual to individual and even in the same individual depending on the duration of diabetes, frequency of hypoglycaemic episodes and overall glycaemic control. If hypoglycaemia is not corrected and blood sugar falls further, it can result in neuroglycopenia with confusion, coma, long-term brain damage and death.

Severity of hypoglycaemia is classified as minor and major depending on whether third party assistance is required (major). Hypoglycaemia is corrected by taking or administering 15–20 g rapidly absorbed glucose (dextrose tablets, gel or solution). In an unconscious patient, i.m. administration of glucagon may be needed, which promotes the breakdown of liver glycogen and release of glucose into the circulation. An alternative is i.v. 50% glucose. Most patients respond rapidly in 5–10 min. Once hypoglycaemia is corrected, patients are advised to take a meal of complex carbohydrate. Prolonged hypoglycaemia can lead to cognitive and intellectual impairment. Patients with hypoglycaemic unawareness should be advised not to drive.

4. Complications of diabetes mellitus

Questions

- How does type 1 diabetes affect life expectancy?
- How is the eye affected in diabetes?

Patients treated with insulin have a reduced life expectancy. The major causes of death are cardiovascular disease (70%), renal failure (10%) and infection (6%). Non-enzymatic glycation of proteins and accumulation of sorbitol are thought to be major factors and blood vessels are key targets. Complications are broadly classified into:

- **microvascular**: characterized by hyaline arteriosclerosis and diffuse thickening of basement membranes (retinopathy, neuropathy, nephropathy)
- **macrovascular**: atherosclerosis indistinguishable from that in non-diabetics occurs at an accelerated rate and at a younger age (ischaemic heart disease, peripheral vascular disease, cerebrovascular disease).

The impact of complications is profound and can lead to visual impairment, renal failure, amputation and functional limitation.

Life expectancy for patients with type 1 and type 2 diabetes is approximately 15 and 5–7 years, respectively, lower than that of the normal population. Aggressive treatment of traditional risk factors such as smoking, hypertension and hyperlipidaemia and good glycaemic control reduce the risk of complications.

Ischaemic heart disease

Mortality from coronary artery disease is two to four times higher in adults with diabetes than those without: the risk of fatal myocardial infarction is double in males and quadruple in females. Diabetes appears to affect the heart in multiple ways:

- coronary artery atherosclerosis: greater tendency for the coronary arteries to be affected by atherosclerosis
- diabetic cardiomyopathy: myocardial dysfunction and accelerated heart failure, contributing factors include severe coronary atherosclerosis, microvascular disease, glycosylation of myocardial proteins and autonomic neuropathy
- autonomic neuropathy affecting the nerve supply to the heart: myocardial ischaemia commonly occurs without symptoms and multivessel atherosclerosis may occur before symptoms promote treatment.

Contributing factors include chronic hyperglycaemia, hyperinsulinaemia, decreased high density lipoprotein cholesterol, elevated triglycerides, increased low density lipoprotein cholesterol and untreated hypertension.

Hypertension

Prevalence of hypertension in type 1 diabetes is approximately 30% and it is often associated with nephropathy. In type 2 diabetes, hypertension is also common and may preceed diagnosis. There may be a genetic predisposition to hypertension in type 2 diabetes through overactivation of the sympathetic nervous system and renin–angiotensin–aldosterone system. All patients with diabetes should have annual blood pressure checks.

Diabetic retinopathy

Diabetes is the most common cause of blindness among those of working age in the UK. All patients with type 1 diabetes have a degree of retinopathy 15–20 years after diagnosis, compared with approximately 60% of individuals with type 2 diabetes. The characteristic lesions of retinopathy include microaneurysms, haemorrhages, exudates and new vessel formation (Fig. 3.4.1). Loss of vision occurs through macular oedema, retinal ischaemia, vitreous haemorrhage, retinal detachment, cataract, ischaemic optic neuropathy and extraocular muscle palsy. Patients with newly diagnosed diabetes can have blurred vision or altering visual acuity from osmotic changes in the fluid content of the lens associated with fluctuation of blood glucose.

Annual retinal screening is recommended. Treatment includes photocoagulation for proliferative retinopathy and vitrectomy for vitreous haemorrhage or retinal detachment.

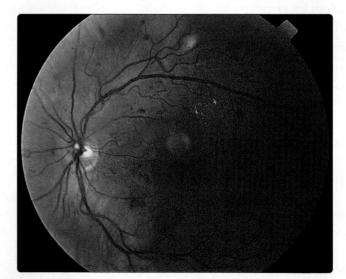

Fig. 3.4.1 Diabetic retinopathy, showing multiple dot and blot haemorrhages. (Reproduced with permission from Douglas G, Nicol F, Robertson C eds 2009 Macleod's Clinical Examination, 12th edn, Churchill Livingstone, Edinburgh.)

Diabetic nephropathy

Diabetic nephropathy is the most common cause of end-stage renal disease in the UK. Overt renal disease may be present at the time of diagnosis in patients with type 2 diabetes, although it usually takes 15–20 years to develop in those with type 1 diabetes. The hallmark of diabetic kidney disease is microalbuminuria, which progresses to proteinuria (24 h albumin loss of 30–300 mg) (Fig. 3.4.2).

All patients with diabetes should be screened annually for microalbuminuria, as it is potentially reversible. Patients with microalbuminuria are at higher risk for cardiovascular disease and should be targeted for aggressive blood pressure reduction, antiplatelet drugs and ACE inhibitors. This can delay the progression of nephropathy and in certain patients even reverse microalbuminuria.

Diabetic neuropathy

Diabetes affects all the nervous system (Fig. 3.4.3). The most common manifestation is sensory peripheral polyneuropathy, which has a characteristic 'glove and stocking' distribution. Combined sensorimotor neuropathy leads to wasting of the intrinsic muscles of the feet, resulting in foot deformity. The lack of sensation, deformity and poor blood supply predispose the foot to ulceration and infection, which may lead to amputation. Painful peripheral neuropathy is difficult to treat, although tricyclic antidepressants, anticonvulsants, carbamazepine or gabapentin can be useful.

Diabetic foot

Foot ulcers develop in 10–15% of diabetic patients at some stage and foot problems are responsible for almost 50% of all diabetes-related hospital admissions. Patients with diabetes should have their feet examined annually. Patients who develop problems should receive regular foot care, education and appropriate foot wear.

Erectile dysfunction

Erectile dysfunction is a common and distressing problem in diabetes. The prevalence increases with age from 6% in diabetic men aged 20–24 years to 52% in men aged 50–59 years. It is an early marker of vascular endothelial dysfunction and an important indicator of increased cardiovascular risk.

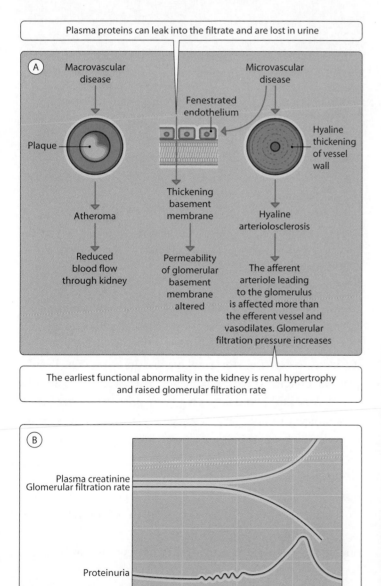

Fig. 3.4.2 Diabetic nephropathy. A, The effect of diabetic angiopathy; B, natural history.

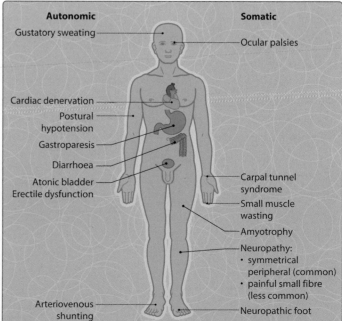

Fig. 3.4.3 Long-term neuropathic complications of diabetes.

5. Metabolic syndrome and hyperlipidaemia

Questions
- What are the criteria used to diagnose metabolic syndrome?
- What is the management of hyperlipidaemia?

Metabolic syndrome

Metabolic syndrome describes a cluster of major risk factors for arteriosclerotic cardiovascular disease:

- raised fasting glucose
- raised blood pressure
- reduced high density lipoprotein (HDL) cholesterol
- raised triglycerides.

Individuals with metabolic syndrome in mid-life are at increased risk of heart failure and stroke and probably dementia.

Epidemiology

Causes of metabolic syndrome include genetic factors, impaired fetal growth and development, childhood obesity and weight gain to overweight in adult life. This often results in high body mass index (BMI) and characteristic elevated waist circumference from accumulation of intra-abdominal fat. These fat cells are metabolically active and release a range of hormones and cytokines, some of which appear to influence sensitivity to insulin in other tissues. Those with metabolic syndrome have approximately double the predictive risk for cardiovascular diseased compared with individuals without the syndrome.

Pathogenesis

Metabolic syndrome is strongly associated with a 'Westernized' lifestyle of physical inactivity and an unlimited supply of high-fat foods. Insulin resistance is a central component of the metabolic syndrome (Fig. 3.5.1). In these patients, glucose uptake in peripheral tissues is reduced and insulin is unable to suppress glucose production by the liver, promote glucose storage and suppress breakdown of fat. Central fat accumulation is a stronger contributing factor than total body fat.

Conditions linked with metabolic syndrome are type 2 diabetes mellitus, polycystic ovary syndrome and non-alcoholic steatohepatitis.

Investigations

The most widely used criteria for metabolic syndrome are:

- increased visceral fat: waist circumference >40 in (>102 cm) in men or >35 in (>88 cm) in women
- fasting glucose >6.1 mmol/l (>1.1 g/l)

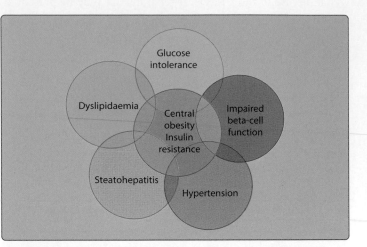

Fig. 3.5.1 Metabolic syndrome. The syndrome is a cluster of interacting conditions with increased risk for type 2 diabetes and cardiovascular disease. Genes, ageing and lifestyles all affect its development.

- blood pressure >130 mmHg/>85 mmHg
- HDL cholesterol: <400 mg/l (1.03 mmol/l) in men, <500 mg/l (1.29 mmol/l) in women
- triglycerides >1.5 g/l (1.7 mmol/l).

An increase in visceral fat accumulation plus any two of the other risk factors confirms the syndrome.

Management

Identifying metabolic syndrome allows early intervention for weight management to prevent cardiovascular disease. Emphasis should be on lifestyle changes to minimize physical inactivity, increase exercise, stop smoking and improve diet. Regular physical exercise (brisk walking for 2–4 h/week) and modest weight loss (approximately 5 kg) can prevent approximately 60% of new cases of diabetes. Indeed quite modest weight loss brings major benefits in all metabolic risk factors for people who are overweight.

Benefits from a 10 kg weight loss in patients initially 100 kg:

- mortality: 20–25% fall in total mortality, 30–40% fall in diabetes-related deaths, 4–50% fall in obesity-related cancer deaths
- blood pressure: 10 mmHg fall in both systolic and diastolic pressure
- diabetes: reduces risk of developing diabetes by >50%, fall of 30–50% in fasting blood glucose, fall of 15% in HbA1c (glycosylated haemoglobin)
- serum lipids: fall of 10% in total cholesterol, fall of 15% in low density lipoprotein (LDL) cholesterol, fall of 30% in triglycerides, increase of 8% in HDL cholesterol.

Antiobesity agents (e.g. orlistat) and hypoglycaemic agents (e.g. metformin and thiazolidinediones) may also have a role.

Hyperlipidaemia

Hyperlipidaemia usually results from a combination of excessive dietary intake and genetic predisposition. Secondary hyperlipidaemia occurs in patients with hypothyroidism, alcohol excess and liver dysfunction, nephrotic syndrome, diabetes mellitus, obesity and drugs, such as steroids, contraceptive pill and thiazide diuretics. Hyperlipidaemia is known to increase the prevalence of atherosclerosis and cardiovascular disease; over 40% of deaths from coronary artery disease are thought to be partly attributable to high lipid levels.

Pathogenesis

Lipids are relatively insoluble and are transported in the bloodstream as lipoproteins. The main types of lipoproteins are chylomicrons, HDL, LDL and intermediate density and very low density lipoproteins. High LDL levels are associated with the development of cardiovascular disease, while HDL has a protective effect.

Clinical features

Hyperlipidaemia is asymptomatic. Most patients are identified during routine screening or further investigation of a cardiovascular event. However, some individuals with inherited disorders of lipids may develop hepatosplenomegaly, pancreatitis or retinal vein occlusion. Individuals with hyperlipidaemia may have palmar, eruptive or tendon xanthomata (fatty deposits over palmar creases, extensor surfaces and tendons (commonly Achilles), respectively; Fig. 3.5.2B). Xanthelasma describes periorbital yellow fatty plaques (Fig. 3.5.2A) and may indicate hyperlipidaemia.

Investigations

Lipids (total, HDL and LDL cholesterol, and triglycerides) should be measured on an overnight fasting blood sample.

Management

Established clinical studies have shown a 34% relative risk reduction in major cardiovascular events in primary prevention and 30% reduction in secondary prevention.

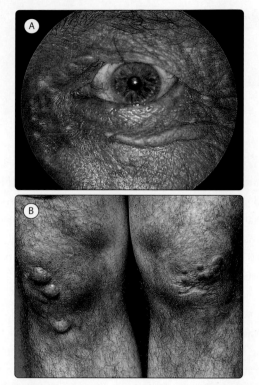

Fig. 3.5.2 Yellowish cholesterol plaques around the eyes (A; xanthelasma) and fatty nodules over the knees (B; eruptive xanthomata). (Reproduced with permission from Douglas G, Nicol F, Robertson C eds 2009 Macleod's Clinical Examination, 12th edn, Churchill Livingstone, Edinburgh.)

Diet and lifestyle. Diet should be low in saturated fats (meat and dairy products) and high in fibre. Monounsaturated and polyunsaturated fats (olive and sunflower oils) should be used for cooking in place of saturated fats. Alcohol consumption should be minimized and weight reduced where necessary.

Drugs. Statins reduce cholesterol synthesis via inhibition of hepatic hydroxymethylglutaryl (HMG) coenzyme A reductase and are more effective than other classes of drug in lowering LDL cholesterol. Statins produce benefits irrespective of the initial cholesterol concentration. Fibrates decrease serum triglycerides. Ezetimibe inhibits intestinal absorption of cholesterol and anion-exchange resins bind bile acids and prevent their reabsorption.

6. Obesity

Questions
- How common is obesity?
- How should obesity be managed?

Obesity is defined as a body mass index (BMI) > 30, where BMI is calculated by weight (kg)/height (m)² (Table 3.6.1). It is widely regarded as a pandemic with potentially disastrous consequences for health. It is associated with an increased risk of multiple conditions (Fig. 3.6.1), including type 2 diabetes (Fig. 3.6.2). It also contributes to the morbidity and mortality from surgical procedures and anaesthesia.

Epidemiology
The prevalence of obesity has increased three-fold since the mid-1980s and in most countries is >15%. Approximately 20% of the adult population is obese in the UK and >30% in the USA. In most of Europe, the prevalence is >20% and is slightly higher in females. Obesity levels are rising in children worldwide.

Pathogenesis
Obesity develops when energy intake exceeds energy expenditure over a long period. Energy balance is usually controlled by short-term signalling of hunger and satiety with hormones derived from the GI tract, long-term signalling of energy stores via leptin and insulin, and control of metabolism. Most obesity develops as a result of modern lifestyles; increased consumption of high-energy foods plus decreased physical activity levels. Often the less affluent seem to be most at risk. Other causes include drugs that increase appetite (e.g. oral steroids) and damage to areas of the brain involved in appetite control (e.g. the hypothalamus).

Clinical features
A careful history can provide useful information: diet, activity, drugs plus weight, height, BMI, waist circumference and cardiovascular risk factors, if indicated.

Investigations
Waist circumference is more directly related to total body fat and the metabolically active visceral fat than BMI.

Management
For effective weight loss, energy intake must be reduced and physical activity increased, ideally through a combination of diet and lifestyle changes. In selected individuals, drugs or surgery can be useful (Figs 3.6.3 and 3.6.4).

Diet
Snacking should be discouraged and smaller portion sizes and limiting the size of plates used may be helpful. Patients should also be advised to avoid having high-energy foods at home, to shop when they are not hungry, and to use a shopping list. Regular meals, particularly breakfast, are important.

Table 3.6.1 RELATIONSHIP BETWEEN BODY MASS INDEX (BMI) AND NUTRITIONAL STATUS

Classification	BMI: non-Asian	BMI: Asian
Underweight	<18.5	<18.5
Normal	18.5–24.9	18.5–22.9
Overweight	25–29.9	23–24.9
Obese	30–40	25–30
Morbidly obese	>40	>30

BMI = weight (kg)/height (m)².

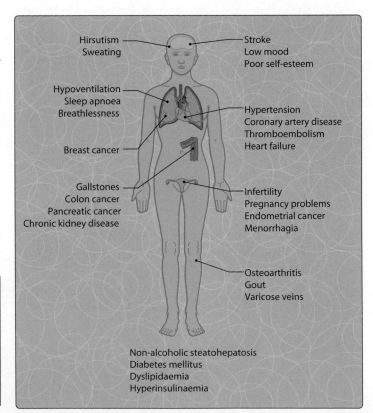

Fig. 3.6.1 Medical consequences of obesity.

Weight-reduction goals and targets should be graded and achievable.

Lifestyle changes

Patients should be encouraged to take more exercise and adopt a healthier overall lifestyle. The main predictors of sustained weight loss are maintenance of high physical activity and regular breakfasts.

Drugs

Drugs are only modestly effective in promoting long-term weight loss (2–4 kg weight loss over 1 year) compared with loss in those not using these agents. Orlistat inhibits pancreatic and gastric lipases, thereby decreasing the hydrolysis of ingested triglycerides and causing malabsorption of 30% of dietary fat. The drug is not absorbed and adverse effects include the passage of loose, oily stools with flatulence and the malabsorption of fat-soluble vitamins.

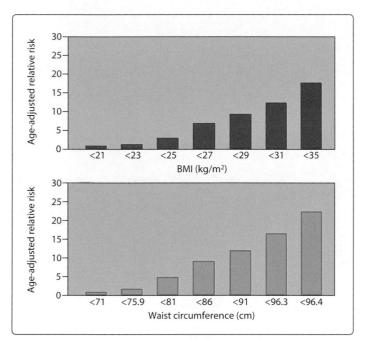

Fig. 3.6.2 Relative risk of developing type 2 diabetes with increasing body mass index (BMI) and waist circumference.

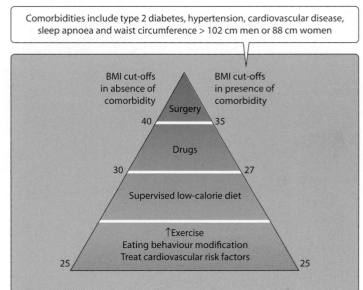

Fig. 3.6.3 Therapeutic options for obesity. BMI, body mass index.

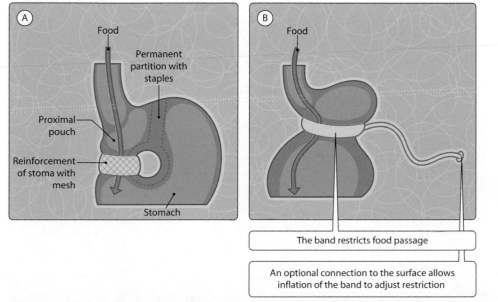

Fig. 3.6.4 Bariatric surgical procedures. A, Vertical banded gastroplasty; B, laparoscopic banding.

Surgery

Motivated patients with a BMI >40 can be considered for bariatric surgery (Fig. 3.6.4). Procedures are either restrictive (reducing dietary intake) or malabsorptive (resulting in nutrient malabsorption). Gastric banding involves placing a prosthetic inflatable band around the upper part of the stomach. It is a relatively simple procedure with low perioperative morbidity and mortality. However, there are risks of infection, erosion and migration of the band. The major cause of operative mortality is pulmonary thromboembolism and, therefore, anticoagulant prophylaxis is essential.

PART IX

Endocrine disorders

John Bevan

The big picture

Endocrinology deals with the synthesis, secretion and action of hormones. The main endocrine glands are the pituitary, thyroid, parathyroids, adrenals and gonads (testes and ovaries) (Fig. 1.1). Endocrinology also involves growth and development, genetics, bone metabolism, late effects of treatment for childhood cancer, fertility and nutrition.

Hormones are chemical messengers secreted directly into the bloodstream to exert their actions on other tissues and organs in the body. They act by binding to specific receptors on or in the target cell. Hormone secretion is either continuous, for example the thyroid hormones (where thyroxine (T_4) has a half life of 7–10 days and triiodothyronine (T_3) of 6–10 h), or intermittent, for example the gonadotrophins (follicle-stimulating hormone (FSH) and luteinizing hormone (LH)), which have pulsatile release from the pituitary depending on the phase of the menstrual cycle.

Although some endocrine glands (e.g. parathyroid glands and pancreas) respond directly to metabolic signals, most are controlled by hormones released from the pituitary gland (Fig. 1.2). Anterior pituitary hormone secretion is controlled by regulators produced in the hypothalamus. Posterior pituitary hormones are synthesized in the hypothalamus, transported down nerve axons and released from the posterior pituitary. A wide variety of molecules act as hormones: peptides (e.g. insulin), glycoproteins (e.g. thyroid-stimulating hormone (TSH)) and amines (e.g. noradrenaline). Some hormones, such as the amines, act on specific cell surface receptors that signal through G-proteins and other transduction mechanisms. Other hormones such as steroids, T_3 and vitamin D bind to specific intracellular receptors that, in turn, bind to DNA to regulate gene transcription.

Patients with endocrine disease present in many ways, reflecting the diverse effects of hormone deficiency and excess:

- hormone excess
  — primary gland overproduction
  — secondary to excess of trophic hormone

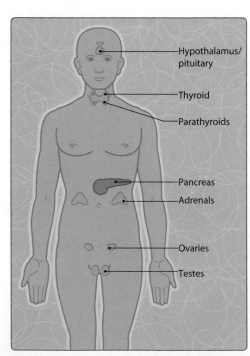

Fig. 1.1 The principal endocrine glands.

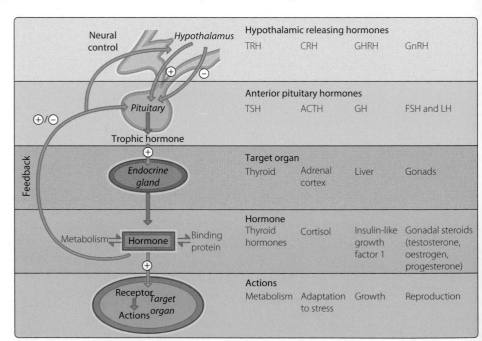

Fig. 1.2 The endocrine axes. TRH, thyrotrophin-releasing hormone; TSH, thyroid-stimulating hormone; thyroid hormones, thyroxine and triiodothyronine; CRH, corticotrophin-releasing hormone; ACTH, adrenocorticotrophic hormone (corticotrophin); GHRH, growth hormone-releasing hormone; GH, growth hormone; GnRH, gonadotrophin-releasing hormone; FSH, follicle-stimulating hormone; LH, luteinizing hormone.

- hormone deficiency
  — primary gland failure
  — secondary to deficient trophic hormone
- hypersensitivity to hormone
  — failure of inactivation of hormone
  — target organ hypersensitivity
- resistance to hormone
  — failure of activation of hormone
  — target organ resistance
- non-functioning tumours.

For many patients, endocrine disease is asymptomatic and detected only by routine biochemical testing. Diagnosis relies on precise biochemical measurements, supported by multimodal imaging techniques. Many endocrine conditions have specific therapies that have been developed from knowledge of basic endocrine physiology and biochemistry. Close links with specialist pituitary, thyroid and adrenal surgical teams are vital for best endocrine outcomes.

Some endocrine conditions are very common. For example, a woman's lifetime risk of thyroid dysfunction is > 5%, and polycystic ovary syndrome affects up to 10% of an increasingly obese young female population. Hypogonadism is surprisingly common in men but often remains undiagnosed (Klinefelter's syndrome occurs in 1:600 men). In contrast, some endocrine disorders are rare but nevertheless potentially life threatening (e.g. Addison's disease and phaeochromocytoma). Other examples include:

- common
  — type 2 diabetes mellitus: 4–8% prevalence (increasing with obesity)
  — primary hypothyroidism: 2% prevalence (5% including subclinical disease), mostly females
  — polycystic ovary syndrome: 6–8% prevalence, depending on definition of the disorder
- moderately common
  — hyperthyroidism: 1% prevalence (80% Graves' disease, 80% in females)
  — type 1 diabetes mellitus: 0.5% prevalence (increasing in children)
  — male hypogonadism: 1–2% prevalence depending on definition

- uncommon
  — hypopituitarism: prevalence 50–100/1 000 000
  — Addison's disease: prevalence 50/1 000 000 (Western world, mostly autoimmune)
  — differentiated thyroid cancer: annual new case incidence of 50/1 000 000
- rare
  — carcinoid tumour: annual new case incidence 20/1 000 000
  — pituitary-dependent Cushing's disease: annual new case incidence 5/1 000 000
  — acromegaly: annual new case incidence 4/1 000 000.

The vast majority of endocrine disorders result either from a tumour arising within endocrine tissues or from an autoimmune reaction that results in tissue destruction.

There are four principles underpinning endocrine diagnosis.

1. Endocrine symptoms are often non-specific so the clinician has to think of an endocrine diagnosis. For example, in a tired patient, thyroid disturbance or adrenal insufficiency should always be considered.
2. In any endocrine situation, ask 'Is there too much hormone being produced?' 'Is there too little being produced?' 'Could a tumour be involved?'
3. If there is too much hormone being produced, a useful endocrine test will assess whether it can be suppressed (e.g. growth hormone suppression following glucose loading in suspected acromegaly). Conversely, if there is too little hormone the endocrine test should evaluate whether it can be stimulated (e.g. Synacthen testing to stimulate cortisol release in suspected Addison's disease).
4. The best endocrine gland imaging modality should be selected. For example, MRI is preferred for the pituitary, CT for the adrenals and ultrasound for the gonads.

Endocrinology is a 'quality of life' speciality: body image, body weight, energy levels and psychological well-being are all commonly affected by endocrine disorders. Remarkably, all of these can be normalized in a hypothyroid patient by T_4 replacement costing less than 20p/day. Other endocrine therapies, such as growth hormone or octreotide, are more expensive but improve life quality and expectancy.

High-return facts

1 **Pituitary** tumours are most commonly benign adenomas. Prolactinoma is the most common functioning pituitary tumour. Acromegaly is caused by growth hormone hypersecretion from a pituitary tumour and develops insidiously. Pituitary tumours can expand and compress surrounding structures. Hypopituitarism is usually caused by a large pituitary tumour compressing the normal gland. Symptoms of anterior hypopituitarism reflect deficiencies of target gland hormones, and treatment is by replacement of these hormones. **Diabetes insipidus** results from deficient secretion of antidiuretic hormone (ADH) from the posterior pituitary. Characteristic features include marked polydipsia (including at night) and polyuria. Treatment of cranial diabetes insipidus involves desmopressin, an orally active analogue of ADH.

2 **Hyperthyroidism** occurs in 2% of the UK female population; 80% is caused by autoimmune Graves' disease. The most common symptoms are weight loss (despite an increased appetite), heat intolerance, sweating, irritability, palpitation and tremor. Atrial fibrillation may be the presenting feature in the elderly. Serum free thyroxine and triiodothyronine are usually both raised; thyroid-stimulating hormone is suppressed and undetectable. Relative triiodothyronine toxicosis occurs in 5–10%. First-line therapy of Graves' disease is a 12–18 month course of the antithyroid drug carbimazole. However, 60% relapse and require definitive treatment with radioiodine or surgery. **Hypothyroidism** occurs in 2% of the population (rising to 5% if subclinical disease is included) and the female: male ratio is 6:1. In iodine-sufficient populations, Hashimoto's thyroiditis is the usual cause. Hypothyroidism should be considered in women with tiredness and weight gain. Asymptomatic patients with raised serum thyroid-stimulating hormone (TSH) and positive thyroid autoantibodies have a 5% annual risk of overt hypothyroidism. Thyroxine is started at a low dose and titrated against TSH. Most hypothyroid women require an increased dose of thyroxine during pregnancy.

3 **Thyroid swellings** include simple diffuse and multi-nodular goitres and solitary thyroid nodules. Fine needle aspiration cytology is the investigation of choice for solitary thyroid nodules. **Thyroid cancer** usually presents as a lump in the neck without associated symptoms. Treatment is total thyroidectomy, usually followed by ablative radioiodine therapy. Overall survival for papillary thyroid cancer is > 90% after 20 years.

4 **Hyperparathyroidism** is the usual cause of hypercalcaemia found in up to 5% of hospitalized patients. Most hyperparathyroid patients require surgical removal of a solitary adenoma. **Hypoparathyroidism** may present several years after thyroid surgery.

5 **Cushing's syndrome** usually results from prolonged oral steroid treatment for non-endocrine illness (e.g. asthma or inflammatory bowel disease). Endogenous Cushing's syndrome is caused by an ACTH-secreting pituitary adenoma or, rarely, a cortisol-secreting adrenal tumour. Clinical features include skin atrophy, spontaneous purpura, proximal myopathy and osteoporosis. Untreated, the 5-year mortality of endogenous Cushing's syndrome approaches 50%. **Addison's disease** is most commonly caused by autoimmune adrenalitis in the developed world but tuberculosis is also a common cause worldwide. Symptoms are typically vague. Treatment is oral hydrocortisone in several doses distributed across the day. **Adrenal tumours** are found incidentally in 5% of abdominal scans. **Conn's syndrome** is primary hyperaldosteronism caused by a tumour of the adrenal cortex and accounts for at least 2% of hypertensive patients. **Phaeochromocytomas** are catecholamine-secreting tumours derived from the adrenal medulla and are much rarer.

6 **Erectile dysfunction** affects 10% of all adult men and over half of those > 70 years. Klinefelter's syndrome is the commonest cause of primary hypogonadism in men. **Amenorrhoea** can be either primary or secondary. Primary amenorrhoea is the failure of menarche to occur by age16 years. Secondary amenorrhoea is disappearance of periods for 6 months or longer in a woman who has previously menstruated. The commonest cause of secondary amenorrhoea is pregnancy.

7 **Infertility** affects 10–15% of all couples. Female factors (e.g. polycystic ovary syndrome, tubal damage) are responsible in 35%, and male factors (mostly idiopathic germ cell failure) in 30%. Both partners should be seen at the first consultation to avoid unnecessary investigations.

1. Pituitary gland disorders

Questions
- What are the clinical features of acromegaly?
- How is the diagnosis of hypopituitarism confirmed?

Secretion from the anterior pituitary is largely regulated by hypothalamic hormones that reach the pituitary through the bloodstream. The posterior pituitary stores hormones, synthesized in the hypothalamic nuclei that pass down axons into it for later release. The two main hormones are oxytocin (which contracts the smooth muscle of the uterus) and antidiuretic hormone (ADH, vasopressin).

Pituitary tumours

Diseases of the pituitary are rare. The most common is a benign adenoma of the anterior pituitary, which may be functioning or non-functioning and if large may cause pressure effects.

Clinical features

Symptoms suggestive of a possible pituitary tumour include:
- prolactinoma (most common): galactorrhoea and secondary amenorrhoea in premenopausal women, reduced libido and erectile dysfunction in men
- acromegaly (growth hormone (GH)): enlargement of hands and feet, jaw protrusion, sweating, snoring, arthralgia, carpal tunnel syndrome, gigantism if before puberty
- Cushing's disease (adrenocorticotrophic hormone (ACTH)): central weight gain, proximal myopathy, spontaneous bruising, low-stress fractures

- headache, visual disturbance ('blinkered' vision or diplopia)
- 'tired all the time' plus low free thyroxine (T_4)/normal thyroid-stimulating hormone (TSH) (TSH deficiency), low sodium (cortisol deficiency) or low/normal follicle-stimulating hormone (FSH) in a postmenopausal woman (hypopituitarism).

Features of acromegaly develop insidiously and if untreated acromegaly may shorten life by 10 years owing to associated hypertension, diabetes mellitus, cardiomyopathy and sleep apnoea.

Pressure effects arise because the pituitary gland is contained within the sella turcica in the base of the skull. Suprasellar extension compressing the optic chiasm produces bitemporal hemianopia (crossing nasal fibres subserving the temporal fields of vision; Fig. 3.1.2). Medical or surgical decompression often results in visual improvement.

Investigations

Serum levels of T_4, cortisol, gonadotrophins (FSH and luteinizing hormone (LH)) and sex steroids (testosterone/oestradiol) should be measured. Elevated prolactin may suggest prolactinoma. Diagnosis of acromegaly rests on the failure of GH to suppress during a glucose tolerance test, plus elevated blood GH-dependent insulin-like growth factor 1 (IGF-1). Gadolinium-enhanced MRI is the preferred imaging modality.

Management

Nearly all prolactinomas respond to dopamine agonists (e.g. cabergoline) and many with acromegaly experience substantial GH/IGF-1 suppression with a somatostatin analogue (e.g. octreotide). Successful hormone lowering is often accompanied by tumour shrinkage. Transsphenoidal surgery is still required for non-functioning and ACTH-secreting tumours. Postoperative radiotherapy is occasionally needed.

Hypopituitarism

Hypopituitarism is usually caused by a large pituitary tumour compressing the normal gland and disrupting control mechanisms. Previous pituitary haemorrhage/infarction (e.g. Sheehan's syndrome, following delivery), severe head injury and cranial irradiation are other causes.

Clinical features

Symptoms of hypopituitarism are caused by deficiencies of target gland hormones and are often non-specific. GH deficiency produces growth failure in children and a syndrome in adults,

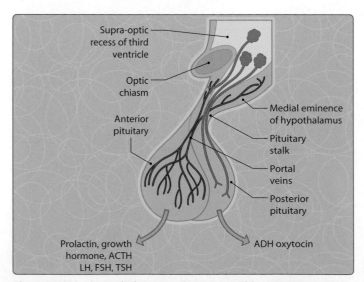

Fig. 3.1.1 The hypothalamus and pituitary. Abbreviations in text.

with reduced exercise capacity and lean body mass, impaired psychological well-being and increased cardiovascular risk.

Investigations

Blood tests include low free T_4 with low or normal TSH, hyponatraemia, normochromic, normocytic anaemia, low testosterone with low/normal FSH/LH (men) and low or premenopausal FSH/LH (women > 50 years).

Dynamic pituitary function tests are used to diagnose ACTH and GH deficiencies; the insulin hypoglycaemia test is the 'gold standard' (Fig. 3.1.3) but cannot be used in patients with heart disease or epilepsy.

Synacthen testing is used to assess cortisol reserve.

Management

Correction of pituitary hormone deficiencies requires replacement of target gland hormones. T_4 is given as a single daily oral dose titrated against serum free T_4, not TSH. Hydrocortisone is given orally two to three times daily to mimic circadian rhythm. In men, testosterone is given by depot i.m. injection or daily topical gel. Sex steroid replacement in women involves the oral contraceptive pill or a 'menopausal' preparation. GH is given by daily s.c. injection and the dose adjusted according to the serum IGF-1 and quality of life scoring. Complex gonadotrophin regimens are needed to treat infertility caused by pituitary disease.

Diabetes insipidus

Cranial diabetes insipidus results from deficient secretion of ADH by the posterior pituitary. Causes include craniopharyngioma, neurosarcoidosis, hypophysitis, head injury, neurosurgery. If a patient is taking lithium, renal resistance to ADH can occur (nephrogenic diabetes insipidus). Characteristic features include marked polydipsia (including during the night) and polyuria (large volumes of light-coloured, dilute urine). Diabetes mellitus, hypokalaemia, hypercalcaemia and renal failure should be excluded. The diagnosis is confirmed by a water deprivation test in an experienced unit since severe water depletion can occur. Diabetes insipidus is confirmed by serum osmolality > 300 mOsm/kg, urine osmolality < 600 mOsm/kg, persistent polyuria and weight loss during deprivation. Cranial diabetes insipidus is confirmed by a rise in urine osmolality to > 600 mOsm/kg after the administration of the vasopressin analogue desmopressin (DDAVP).

Long-term treatment of cranial diabetes insipidus involves replacement of ADH using DDAVP, given orally or intranasally.

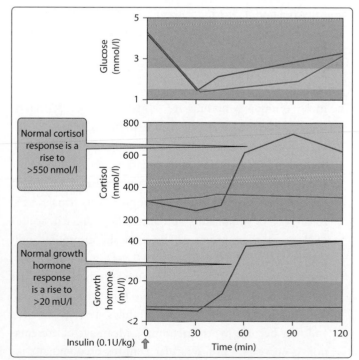

Fig. 3.1.3 The insulin hypoglycaemia test uses a bolus of insulin to cause hypoglycaemia (should be < 2.2 mmol/l) and then responses are followed. The normal response is given in green and the response in hypopituitarism is in red. The normal response ranges are given as pale blue bands.

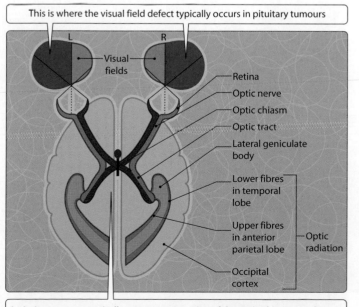

Fig. 3.1.2 Optic pathways and mechanism of bitemporal hemianopia.

2. Hyper- and hypothyroidism

Questions
- What are the clinical features of hyperthyroidism?
- How common is hypothyroidism?

The thyroid secretes three main hormones: thyroxine (T_4), tri-iodothyronine (T_3) (the thyroid hormones) and calcitonin (see Part VII, Ch. 2). T_4 and T_3 are critically important for normal growth and development and energy metabolism. Synthesis of the thyroid hormones requires a supply of iodide. Thyroid disease is common. Significant non-thyroidal illness (e.g. infection or surgery) also affects thyroid function tests (e.g. reduced free T_3 and thyroid-stimulating hormone (TSH)). Features that should prompt testing include tired all the time, weight change, change in bowel habit, thirst, sweating, hyponatraemia, carpal tunnel syndrome, anxiety or depression, menstrual disturbance, goitre, atrial fibrillation and macrocytosis.

Hyperthyroidism

Hyperthyroidism occurs in 2% of the UK female population and is 10 times more common in females than in males. The annual incidence of new cases is 3/1000 in females. Most result from Graves' disease (80%), multinodular goitre (10%) or an autonomous thyroid nodule (toxic adenoma: 5%). Less common causes include destructive thyroiditis (viral or autoimmune) and drugs (e.g. amiodarone).

Clinical features

The most common symptoms are shown in Fig. 3.2.1. Atrial fibrillation may be the presenting feature in the elderly.

Graves' disease. Typically there is diffuse thyroid enlargement, thyroid ophthalmopathy (inflammation and swelling of the extraocular muscles) and (rarely) pretibial myxoedema. It occurs at any age but most commonly affects females aged 20–50 years. Stimulatory autoantibodies directed against TSH receptors are produced by genetically susceptible individuals (*HLA-B8*, *HLA-DR3* and *HLA-DR2* in Caucasians) and lead to increased thyroid hormone synthesis and goitre formation. The natural history varies (Fig. 3.2.2).

Toxic multinodular goitre. Benign nodules develop with age and may become hyperfunctioning. Mean age of presentation is 60 years. Cardiovascular features predominate, including atrial fibrillation and heart failure.

Toxic adenoma. Most nodules are palpable and the rest of the thyroid atrophic and impalpable: diagnosis can only be made with certainty using scintigraphy (Fig. 3.2.3).

Investigations

Serum free T_4 and T_3 are usually both raised, but relative T_3 toxicosis occurs in 5–10%. TSH is suppressed and undetectable. Older patients with comorbidities (e.g. ischaemic heart disease) may present with lower thyroid hormone levels. Thyroid scintiscans distinguish the main causes.

Management

Graves' disease. First-line therapy is a 12–18 month course of carbimazole, which reduces thyroid hormone synthesis. Side-effects include rash (2%) and agranulocytosis (0.1%). Definitive treatment using either radioiodine or thyroidectomy can be offered to the 60% who relapse after carbimazole. Graves' ophthalmopathy is more common in smokers and may be exacerbated by radioiodine therapy.

Toxic multinodular goitre. Radioiodine is the treatment of choice: the risk of subsequent hypothyroidism is lower than in Graves' disease because a multinodular gland is more resistant to radiation. Long-term, low-dose carbimazole may be appropriate for frail elderly patients.

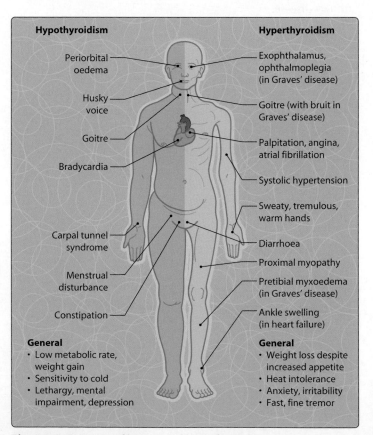

Fig. 3.2.1 Features of hyper- and hypothyroidism.

Toxic adenoma. Radioiodine is effective and has a relatively low risk of hypothyroidism since atrophic thyroid cells take up little isotope and regain function after the nodule has been treated. Partial thyroidectomy is an alternative approach.

Hypothyroidism

Thyroid failure occurs in 2% of the population, with a female: male ratio of 6:1. This rises to 5% if subclinical hypothyroidism is included (normal free T_4 and raised TSH). Autoantibodies against thyroid peroxidase are found in 10% of women > 60 years. Neonatal screening shows an incidence of 1/3000 births.

In iodine-sufficient populations, over 90% of hypothyroidism is caused by **Hashimoto's thyroiditis** or radioiodine or surgical treatment for hyperthyroidism. Congenital hypothyroidism results from thyroid agenesis, hypoplastic glands or a defect in thyroid hormone synthesis (dyshormonogenesis). Drug-induced hypothyroidism occurs in patients on long-term lithium or amiodarone.

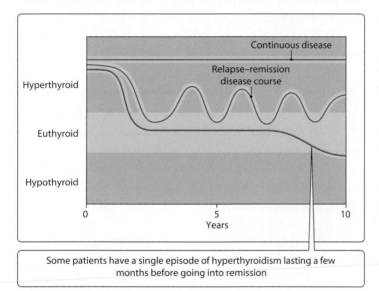

Some patients have a single episode of hyperthyroidism lasting a few months before going into remission

Fig. 3.2.2 The variable natural history of Graves' disease.

Clinical features

Common symptoms are shown in Fig. 3.2.1. Other features, such as pericardial/pleural effusions, ascites, cerebellar ataxia and psychosis, are rare.

Investigations

In primary hypothyroidism, serum free T_4 is low and TSH elevated. If TSH is not raised, secondary hypothyroidism from hypothalamo-pituitary disease should be considered. Thyroid peroxidase autoantibodies suggest autoimmune thyroiditis.

Management

Thyroxine is usually started at a low dose of 50 μg daily, increasing to 100 μg after 2 weeks. Replacement should be started cautiously in patients with ischaemic heart disease (e.g. 25 μg daily). Subsequent dose titrations should be made against serum TSH. T_4 is converted to T_3 in tissues by deiodinase and there is no additional benefit from combined T_4 and T_3 replacement. Most patients are treated adequately with 100–150 μg daily; doses > 200 μg suggest poor compliance or T_4 malabsorption (e.g. in coeliac disease). Symptom improvement usually occurs within 2–3 weeks and complete recovery after 3 months. Asymptomatic patients with raised TSH and positive thyroid autoantibodies have a 5% annual risk of clinical hypothyroidism; most should receive thyroxine.

In pregnancy, most hypothyroid women require an increased thyroxine dose (50–100 μg increment). Adequate serum levels of thyroid hormones during pregnancy are important for the child's neuropsychological development. Pregnancy may also unmask previously unsuspected autoimmune thyroid disease in euthyroid women with positive thyroid peroxidase antibodies.

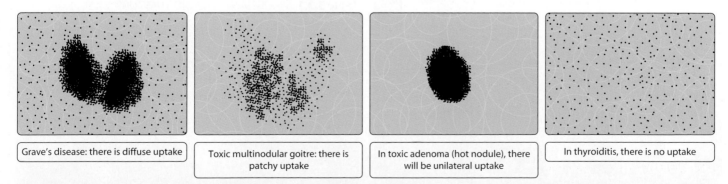

Grave's disease: there is diffuse uptake

Toxic multinodular goitre: there is patchy uptake

In toxic adenoma (hot nodule), there will be unilateral uptake

In thyroiditis, there is no uptake

Fig. 3.2.3 Thyroid scintiscans. The three most common causes of hyperthyroidism are Graves' disease (80%), toxic multinodular goitre (10%) and toxic adenoma (5%).

3. Thyroid swellings and cancer

Questions
- What types of thyroid swelling are there?
- What is the management of thyroid cancer?

Simple goitre

Simple goitre is defined as diffuse or multinodular thyroid enlargement that occurs with no known cause (Fig. 3.3.1). Patients are euthyroid, mostly female and may have a family history of goitre. **Simple diffuse goitre** often presents during pregnancy. Autoantibodies are negative and no treatment is required. The goitre commonly regresses with time but the gland become multinodular over several decades. **Simple multinodular goitre** can be very large with mediastinal extension, and may cause stridor or dysphagia. Approximately 30% of patients develop biochemical hyperthyroidism. Even very large goitres can be shrunk successfully with high-dose radioiodine; surgery is an alternative approach.

Solitary thyroid nodule

It is important to determine whether nodules are benign (e.g. cyst or colloid nodule) or malignant. Extremes of age and a past history of neck irradiation increase the probability of malignancy. Fine needle aspiration cytology (FNAC) is the investigation of choice and will differentiate benign (80%) from suspicious or malignant nodules (20%). It cannot distinguish between follicular adenoma and cancer. It is important to check thyroid function and consider the possibility of a toxic adenoma, which is virtually always benign.

Thyroid cancer

Thyroid cancer is the commonest endocrine malignancy but accounts for <1% of all cancers. Most arise from thyroid hormone-synthesizing cells and are well differentiated (Table 3.3.1). Papillary cancers spread to regional lymph nodes and carry a better prognosis than follicular cancers, which undergo blood-borne spread. Medullary tumours arise from thyroid C-cells, secrete calcitonin and are familial in 25%.

Most thyroid cancers present as a lump in the neck without associated symptoms. Undifferentiated anaplastic tumours are locally invasive and commonly cause stridor and recurrent laryngeal nerve palsy.

Management

Treatment is total thyroidectomy for most thyroid cancers, usually followed by radioiodine therapy. Since thyroid-stimulating hormone acts as a thyroid growth stimulator, its secretion needs to be suppressed by thyroxine (150–200 µg daily). Follow-up is by measuring thyroid-specific protein (thyroglobulin) and whole-body isotope scanning using radioiodine. Thyroid lymphoma can occur with Hashimoto's thyroiditis and usually responds dramatically to radiotherapy.

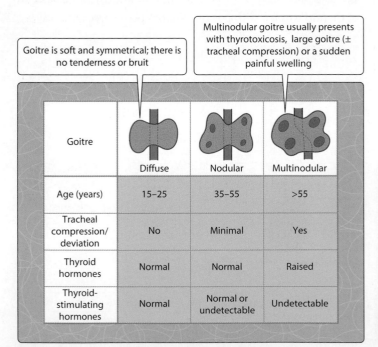

Fig. 3.3.1 Features of different types of goitre.

Table 3.3.1 MALIGNANT THYROID TUMOURS

Type	Frequency (%)	Age (years) at presentation	Survival, 20-year (%)
Papillary	70	20–40	95
Follicular	10	40–60	60
Undifferentiated, anaplastic	5	> 60	< 1
Medullary carcinoma	5–10	> 40	50
Lymphoma	5–10	> 60	10

4. Parathyroid gland disorders

Questions
- How is hyperparathyroidism diagnosed?
- What are the clinical features of hypoparathyroidism?

Calcium homostasis

Serum calcium is regulated by parathormone (PTH) and activated vitamin D_3, with a minor contribution from calcitonin (Fig. 3.4.1). Since approximately 40% of serum calcium is bound to albumin, total serum calcium should be adjusted for albumin (add/subtract 0.02 mmol/l for every 1 g/l of albumin below/above 40 g/l).

Hypercalcaemia is found in 5% of inpatients and is usually caused by hyperparathyroidism (primary or tertiary) or malignancy (PTH-related protein production, myeloma, bony metastases). Secondary hyperparathyroidism occurs in coeliac disease or chronic kidney disease. It is associated with hypocalcaemia not hypercalcaemia. Other less-common causes of hypercalcaemia are vitamin D intoxication, sarcoidosis and familial hypocalciuric hypercalcaemia. Rare causes are immobilization, thiazide diuretics, thyrotoxicosis and Addison's disease. **Hypocalcaemia** is much less common and usually caused by vitamin D deficiency.

Hyperparathyroidism

The female:male ratio is 3:1 for hyperparathyroidism and most patients are >50 years. The primary form is caused by a solitary parathyroid adenoma in > 90%, multiple adenomata (4%), nodular hyperplasia (5%) and cancer (<1%). Hyperparathyroidism may be part of **multiple endocrine neoplasia syndromes** (MEN1 and 2a). Chronic renal disease and long-standing vitamin D deficiency lead to secondary hyperparathyroidism (parathyroid gland hyperplasia in response to hypocalcaemia), which may progress to tertiary hyperparathyroidism (autonomous adenomata).

Clinical features

Most patients are identified by 'routine' blood tests, and rarely by 'moans' (depression), 'bones' (parathyroid bone disease) and 'abdominal groans' (hypercalcaemia or renal colic). Symptoms of hypercalcaemia include thirst, polyuria, lethargy, anorexia, nausea, constipation, drowsiness and impaired cognition. Severe dehydration may be present.

Investigations

Calcium, albumin, phosphate (low) and PTH are measured in a fasting, morning blood sample (inappropriately raised PTH in the presence of hypercalcaemia). A 24 h urinary calcium excretion is usually upper normal or high. Baseline bone densitometry should assess for secondary osteoporosis. Concordance between ^{99m}Tc-sestamibi (methoxyisobutylisonitrile) uptake and ultrasound scanning is used for localization of the glands prior to parathyroid adenomectomy.

Management

Severe hypercalcaemia requires emergency treatment with i.v. saline and bisphosphonate (e.g. i.v. pamidronate). Parathyroid adenoma can be resected. For hyperplasia, all the parathyroid glands can be removed with autotransplantation of parathyroid tissue to the forearm, for later removal if hypercalcaemia recurs.

Hypoparathyroidism

The usual cause of hypoparathyroidism is damage to the glands or blood supply during thyroid surgery. Functional hypoparathyroidism occurs in severe magnesium deficiency.

Clinical features

Low calcium induces neural excitability, with distal tingling and carpopedal spasm. Trousseau's sign may reveal latent tetany (carpal muscle spasm after blood pressure cuff inflation above arterial blood pressure for 3 min). Investigations are as for hyperparathyroidism (PTH low or inappropriately normal in the presence of hypocalcaemia).

Management

Severe hypocalcaemic tetany requires i.v. infusion of 10% calcium gluconate. Magnesium supplements may also be required. Oral 1α-hydroxycholecalciferol (alfacalcidol) is used long term.

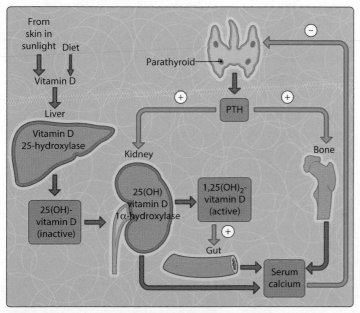

Fig. 3.4.1 Calcium homeostasis PTH, parathormone.

5. Adrenal gland disorders

Questions
- What are the clinical features of Cushing's syndrome?
- How is a diagnosis of Addison's disease confirmed?

Cushing's syndrome

Iatrogenic Cushing's syndrome is usually caused by prolonged oral steroids. Severe depression or alcoholism may cause abnormal cortisol metabolism and a pseudo-Cushingoid state. Endogenous Cushing's syndrome results from cortisol hyper-secretion. This can occur from excess adrenocorticotrophic hormone (ACTH) production (from a pituitary adenoma (incidence only 2/1 000 000) or ectopic ACTH secretion by other tumour types, e.g. carcinoid) or rarely from excess cortisol secretion (usually a benign adrenal adenoma).

Clinical features

Hypercortisolism causes tissue breakdown (atrophy of skin, muscle and bone), sodium retention (hypertension, heart failure) and insulin antagonism (diabetes mellitus) (Fig. 3.5.1).

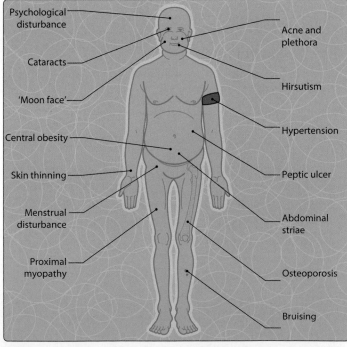

Psychological disturbance
Cataracts
'Moon face'
Central obesity
Skin thinning
Menstrual disturbance
Proximal myopathy

Acne and plethora
Hirsutism
Hypertension
Peptic ulcer
Abdominal striae
Osteoporosis
Bruising

Fig. 3.5.1 Features of Cushing's syndrome.

Investigations

There are two main steps:

- measurement of 24 h urinary free cortisol excretion or an overnight dexamethasone suppression test: failure of serum cortisol to suppress confirms hypercortisolism
- plasma ACTH measurement, prolonged dexamethasone suppression and corticotrophin-releasing hormone stimulation tests, plus appropriate radiology.

In ACTH-dependent disease and equivocal test results, inferior petrosal sinus blood sampling may be necessary to confirm the pituitary as the source of ACTH.

Management

Pituitary adenoma is treated by selective transsphenoidal adenomectomy. Primary adrenal tumours may be removed by laparoscopy although adrenal function often takes many months to recover. In ectopic ACTH production, the primary tumour should be removed. Untreated, the 5-year mortality of endogenous Cushing's syndrome approaches 50%, through vascular disease and susceptibility to infection.

Addison's disease

Destruction of the adrenal cortex leads to combined glucocorticoid (cortisol) and mineralocorticoid (aldosterone) deficiencies. Autoimmune adrenalitis causes > 80% of cases in the developed world but tuberculosis is the most common cause worldwide. Other rarer causes of adrenal insufficiency include adrenal haemorrhage in disseminated intravascular coagulation or adrenal vein thrombosis in antiphospholipid syndrome.

Clinical features

Symptoms are non-specific and include:

- disproportion between illness severity and the degree of circulatory collapse
- postural dizziness and syncope (postural hypotension)
- pigmentation (skin creases, buccal mucosa, recent scars): not in all patients
- vitiligo (an associated autoimmune condition)
- unexplained hypoglycaemia (reduced insulin antagonism)
- unexplained vomiting or diarrhoea
- hyponatraemia (often with raised serum potassium ions)
- other endocrine features (amenorrhoea, body hair loss)
- associated type 1 diabetes mellitus, thyroid disease, pernicious anaemia or coeliac disease
- refractory depression.

Investigations

In untreated Addison's disease, serum sodium is usually low and potassium elevated (from aldosterone deficiency). If a random serum cortisol is >700 nmol/l, Addison's disease is unlikely; further testing is required if it is <700 nmol/l. Synacthen (synthetic analogue of ACTH) test shows reduced or absent cortisol increment (Fig. 3.5.2). Raised basal ACTH before Synacthen confirms primary adrenal insufficiency. Adrenal autoantibodies are present in 70% of autoimmune disease. Thyroid function tests commonly show compensated hypothyroidism that normalizes after hydrocortisone replacement (thyroxine treatment is potentially hazardous in untreated Addison's disease and may precipitate adrenal crisis).

Management

In an acute Addisonian crisis, patients need i.v. saline and hydrocortisone. The hydrocortisone dose is subsequently tapered over a few days and continued orally. Steroid education and self-care are important (Box 3.5.1). Patients with primary adrenal failure require additional mineralocorticoid replacement with fludrocortisone. Patients with autoimmune Addison's should be screened for other endocrinopathies.

Adrenal tumours

'Incidentalomas'. Incidental adrenal swellings are revealed by 5% of abdominal CT/MRI. Most are small (<2 cm), lipid-rich, non-functioning adenomas. If the patient is hypertensive, hypokalaemic or diabetic, serum electrolytes, renin/aldosterone and 24 h urinary free cortisol and catecholamines should be checked. Endocrine-active lesions should be surgically removed. Lesions <2 cm in diameter with negative endocrine tests do not require follow-up. Lesions >5 cm in diameter have a risk of malignancy and should be removed.

Hyperaldosteronism (Conn's syndrome). Conn's syndrome usually occurs in a hypertensive woman aged 40–70 years with a unilateral adrenal adenoma (<2.5 cm) on imaging. Primary hyperaldosteronism accounts for at least 2% of hypertensive patients. There is sodium retention and hypokalaemic alkalosis. Serum potassium is normal in approximately 25% and renin/aldosterone measurement is necessary for precise diagnosis. Hypertension is cured in 70% after surgical removal. An aldosterone antagonist (spironolactone or eplerenone) can be used in bilateral disease.

Phaeochromocytoma. These catecholamine-secreting tumours derive from the adrenal medulla (Fig. 3.5.3); paragangliomas are related tumours derived from extra-adrenal neural crest-derived tissues. Phaeochromocytomas account for <0.1% of those with hypertension. Patients present with paroxysmal headache, sweating, palpitation, fear, tremor, extreme pallor and hypertension. Diagnosis is established by raised plasma and urinary catecholamine levels in combination with positive radionuclide imaging with ^{123}I-mIBG. Most phaeochromocytomas are benign and solitary; cure is achieved with surgical removal. Phaeochromocytomas/paragangliomas are known as the '10% tumours': 10% are extra-adrenal, 10% malignant, 10% multiple (both adrenals), 10% associated with diabetes mellitus and 10% familial (e.g. multiple endocrine neoplasia type II).

BOX 3.5.1 IMPORTANT SELF-CARE ADVICE FOR PATIENTS ON ORAL STEROIDS

- Never miss steroid doses
- Double the hydrocortisone dose in event of intercurrent illness (e.g. infection)
- If severe vomiting or diarrhoea, call for urgent medical assistance (or administer parenteral hydrocortisone)
- Wear a Medic-Alert device
- Carry an up-to-date steroid card
- Carry hydrocortisone in hand luggage.

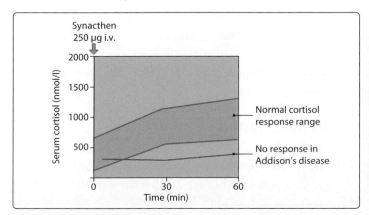

Fig. 3.5.2 A short Synacthen test.

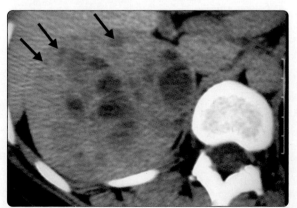

Fig. 3.5.3 CT of the abdomen showing a large phaeochromocytoma (arrows) adjacent to a lumbar vertebra.

6. Reproductive system disorders

Questions
- What are the causes of erectile dysfunction?
- How should premature ovarian failure be managed?

The male system: erectile dysfunction

Figure 3.6.1 shows the production and role of male sex hormones.

Erectile dysfunction (ED) affects 10% of all adult men and over half of those > 70 years. It may occur through several mechanisms:
- libido reduced
  — hypogonadism: either primary (Klinefelter's syndrome (47XXY), the commonest cause of male hypogonadism (1:600 males); orchitis; chemotherapy; radiotherapy; trauma; varicocele) or secondary (hypopituitarism, hyperprolactinaemia, Kallmann's syndrome (isolated gonadotrophin deficiency), haemochromatosis)
  — depression and major psychiatric illness

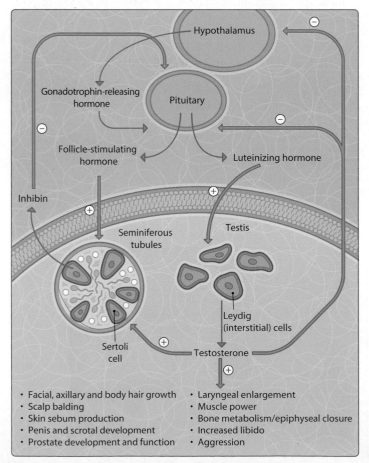

- libido intact
  — psychological problems (stress, anxiety)
  — drugs (beta-blockers, benzodiazepines, alcohol, heroin)
  — vascular insufficiency (atherosclerosis, diabetes)
  — neurological disorders (peripheral neuropathy, diabetes, multiple sclerosis)
  — penile abnormalities (Peyronie's disease).

Clinical features

A detailed history is essential and includes sexual history (presence of morning erections), symptoms of hypogonadism (reduced libido), past medical history (diabetes, vascular disease, neurological problems, psychological illness) and drug and social history (alcohol, 'recreational' drugs). Signs of hypogonadism include fine skin, sparse sexual hair, reduced testicular size and consistency.

Investigations

Assays include early morning serum testosterone (testosterone has a circadian variation), prolactin, luteinizing hormone (LH) and follicle-stimulating hormone (FSH) (LH and FSH raised in primary hypogonadism). Secondary causes are excluded by thyroid function tests, fasting glucose, liver function tests, lipids and ferritin (haemochromatosis). Klinefelter's syndrome can be confirmed by karyotyping.

Management

The underlying disorder should be treated (including psychosexual therapy) and, if possible, any drugs implicated withdrawn. Men with hypogonadism and/or hyperprolactinaemia may require androgen replacement and dopamine agonists. Oral phosphodiesterase inhibitors (e.g. sildenafil) amplify the vasodilatory action of nitric oxide and thus the erectile response to sexual stimulation. They should be used with caution in men with recent stroke or ischaemic heart disease and cannot be used with nitrates; headache and colour vision disturbance are common side-effects. Other treatments include intracavernous prostaglandin injections, vacuum devices and inflatable penile implants.

The female system: amenorrhoea

Oligomenorrhoea is the reduction in menses to < 9/year. **Primary amenorrhoea** is the failure of menarche to occur by the age of 16 years. **Secondary amenorrhoea** is disappearance of periods for ≥ 6 months in a woman who has previously menstruated.

Fig. 3.6.1 Production and role of male sex hormones.

Pathogenesis

Causes of primary amenorrhoea include congenital abnormalities of Mullerian development and genetic conditions, for example Turner's (45XO) or Kallmann's (isolated gonadotrophin deficiency) syndromes. Pregnancy and the menopause are the commonest causes of secondary amenorrhoea. Other causes are:

- hypothalamic dysfunction: craniopharyngioma, anorexia nervosa, excessive exercise
- pituitary disease: macroadenoma, hyperprolactinaemia
- ovarian disorders: polycystic ovary syndrome (PCOS), autoimmune
- other endocrine diseases: hypo- and hyperthyroidism, Cushing's syndrome, congenital adrenal hyperplasia
- major systemic disease: rheumatoid disease, Crohn's disease, chronic renal disease, depression.

Clinical features

Features depend on age and the underlying cause. Oestrogen-deficiency symptoms (flushes, sweating, emotional lability) accompany ovarian failure at any age not just at the natural menopause. Premature menopause is defined as primary ovarian failure before 40 years of age. Weight loss and preoccupation with exercise suggests an underling eating disorder. Weight gain may suggest PCOS (hirsutism, acne and long-standing oligomenorrhoea), hypothyroidism or, more rarely, Cushing's syndrome or a hypothalamic tumour.

Investigations

Pregnancy should be excluded in women of reproductive age. Serum FSH and LH will be high in primary ovarian failure. Serum oestradiol will be low in primary or secondary ovarian failure. Serum prolactin is high in prolactinoma (Fig. 3.6.3). Pelvic ultrasound of the ovaries shows peripheral cysts and increased stroma in PCOS. Bone densitometry should be assessed in women with low oestrogen levels for > 1 year.

Management

Women with premature ovarian failure require sex hormone replacement to relieve symptoms and prevent osteoporosis. Women with PCOS are usually overweight and insulin resistant. Effective weight loss is required. Treatment with an insulin-sensitizing agent (e.g. metformin) increases ovulatory menses, reduces ovarian androgen secretion and may reduce the risk (six times increase) of type 2 diabetes mellitus. Hirsutism in PCOS is treated with the oral contraceptive (reduces LH drive to the ovaries), testosterone antagonists (e.g. spironolactone) and topical eflornithine cream. Cosmetic approaches such as waxing and electrolysis are also helpful.

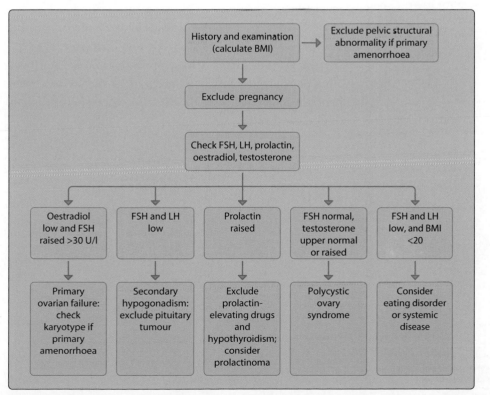

Fig. 3.6.2 Diagnostic approach to amenorrhoea. BMI, body mass index; LH, luteinizing hormone; FSH, follicle-stimulating hormone.

7. Infertility

Questions
- What are the causes of infertility?

Figure 3.7.1 shows the production and role of sex hormones in the female cycle thus releasing an egg and preparing the uterus for a potential embryo.

Infertility is defined as failure of pregnancy to occur after 1 year of unprotected, regular (twice weekly) sexual intercourse. It affects 10–15% of all couples. Female factors (e.g. PCOS, tubal damage) are responsible in 35% of cases, male factors (mostly idiopathic germ cell failure) in 30% and combined factors in 20%; infertility remains unexplained in 15%.

Causes of infertility in women:
- anovulation (PCOS, hyperprolactinaemia, pituitary disease, systemic illness)
- tubal defects (chlamydial infection, endometriosis, surgery)
- uterine abnormalities (congenital, adhesions, fibroids).

Causes of infertility in men:
- primary gonadal failure
- secondary gonadal failure
- genital tract abnomalities (congenital, surgical)
- drugs (steroids, alcohol)
- systemic illness (e.g. Crohn's disease).

Assessment

Both partners should be seen at the first consultation to avoid delay and unnecessary investigations.

A careful menstrual history is vital. Oligomenorrhoea suggests that menstrual cycles are anovulatory. This can be confirmed by measuring serum progesterone on day 21 of the cycle (and sometimes on days 28 and 35): < 20 nmol/l suggests anovulation. Other investigations are similar to those described above for secondary amenorrhoea (Fig 3.6.2, p. 225). If the woman has regular menses and her partner has a normal seminal analysis, further gynaecological assessment of tubal patency is necessary.

The man should be examined for any testicular abnormality or varicocele, and a sample submitted for seminal analysis. If the sperm count is reduced, blood should be taken for testosterone, prolactin, LH and FSH. If the sole abnormality is a raised FSH, irreversible germ cell failure is likely to be present.

Management

Management is complex and depends on the underlying cause. Some causes can be treated effectively with endocrine therapies, for example the treatment of hyperprolactinaemic amenorrhoea with a dopamine agonist (e.g. cabergoline) and the treatment of gonadotrophin deficiency in either sex with gonadotrophin-replacement therapy.

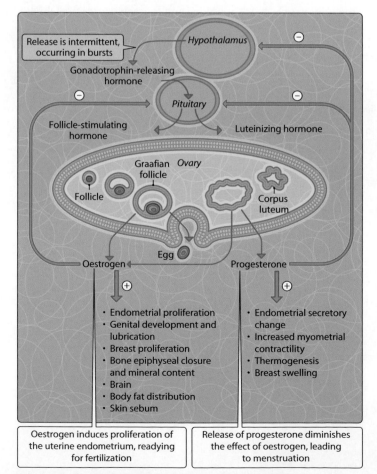

Fig. 3.7.1 Production and role of female sex hormones.

Musculoskeletal disorders

Vinod Kumar and Neil Basu

The big picture

Rheumatology covers disorders affecting joints, bones, soft tissues and muscles (Figs 1.1 and 1.2). Some conditions, such as osteoarthritis, rheumatoid arthritis and osteoporosis, are very common, while others are rare. Soft tissue disorders may be localized while others have multisystem involvement (e.g. systemic lupus erythematosus). Many of these multisystem conditions are autoimmune diseases, although their precise trigger and pathophysiology remain unknown.

There is a wide variety of conditions that cause joint pain (Table 1.1), and it can often be helpful to note how many joints are involved (Table 1.2). The prevalence and sex predominance of various musculoskeletal disorders are shown in Table 1.3.

Morbidity

Pain and disability are common with many of musculoskeletal conditions. In the Western world they cause more functional limitation than any other group of disorders. They rank second to respiratory diseases as a cause of short-term illness but are the most common cause of long-term absence from work. Osteoarthritis and rheumatoid arthritis account for 3.5% of disability-adjusted life-years lost in the UK. Approximately 20% of UK primary care consultations are related to musculoskeletal problems.

Mortality

Patients with rheumatoid arthritis have reduced life expectancy of approximately 7 years because of cardiovascular problems. Osteoporosis does not directly cause death but mortality is increased following hip fractures. There is a significant increase in both morbidity and mortality in patients with connective tissue diseases (e.g. systemic lupus erythematosus, polymyositis and vasculitis) partly because of potentially toxic treatment regimens including immunosuppressive agents.

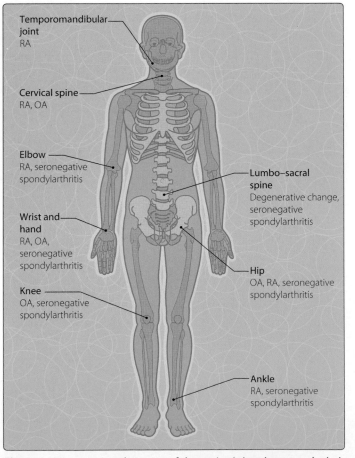

Fig. 1.1 Common involvement of the major joints in musculoskeletal disease. RA, rheumatoid arthritis; OA, osteoarthritis.

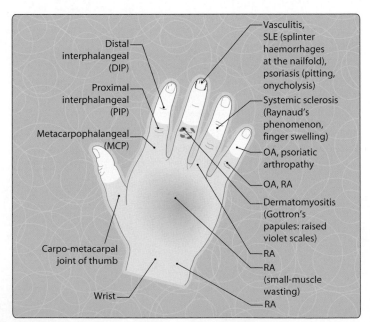

Fig. 1.2 Involvement of the joints and soft tissues of the hand in musculoskeletal disorders. RA, rheumatoid arthritis; OA, osteoarthritis; SLE, systemic lupus erythematosus.

Table 1.1 CAUSES OF JOINT PAIN (ARTHRALGIA)

Type and causes	Examples
Generalized	
Infective	Viral, e.g. rubella, mumps, hepatitis B Bacterial, e.g. staphylococcal, tuberculosis
Postinfective	Rheumatic fever, reactive arthritis
Inflammatory	Rheumatoid arthritis, systemic lupus erythematosus, ankylosing spondylitis, systemic sclerosis
Degenerative	Osteoarthritis
Tumour	Primary, e.g. osteosarcoma, chondrosarcoma Metastatic, e.g. from lung, breast, prostate
Crystal formation	Gout, pseudogout
Trauma	Road traffic accidents, falls, etc.
Miscellaneous	Fibromyalgia, hypermobility syndromes
Localized	
Trauma	Sports injuries
Tendonitis	Shoulder rotator cuff capsulitis, Achilles tendonitis
Enthesopathies	Tennis elbow, golfer's elbow
Bursitis	Trochanteric bursitis
Nerve entrapment	Carpal tunnel syndrome

Incidence and prevalence

The WHO has indicated that the prevalence of musculoskeletal conditions is expected to rise rapidly with increases in life expectancy. Almost one-quarter of Europeans suffer some form of rheumatism or arthritis. The prevalence of rheumatoid arthritis varies between 0.3 and 2% in developed countries, whereas it is far less common in Africa. It is estimated that 10% of the world's population who are >60 years have significant problems that can be attributed to osteoarthritis. Osteoporosis is reaching epidemic proportions in all countries as more than one in four women by age 70 will have sustained at least one osteoporotic fracture.

Table 1.2 JOINT INVOLVEMENT IN ARTHRITIS

No. joints involved	Type	Examples
Single joint (monoarthritis)	Infective	*Staphylococcus aureus, Salmonella* spp., *Neisseria gonorrheae*, tuberculosis
	Traumatic	Sport injury
	Bleeding disorder	Haemarthrosis/haemophilia A
	Post-traumatic	
	Degenerative	Charcot joint e.g. diabetes
	Metabolic	Gout, pseudogout
2–4 joints (oligoarthritis)	Degenerative	Osteoarthritis
	Inflammatory	Reactive arthritis, psoriatic arthritis, sarcoidosis
> 4 joints (polyarthritis)	Inflammatory	Rheumatoid arthritis, systemic lupus erythematosus
	Non-inflammatory	Bacterial: Lyme disease Viral: rubella, mumps, hepatitis B
	Metabolic	Haemochromatosis

Table 1.3 PREVALENCE AND SEX RATIO OF MUSCULOSKELETAL DISORDERS

	Prevalence (%)	Sex ratio
Non-inflammatory		
Osteoarthritis: knee	10	F > M
Osteoarthritis: hip	4	Equal
Osteoporosis	15	F > M
Neck and back pain	20	Equal
Fibromyalgia	3	F > M
Inflammatory		
Rheumatoid arthritis	1–2	F > M
Gout	1	M > F
Seronegative spondyloarthritis	0.8	Equal
Polymyalgia rheumatica	0.04	F > M
Connective tissue disorders	0.02	F > M

High-return facts

1 Arthritis is an umbrella term encompassing different types of inflammatory arthritis (e.g. rheumatoid arthritis) and degenerative arthritis (e.g. osteoarthritis). The history and pattern of joint involvement are important in differentiating between each type. **Osteoarthritis** is very common. It can affect any joint, but most commonly affects the small joints of hands and feet and weight-bearing joints (hips and knees). Although slowly progressive, it can cause significant pain, morbidity and reduced mobility. Extra-articular manifestations do not occur. Radiographs show joint space narrowing, subchondral sclerosis and osteophytes. Treatment is with analgesia and NSAIDs; in severe joint disease, surgical replacement can relieve pain and improve mobility.

2 **Rheumatoid arthritis** is the most common autoimmune inflammatory arthritis and has a peak age of onset of 30–55 years. Small joint stiffness, swelling and tenderness in the hands and feet are common and rheumatoid factor (IgM antibody) is positive in approximately 70%. Although NSAIDs provide pain relief, they do not prevent progressive joint damage. Early treatment with disease-modifying antirheumatic drugs may improve long-term prognosis. Rheumatoid arthritis is a systemic disease and is associated with a wide variety of extra-articular manifestations.

3 **Systemic lupus erythematosus** is a multisystem autoimmune disorder principally affecting premenopausal women. Skin rash, lung, kidney and joint involvement are common. Antinuclear antibodies, which are present in 95%, and double-stranded DNA antibodies are characteristic. Hydroxychloroquine, steroids and immunosuppressants are sometimes required. **Scleroderma** is characterized by excessive collagen deposition, resulting in thickened skin. Three main subgroups have been identified. Localized disease (morphoea) typically involves patches of skin alone and has a good prognosis. Limited cutaneous disease involves thickening of the face and skin of the distal limbs and is associated with long-standing Raynaud's phenomenon. Soft tissue calcification, gastro-oesophageal reflux and pulmonary hypertension can be long-term complications. Diffuse cutaneous disease (**systemic sclerosis**) presents relatively acutely with a short history of Raynaud's phenomenon, generalized skin thickening and potentially fatal complications of renal and pulmonary fibrosis. Response to treatment is usually poor.

4 **Sjögren's syndrome** is characterized by dry eyes and mouth. Multiorgan involvement is less common, although affected patients have an increased risk of lymphoma. **Polymyositis** and **dermatomyositis** are autoimmune inflammatory muscle disorders and can be associated with underlying cancer; patients present with proximal muscle weakness. A heliotropic rash and Gottron's papules are characteristic of dermatomyositis. Blood levels of the muscle enzyme creatinine kinase are high and there are typical features on muscle biopsy. Management is with oral steroids and immunosuppressants.

5 **Polymyalgia rheumatica** and **giant cell arteritis** are associated with large-vessel vasculitis. They affect those > 50 years and are associated with weight loss, night sweats, depression and anorexia. Polymyalgia rheumatica causes proximal muscle stiffness, while giant cell arteritis may result in headache and occasionally visual loss. Both respond rapidly to oral steroids. **Behçet's syndrome** is a vasculitis with the classical triad of recurrent oral ulcers, genital ulcers and iritis. It is more common in Mediterranean, Middle East and Far East populations and occurs in those aged 20–40 years. **Wegener's granulomatosis** is an autoimmune vasculitis typically affecting small vessels. It often presents with respiratory or renal disease. Anti-neutrophilic cytoplasmic antibodies (ANCA) are thought to play a key pathogenic role. **Polyarteritis nodosa** is a rare systemic vasculitis with microaneurysms in small and medium-sized blood vessels. The skin, peripheral nerves, gut and kidney are particularly prone to damage. It is associated with hepatitis B infection. Systemic symptoms include weight loss, fevers, myalgia and arthralgia.

6 The **spondyloarthritides** are a group of related conditions involving the sacroiliac joints and axial skeleton. They are strongly associated with *HLA-B27*. The most common is **ankylosing spondylitis**. Low-back pain is the usual presenting symptom; in early disease, radiographs may be normal but later they may reveal features such as bamboo spine. Prognosis varies but regular physiotherapy and NSAIDs may be beneficial in progressive disease. **Reactive arthritis** presents as either mono- or oligoarthritis of large joints 1–3 weeks after a genitourinary or enteric infection. Symptoms usually respond to rest and NSAIDs. Individuals carrying *HLA-B27* are at risk of developing seronegative spondyloarthropathy following reactive arthritis. **Psoriatic arthritis** has some similarities to rheumatoid arthritis but is genetically and clinically different. Significant disability is rare in psoriatic arthritis but progressive disease warrants treatment with disease-modifying drugs such as methotrexate.

7 **Pseudogout** usually affects one joint, most commonly the knee. Acute joint inflammation follows deposition of calcium pyrophosphate dihydrate crystals. Intra-articular steroid injections provide rapid improvement but no maintenance treatment is required. **Gout** also usually affects one joint, most commonly the first metatarsophalangeal joint. Acute joint inflammation is initiated by deposition of uric acid crystals. Although hyperuricaemia is almost always present, high levels of uric acid in serum may be found without the disease. In chronic gout, acute attacks are polyarticular and tophi (deposits of urate) occur in the pinnae of the ear, fingers and toes. NSAIDs, colchicine and steroids are useful in acute episodes. Following two episodes of gout, the xanthine oxidase inhibitor allopurinol should reduce serum uric acid levels and prevent further attacks.

8 **Septic arthritis** usually affects one joint. Bacterial infection of a joint, often following bacteraemia, results in inflammation and an effusion. Septic arthritis presents with acute pain, swelling, redness, warmth and tenderness of the affected joint. Synovial fluid culture is positive in 90% and the most common organisms found are streptococci and staphylococci. Management involves joint immobilization and prolonged i.v. antibiotics followed by oral antibiotics.

9 **Fibromyalgia** is the most common cause of widespread musculoskeletal pain, particularly of the neck and back, affecting 2–3% of the adult population. Pathogenesis is not established and its diagnosis is based on the clinical finding of acute tenderness at specific sites. The pain is unresponsive to usual treatments (simple analgesia and NSAIDs). Management includes education and reassurance. Occasionally low-dose antidepressants can be effective.

10 **Osteoporosis** is a worldwide health problem particularly in postmenopausal women. Associated factors include premature menopause, cigarette smoking, low body mass index, steroid use, thyrotoxicosis, alcohol abuse and immobility. Although osteoporosis is often asymptomatic, complications such as hip and spine fractures are associated with significant morbidity and mortality. The diagnosis can be confirmed by bone mineral density scanning. Lifestyle modification, hormone replacement therapy, calcium supplements and bisphosphonates can reduce the risk of fracture.

11 **Paget's disease** is a localized bone disorder characterized by increased osteoclastic and osteoblastic activity, leading to mechanically weak bone. Characteristic findings include bowing in long bones, enlarged skull, erythema and increased warmth over the affected area. Complications include pathological fracture, high-output heart failure, deafness and, rarely, sarcomatous change. Treatment is usually not required, but bisphosphonates are sometimes used. **Osteogenesis imperfecta** is caused by deficiency in type 1 collagen synthesis. This results in abnormal bone formation and reduced bone matrix with secondary undermineralization. It may involve other tissues such as ligaments, eyes and teeth. **Osteomyelitis** is bacterial infection of bone. Bacteria may reach bone via the bloodstream, by contiguous spread or direct implantation, with resulting local oedema, redness, heat and tenderness. The ends of long bones are most frequently involved. Diagnosis requires a high index of clinical suspicion and can be confirmed by isotope bone scanning. Bone penetration by most antibiotics is poor and a prolonged i.v. course is necessary.

12 **Amyloidosis** is a systemic disease caused by deposition of an insoluble protein within various organs including the kidney, liver and spleen. It is associated with chronic conditions such as rheumatoid arthritis and bronchiectasis. Diagnosis is made by demonstrating amyloid protein deposits stained with Congo red in biopsy specimens. Prognosis for systemic amyloidosis is poor. **Relapsing polychondritis** causes episodic inflammation of multiple cartilagenous structures. The ears, nose and respiratory tract are principally affected. Vasculitis is often present. There is no effective treatment.

1. Osteoarthritis

Questions
- What joints are commonly affected in osteoarthritis?
- How is osteoarthritis managed?

Osteoarthritis is characterized by cartilage loss and periarticular bone reaction of joints. It is the most common joint disorder but progresses very slowly. It is often found in the elderly although it may present earlier in life if there is a previous joint injury or abnormal articular contour. Osteoarthritis is not life threatening, but it can cause severe pain and loss of mobility and independence.

Epidemiology
At some time in their life, 3–6% of the general population will be affected by osteoarthritis and, by 55 years of age, approximately 15% of the population will have symptomatic osteoarthritis of the knee. Women may have more severe arthritis than men.

Pathogenesis
Osteoarthritis affects the entire joint but especially the cartilage (Fig. 3.1.1). The pathogenesis is complex and involves cartilage degradation initiated by either abnormal biomechanical forces on the joint or abnormalities in cartilage. The process is mediated by enzymes, metalloproteinases and cytokines. Risk of osteoarthritis is increased by genetic factors, particularly in nodal osteoarthritis, altered joint surfaces (e.g. in epiphyseal

dysplasia), previous trauma, obesity, age and certain occupations (hip osteoarthritis in farmers). Factors predisposing to osteoarthritis are shown in Table 3.1.1.

Clinical features
Although osteoarthritis can affect any joint, including those in the spine, it most commonly involves the distal interphalangeal joints, hips and knees (Fig. 3.1.2). The classic symptom is pain

Table 3.1.1 FACTORS PREDISPOSING TO OSTEOARTHRITIS (OA)

Factor	Comments
Heredity	Familial tendency to develop nodal and generalized OA
Gender	Polyarticular OA is more common in post-menopausal women
Sport	Repetitive use and injury can cause lower limb OA
Occupation	OA develops in the hip, knee and shoulder of miners, the hands of cotton workers and the hips of farmers
Childhood	Early OA of the hip occurs in acetabular dysplasia and dislocation of the hip, Perthes' disease, slipped femoral epiphysis and osteonecrosis of the femoral head
Preexisting joint disease	Rheumatoid arthritis, gout, septic arthritis, Paget's disease, haemochromatosis
Obesity	Particularly of knee and hip
Trauma	Particularly fracture through a joint

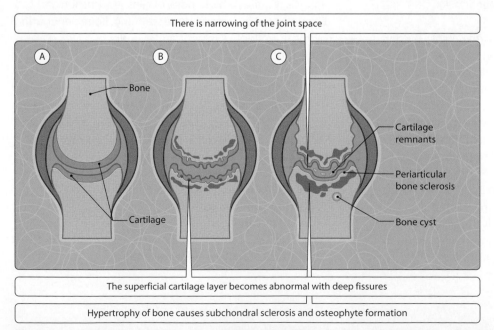

There is narrowing of the joint space

A — Bone

Cartilage remnants

Periarticular bone sclerosis

Cartilage

Bone cyst

The superficial cartilage layer becomes abnormal with deep fissures

Hypertrophy of bone causes subchondral sclerosis and osteophyte formation

Fig. 3.1.1 Joint changes found in osteoarthritis. A, Normal joint; B, gradual disintegration of the joint; C, radiographic changes in an affected joint.

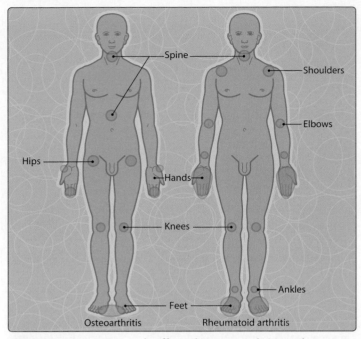

Fig. 3.1.2 Joints commonly affected in osteoarthritis and rheumatoid arthritis. Joint involvement is usually bilateral and symmetrical in both.

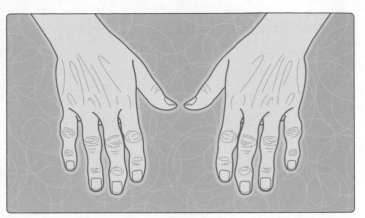

Fig. 3.1.3 Heberden's nodes (distal interphalangeal joints) and Bouchard's nodes (proximal interphalangeal joints) in osteoarthritis.

on exertion or movement in the affected joint that is relieved by rest; as the disease progresses, pain also occurs at rest.

Examination may reveal bony swelling in the small joint of the hands (Heberden's nodes in the distal interphalangeal joints and Bouchard's nodes in proximal interphalangeal joints; Fig. 3.1.3); those with these bony swellings carry a higher risk of developing hip, knee and spine arthritis. Other typical features are joint deformity, crepitus (grating or creeping sensation on movement of the joint), stress pain and restricted joint movement.

Investigations

Laboratory investigations are usually not helpful. Radiography shows joint space narrowing, subchondral sclerosis and osteophyte formation in advanced stages. It is common to see discordance between symptoms and radiograph findings.

Management

Non-pharmacological strategies play an important role, such as education on protection of the joint (e.g. provision of a walking stick), weight loss and exercises to strengthen muscles. There is no effective medical treatment that can limit progression of the disease, but complementary treatments such as glucosamine and chondroitin supplements may reduce pain and improve mobility in osteoarthritis of the knee. Paracetamol and NSAIDs have some value in symptomatic pain relief.

Surgical procedures such as joint replacement or fusion offer complete pain relief in the majority of patients but are limited to large joints such as hips and ankles. Surgery should be reserved for severe symptomatic disease, as risks may outweigh benefits.

2. Rheumatoid arthritis

Questions
- What are the main articular and non-articular features of rheumatoid arthritis?
- What are the main treatment options?

Rheumatoid arthritis (RA) is a chronic inflammatory disorder primarily affecting joints, but it can affect most body systems. If untreated or poorly controlled, it can lead to serious morbidity and premature death.

Epidemiology

The prevalence of RA is 1–2% and incidence varies between 2 and 3/10 000 population. Disease incidence is highest between 30 and 55 years but it is well recognized in children and the elderly. It is more common in females, with a female to male ratio of 3:1.

Pathogenesis

The cause of RA is not known but interaction between genetic factors, sex hormones and infection may trigger an autoimmune process causing inflammation in joints and other organs. First-degree relatives of individuals with RA have a higher disease frequency; however, disease concordance is only approximately 20% in monozygotic twins, indicating that non-genetic factors play a role. Individuals with a genetic predisposition may develop RA following exposure to stimuli such as infection.

Clinical features

RA presents with typical features of joint inflammation, which include early morning stiffness, pain and swelling. Although RA typically affects metacarpophalangeal and proximal interphalangeal joints in the hands (Fig. 3.2.1), and metatarsophalangeal joints in the feet, it can involve any other joint. Swelling around joints may be caused by synovitis, and palpation may reveal heat, tenderness and a reduced range of joint movement. In poorly controlled arthritis, swan-neck, Boutonnière's and mallet deformities of the fingers, with small muscle wasting of the hand, can develop (Figs 3.2.1 and 3.2.2). In long-standing disease, generalized muscle wasting may occur, resulting in reduced or loss of function. Multiple and symmetrical joint involvement may help to differentiate it from other types of inflammatory arthropathy.

Constitutional symptoms such as fatigue, malaise, anorexia, weakness and low-grade fever may be present. Other features include painless, subcutaneous nodules over the extensor surface of the forearms and knees. Rheumatoid factor is usually positive in the presence of rheumatoid nodules. Patients may complain

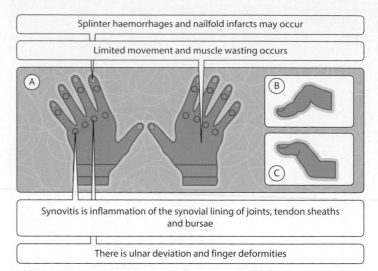

Fig. 3.2.1 Rheumatoid arthritis in the hand. A, Patterns of hand involvement; B, Boutonnière's deformity; C, swan-neck deformity.

Splinter haemorrhages and nailfold infarcts may occur

Limited movement and muscle wasting occurs

Synovitis is inflammation of the synovial lining of joints, tendon sheaths and bursae

There is ulnar deviation and finger deformities

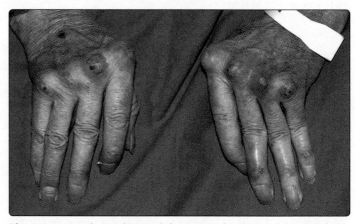

Fig. 3.2.2 Hands in advanced rheumatoid arthritis showing ulnar deviation.

of many other symptoms depending on involvement of other systems (Fig. 3.2.3). Clinical features that tend to be associated with a poorer prognosis include male sex, smoking, high titre of rheumatoid factor, rheumatoid nodules, and joint erosions on radiography at the time of diagnosis.

Investigations

Although there is no single diagnostic test, investigations are important in the assessment of arthritis and are widely used as aids—along with clinical features—to confirm the diagnosis:

- CRP and ESR are usually raised
- FBC may show anaemia, thrombocytosis and mild leukocytosis
- rheumatoid factor (IgM) is raised in approximately 70% of patients (less frequently with early disease)

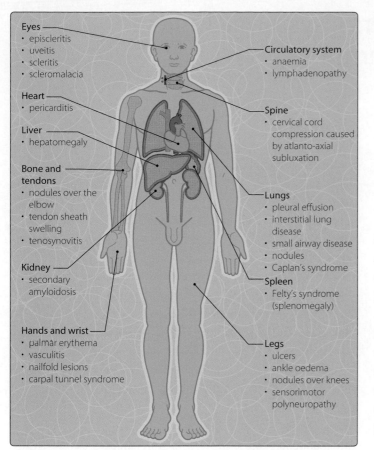

Eyes
- episcleritis
- uveitis
- scleritis
- scleromalacia

Heart
- pericarditis

Liver
- hepatomegaly

Bone and tendons
- nodules over the elbow
- tendon sheath swelling
- tenosynovitis

Kidney
- secondary amyloidosis

Hands and wrist
- palmar erythema
- vasculitis
- nailfold lesions
- carpal tunnel syndrome

Circulatory system
- anaemia
- lymphadenopathy

Spine
- cervical cord compression caused by atlanto-axial subluxation

Lungs
- pleural effusion
- interstitial lung disease
- small airway disease
- nodules
- Caplan's syndrome

Spleen
- Felty's syndrome (splenomegaly)

Legs
- ulcers
- ankle oedema
- nodules over knees
- sensorimotor polyneuropathy

Fig. 3.2.3 Extra-articular manifestations of rheumatoid arthritis.

- anti-nuclear antibodies are detected in 40% of patients
- newer autoantibodies such as anti-cyclic citrullinated protein (CCP) have higher specificity than rheumatoid factor and the presence of both anti-CCP and rheumatoid factor is highly specific for the diagnosis
- plain radiographs of hands and feet may show peri-articular osteopenia and soft tissue swelling; joint erosions, joint space narrowing and joint destruction may become more obvious as the disease advances.

The American College of Rheumatology has a set of criteria for the diagnosis of RA. Four criteria must have been present for at least 6 weeks for the diagnosis (criteria 2–5 must be noted by a physician).

1. Morning stiffness lasting more than an hour
2. Soft tissue swelling or effusion in at least three joints
3. One swollen area in wrist, metacarpophalangeal joint or proximal interphalangeal joint
4. Symmetric arthritis
5. Rheumatoid nodules
6. Positive rheumatoid factor in serum
7. Radiographic changes in hands or feet consistent with rheumatoid arthritis.

Management

A multidisciplinary team approach is required and includes education, pain control, occupational therapy and physiotherapy. Joint replacement may be required in advanced stages of disease.

Simple analgesics such as paracetamol are often used to control pain. NSAIDs are widely used as they have both analgesic and anti-inflammatory properties, although they fail to alter the natural history of the disease. Differences in anti-inflammatory efficacy between preparations are small, although there is often considerable variation in tolerability, response and adverse effect profile (such as peptic ulceration).

Disease-modifying antirheumatic drugs (DMARDs) are now used early after diagnosis and may slow progression of disease and prevent joint damage. Up to 6 months of treatment is required before a therapeutic response can be expected and DMARDs may also improve extra-articular features of RA such as vasculitis. Drugs such as sulfasalazine, methotrexate and leflunomide can be used as first-line DMARDs. The availability of biological treatments such as agents blocking tumour necrosis factor alpha (e.g. infliximab and etanercept) and the anti-B cell agent rituximab has revolutionized the treatment of RA, although they are currently reserved for severe arthritis. Systemic steroids provide fairly immediate relief of symptoms and may prevent joint damage in the short term, although long-term use should be avoided because of adverse effects.

3. Connective tissue disorders I: systemic lupus erythematosus and scleroderma

Questions
- What are the features of systemic lupus erythematosus?
- How does scleroderma affect the skin?
- What other organs can scleroderma affect?

Systemic lupus erythematosus

Systemic lupus erythematosus (SLE) is a chronic autoimmune disorder that causes a variety of features (Fig. 3.3.1).

Epidemiology

Although principally a disease of premenopausal women, SLE can affect individuals of any age. The prevalence in the UK is approximately 28/100 000, with an annual incidence of 4/100 000. The female:male ratio is 9:1, and there is greater prevalence and severity among Afro-Caribbeans.

Pathogenesis

An excess production of autoantibodies, in particular antinuclear antibodies (ANA), leads to organ damage by way of antigen-complex formation and inflammatory cascades. These autoantibodies affect a variety of organs.

Clinical features

SLE should be considered in individuals presenting with multiple non-specific complaints, especially if there is no obvious cause.

Investigations

Typical features and the presence of certain autoantibodies, particularly ANA, make the diagnosis. Up to 95% of individuals with SLE develop ANA (ANA can also be found in 20% of normal individuals); more specific autoantibodies such as double-stranded DNA and extractable nuclear antigens (e.g. Sm, Ro and La) are not as sensitive but add significant weight to the diagnosis. Anti-phospholipid antibodies are sometimes present. Low complement C3 and C4 levels indicate active disease. Renal biopsy can provide vital information on the type and severity of involvement. Other investigations are given in Table 3.3.1.

Management

Most patients require simple analgesics and NSAIDs for symptomatic relief; others need more potent anti-inflammatory drugs such as steroids and hydroxychloroquine. Cytotoxic agents (e.g. cyclophosphamide) and the anti-B cell monoclonal antibody rituximab are often required in renal disease or for those with severe neurological involvement. Once disease remission is achieved, less-toxic immunosuppressants such as azathioprine or methotrexate may be used.

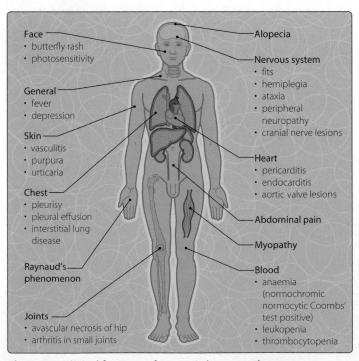

Fig. 3.3.1 Clinical features of systemic lupus erythematosus.

Face
- butterfly rash
- photosensitivity

General
- fever
- depression

Skin
- vasculitis
- purpura
- urticaria

Chest
- pleurisy
- pleural effusion
- interstitial lung disease

Raynaud's phenomenon

Joints
- avascular necrosis of hip
- arthritis in small joints

Alopecia

Nervous system
- fits
- hemiplegia
- ataxia
- peripheral neuropathy
- cranial nerve lesions

Heart
- pericarditis
- endocarditis
- aortic valve lesions

Abdominal pain

Myopathy

Blood
- anaemia (normochromic normocytic Coombs' test positive)
- leukopenia
- thrombocytopenia

Table 3.3.1 INVESTIGATIONS USED TO ASSESS ORGAN INVOLVEMENT IN SYSTEMIC LUPUS ERYTHEMATOSUS

System	Investigation
Central nervous system	MRI, lumbar puncture
Respiratory	Chest radiography and high-resolution CT, pulmonary function tests
Cardiac	ECG, echocardiogram
Renal	U&Es, renal ultrasound, isotope glomerular filtration rate, urine protein: creatinine ratio
Haematological	FBC, Coombs' tests, reticulocyte count, lupus anticoagulant, anti-phospholipid antibodies, bone marrow aspirate

U&Es, urea and electrolytes; FBC, full blood count.

The overall 10-year survival has increased to approximately 90% with modern immunosuppressants. Interventions vary from simple lifestyle advice (avoiding stress and sun exposure) to potentially toxic chemotherapy regimens.

Scleroderma

Scleroderma is a chronic autoimmune disease characterized by excessive collagen deposition. Three main subgroups have been defined (localized, limited cutaneous and diffuse cutaneous) with variable clinical courses. The systemic form (**systemic sclerosis**) can be fatal through damage to the heart, kidney, lung or intestine.

Epidemiology

Scleroderma is a rare worldwide disease with a female preponderance (3:1). Several environmental factors have been implicated in its development, including hydrocarbons (e.g. vinyl chloride), epoxy resins and silica. Prognosis varies with disease subgroups: a normal lifespan in localized disease, 71% and 21% 10-year survival rate in limited and diffuse cutaneous disease, respectively.

Pathogenesis

The inflammatory response is thought to be autoimmune and leads to excess collagen production and fibrosis. Skin, small blood vessels, lungs, GI tract and kidneys are particularly vulnerable to damage, resulting in several clinical manifestations.

Clinical features

Localized disease (morphoea) results in a skin rash only. It is usually asymptomatic but can be painful and associated with localized arthralgia. In limited cutaneous disease, Raynaud's phenomenon is normally present for several years before skin changes are noted. The skin changes, swelling and thickening, are limited to the face and distal limbs.

Diffuse cutaneous disease can present acutely, often with a short history of Raynaud's phenomenon. Skin swelling can be painful and affects the entire body. Polyarthalgia, myalgia and fatigue are prominent in early disease. Damage can occur within 1–2 years of diagnosis and results in poor mobility from severe skin tightening and contractures. Other features include:

- dyspepsia from oesophageal dysmotility
- painful skin lesions related to calcium deposition
- breathlessness secondary to pulmonary fibrosis
- headaches and blurred vision from malignant hypertension
- weight loss from intestinal involvement.

Table 3.3.2 TREATMENT OF SCLERODERMA

Disease process	Treatment
Raynaud's phenomenon	Gloves, calcium channel blockers, prostacyclin
Renal	ACE inhibitors
Pulmonary arterial hypertension	Bosentan, sildenafil, warfarin
Small bowel bacterial overgrowth	Cyclical antibiotics
Gastro-oesophageal reflux	Proton pump inhibitors
Arthalgia	NSAIDs
Interstitial lung disease	Prednisolone, cyclophosphamide

In limited cutaneous disease, finger swelling results in a 'sausage like' appearance and progresses to skin thickening. Facial skin stiffening results in puckering of the mouth and 'beaking' of the nose. Small, dilated blood vessels become pronounced over the face and hands (telangiectasia). Calcium deposition occurs at the finger tips and can ulcerate and become infected.

In diffuse cutaneous disease, regular blood pressure monitoring is needed in an attempt to prevent end-organ damage. Fine bibasal crackles may indicate interstitial lung disease. Skin swelling and later thickening are rapidly progressive and can be complicated by tendon friction rubs and ulceration. Although joint pain is a common complaint, synovitis is seldom seen.

Investigations

ANA are found in 80% of patients; anti-topoisomerase I (Scl-70) antibodies are specific and predictive for diffuse cutaneous scleroderma. Anti-centromere antibodies are found in more limited disease. Chest radiograph and pulmonary function tests identify and monitor respiratory complications. High-resolution CT of the chest will detect interstitial lung disease and echocardiography detects pulmonary hypertension. Upper GI involvement can be assessed by barium swallow. Hydrogen breath tests are useful in diagnosing bacterial overgrowth, a complication of small bowel involvement.

Management

Scleroderma remains a therapeutic challenge (Table 3.3.2). Disease-modifying agents such as methotrexate, D-penicillamine and azathioprine are occasionally used to slow generalized disease progression.

4. Connective tissue disorders II: Sjögren's syndrome, polymyositis and dermatomyositis

Questions
- What is Sjögrens syndrome?
- What conditions are associated with it?
- How are polymyositis and dermatomyositis diagnosed?

Sjögren's syndrome

Sjögren's syndrome (or keratoconjunctivitis sicca) is characterized by the combination of dry eyes (xeropthalmia) and mouth (xerostomia) and is often associated with systemic features (Fig. 3.4.1).

Epidemiology

Sjögren's syndrome is a relatively common autoimmune disorder associated with rheumatoid arthritis and systemic lupus erythematosus. The female to male ratio is 9:1. Patients usually present in their fifth or sixth decade. The disease is slowly progressive and a normal lifespan is expected.

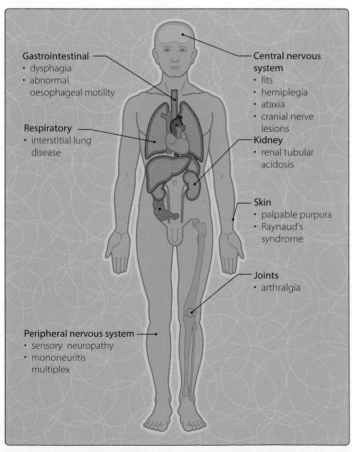

Fig. 3.4.1 Systemic manifestations of Sjögren's syndrome.

Gastrointestinal
- dysphagia
- abnormal oesophageal motility

Respiratory
- interstitial lung disease

Peripheral nervous system
- sensory neuropathy
- mononeuritis multiplex

Central nervous system
- fits
- hemiplegia
- ataxia
- cranial nerve lesions

Kidney
- renal tubular acidosis

Skin
- palpable purpura
- Raynaud's syndrome

Joints
- arthralgia

Pathogenesis

The aetiology is unknown although hormonal imbalance, genetic predisposition and infection may be implicated. It is thought to have an autoimmune basis, with activated lymphocytes migrating to and damaging glandular tissue, particularly tear and salivary glands.

Clinical features

Sjögren's syndrome often presents as itchy/gritty eyes and/or difficulty eating dry food. Other mucosal surfaces can be involved; sexual problems can reflect vaginal dryness, and hoarse voice suggests tracheal involvement. Systemic features such as arthalgia, myalgia and fatigue are common. Patients complaining of breathlessness, rashes, night sweats or weight loss should be assessed for more serious complications.

Eye examination is usually normal although opacities and ulcers can be present. Poor dentition can occur because of the reduced production of saliva and an increased bacterial load. Parotid gland enlargement can be an intermittent finding. Arthritis is normally non-erosive, polyarticular and symmetrical. Sensory peripheral neuropathy is common and mononeuritis multiplex and palpable purpura are suggestive of associated vasculitis. Persisting lymphadenopathy should be taken seriously, as Sjögren's syndrome is associated with an increased risk of lymphoma.

Investigations

Schirmer's tear test involves the application of a strip of sterilized blotting paper under the eyelid for 5 min to measure tear production. If the paper is moistened to < 10 mm, defective tear production is present. Reduced salivary function can be established with salivary scintigraphy or parotid sialography.

Lip biopsy can reveal characteristic lymphocytic infiltration. Rheumatoid factor is frequently positive. Anti-Ro and anti-La antibodies are found in 70% of patients.

Management

Artificial tears and saliva are usually sufficient to treat dry eyes and mouth. Arthalgia often responds well to NSAIDs, although hydroxychloroquine may be required in resistant disease. More potent immunosuppressants such as cyclophosphamide, methotrexate and prednisolone are considered if severe multi-organ involvement is present.

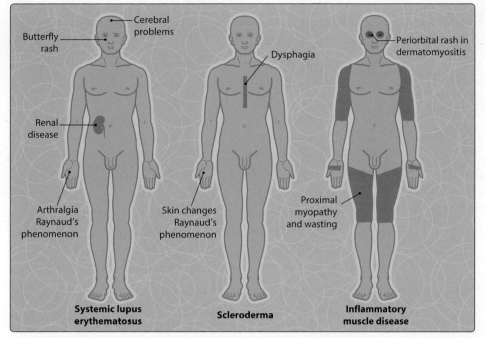

Fig. 3.4.2 Clinical features that may help to distinguish different connective tissue disorders.

Polymyositis and dermatomyositis

Polymyositis and dermatomyositis are examples of inflammatory muscle diseases. Adult dermatomyositis can be associated with a wide variety of cancers, with a relative risk of 2.4 in males and 3.4 in females.

Epidemiology

This rare group of disorders affect 6–8/1 000 000 of the population, with varying degrees of severity. Polymyositis is a disease of middle age, whereas dermatomyositis affects children and the elderly.

Pathogenesis

The aetiology of these conditions is uncertain, although autoimmunity plays some role.

Clinical features

Patients typically present with an insidious onset of weakness of proximal limbs and trunk characterized by difficulty climbing stairs or standing from a sitting position (Fig. 3.4.2). A significant proportion also complains of muscle pain and fatigue. Muscles are not tender on palpation.

Dermatomyositis is associated with skin lesions characterized by a blue/purple discoloration of the upper eyelids (heliotrope rash), and raised violet scales over the knuckles (Gottron's papules). Polymyositis is occasionally associated with interstitial lung disease.

Investigations

Muscle enzymes, particularly creatine kinase, are raised in serum, although other causes should be excluded. Electromyography can detect impaired electrical impulses associated with inflamed muscle. Polymyositis and dermatomyositis have distinct histological appearances on muscle biopsy.

When associated malignancy is suspected, further investigations such as abdominal ultrasound and chest radiograph are necessary. High-resolution CT of the chest is required in patients suspected of having interstitial lung disease complicating polymyositis.

Management

Immunosuppressants such as tapering doses of oral steroids are effective in mild disease. Immunoglobulin infusions, azathioprine and methotrexate are used for more resistant disease.

5. Systemic inflammatory disorders and vasculitides

Questions
■ What are the clinical features of polymyalgia rheumatica?
■ What are the clinical features of giant cell arteritis?
■ What is Behçet's syndrome?
■ What are the clinical features of Wegener's granulomatosis?

Vasculitis is defined as inflammation in or through blood vessel walls. The vasculitides are often classified on the size of vessel affected (Fig. 3.5.1) but there is often some overlap and other conditions may show some vasculitis.

Behçet's syndrome

Behçet's syndrome has a typical triad of recurrent oral ulcers, genital ulcers and iritis. It is more common in the Mediterranean, Middle East and Far East and rare in Europe. It usually occurs in the third and fourth decades with equal sex preponderance. Aetiology is not known but it is typically associated with *HLA-B5*. Diagnosis is based upon clinical features. It can be easily confused with reactive arthritis, Steven–Johnson syndrome and inflammatory bowel disease with skin and eye manifestations. Steroids are the mainstay of treatment.

Wegener's granulomatosis

Wegener's granulomatosis is a multisystem autoimmune disease causing inflammation of small blood vessels. It is rare and invariably fatal if not treated. Increased awareness and effective immunosuppressives has resulted in a 75% 5-year survival.

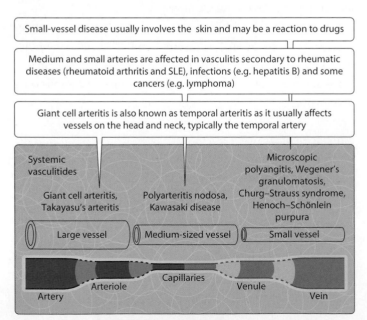

Small-vessel disease usually involves the skin and may be a reaction to drugs

Medium and small arteries are affected in vasculitis secondary to rheumatic diseases (rheumatoid arthritis and SLE), infections (e.g. hepatitis B) and some cancers (e.g. lymphoma)

Giant cell arteritis is also known as temporal arteritis as it usually affects vessels on the head and neck, typically the temporal artery

Systemic vasculitides

Giant cell arteritis, Takayasu's arteritis

Polyarteritis nodosa, Kawasaki disease

Microscopic polyangitis, Wegener's granulomatosis, Churg–Strauss syndrome, Henoch–Schönlein purpura

Large vessel   Medium-sized vessel   Small vessel

Artery   Arteriole   Capillaries   Venule   Vein

Fig. 3.5.1 Vessels affected by vasculitides.

Respiratory tract manifestations include sinusitis, subglottic stenosis, pulmonary haemorrhage and cavitation. Renal biopsy reveals crescentic glomerulonephritis. There may be skin rashes and cartilage destruction, causing a collapsed nasal bridge.

Chest radiograph may show cavitation, interstitial changes or patchy consolidation after haemorrhage. Bronchoscopy may show subglottic stenosis and airway narrowing. Tissue biopsy confirming appearances of granulomatous disease and necrotizing vasculitis is usually required to confirm the diagnosis.

Blood and protein on urine dipstick, abnormal U&E and creatinine all may indicate renal involvement. Proteinase 3-specific anti-neutrophilic cytoplasmic antibodies (ANCA) play a key pathogenic role and are positive in 85% of affected individuals.

Generalized and organ-threatening disease requires cyclophosphamide and high-dose steroids to induce remission. This is effective in up to 90%, although plasma exchange, immunoglobulins and the anti-B cell monoclonal antibody rituximab have been used. Remission of early localized disease can be induced with methotrexate. Most patients require long-term immunosuppression (e.g. with azathoprine or methotrexate), although relapses are frequent.

Other ANCA-associated vasculitides

Microscopic polyangiitis typically presents with rapidly progressive glomerulonephritis and pulmonary alveolar haemorrhage. Haemoptysis may be the presenting symptom. Perinuclear p-ANCA is usually positive. **Churg–Strauss syndrome** consists of a triad of skin lesions (purpura or nodules), mononeuritis multiplex and blood eosinophilia on a background of poorly controlled asthma. Pulmonary infiltrates may be evident on chest radiograph and mesenteric vasculitis can cause abdominal symptoms. Either c-ANCA or p-ANCA is found in about 40% of cases.

Polyarteritis nodosa

Polyarteritis nodosa is a rare systemic vasculitis that produces microaneurysms in small and medium-sized blood vessels. Subsequent thrombosis and rupture can lead to haemorrhage and infarction of end-organs. Pathogenesis may relate to immune-complex deposition and viruses, in particular hepatitis B, are strongly linked.

Patients present insidiously with weight loss, fevers, myalgia and arthralgia. The skin, peripheral nerves, gut and kidneys are particularly sensitive to damage (Fig. 3.5.2).

Diagnosis relies on typical clinical features with histology. If biopsy is not possible, radiological evidence of microaneuyrsms is supportive (e.g. renal and coeliac axis angiograms).

Antiviral therapies are the mainstay of treatment of polyarteritis nodosa associated with hepatitis B. High-dose steroids

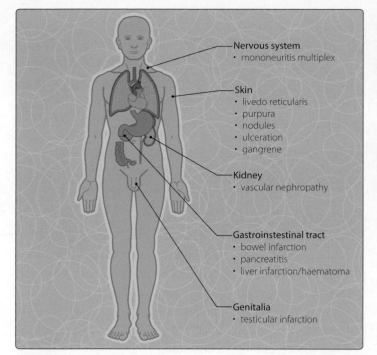

Fig. 3.5.2 Organ involvement in polyarteritis nodosa.

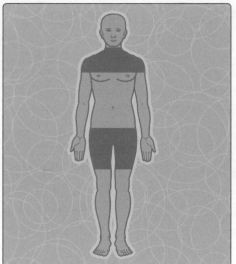

Fig. 3.5.3 Areas of pain in polymyalgia rheumatica.

and cyclophosphamide may be effective. Without intervention, 5-year survival is only 10% but this rises to 80% with treatment. Relapse rates are low in comparison with other vasculitic disorders.

Polymyalgia rheumatica

Polymyalgia rheumatica presents with an abrupt onset of shoulder and hip girdle pain (Fig. 3.5.3). Associated symptoms include significant early morning stiffness lasting several hours, weight loss, night sweats, depression and anorexia. Muscle power is preserved, although muscle tenderness can be present. There is no diagnostic test but a typical clinical presentation in individuals over the age of 50 years is highly suggestive. Prompt resolution of symptoms following a low dose of steroid confirms the diagnosis.

The main differential diagnoses are rheumatoid arthritis, inflammatory muscle disease, osteoarthritis, rotator cuff lesions, infection, malignancy (e.g. multiple myeloma), fibromyalgia and giant cell arteritis.

ESR and CRP are always raised. Serum alkaline phosphatase and gamma-glutamyl transpeptidase are often raised. A normochromic normocytic anaemia may occur. Temporal artery biopsy shows inflammation in only 10–30%.

Treatment with a reducing course of oral steroid is very effective. A typical starting dose is 15 mg/day, with treatment often required for 2–3 years. Steroid-sparing agents such as methotrexate and azathioprine are occasionally required if symptoms persist on tapering the steroid dose.

Giant cell arteritis

Giant cell arteritis is a distinct entity to polymyalgia rheumatica, although approximately 25% of patients develop symptoms in keeping with polymyalgia at some point. It affects 20/100 000 of North Europeans over the age of 50 years. The temporal arteries are typically affected, although a significant minority experiences involvement of the main aortic root branches.

Presenting symptoms include visual disturbance, temporal tenderness, jaw claudication, night sweats and fever. Irreversible blindness can result if treatment is not promptly instituted. Clinical examination often reveals tender, pulseless temporal arteries. The scalp can be tender to touch and on brushing hair. Optic ischaemia is suggested by visual field defects and optic disc oedema.

Diagnosis requires three of five criteria:

- age ≥ 50 years
- new headache
- abnormality of the temporal arteries
- ESR > 50
- temporal artery histology in keeping with giant cell arteritis.

Temporal artery biopsy revealing granulomatous arteritis is diagnostic, although a negative biopsy does not exclude it. This should be performed within 14 days of starting high-dose steroids. ESR and CRP are invariably raised.

Confirmation of diagnosis should not delay treatment. High-dose prednisolone (1 mg/kg) should be started immediately and gradually reduced according to symptoms and ESR/CRP. As with polymyalgia rheumatica, back titration of oral steroids can take several years, although relapses are less common.

6. Seronegative arthritides

Questions
- How does ankylosing spondylitis affect the spine?
- What are the extra-articular features of ankylosing spondylitis?
- What infections result in reactive arthritis?

Reactive arthritis

Reactive arthritis is an acute, non-infectious arthritis that can follow a genitourinary or GI infection. It is slightly more common in males and most often occurs between 20 and 40 years of age.

Pathogenesis

The most common triggers are enteric infections caused by *Shigella*, *Salmonella* and *Campylobacter* spp. or *Chlamydia* infection of the genitourinary tract.

Clinical features

Joint inflammation usually starts 2–4 weeks after an episode of diarrhoea or genitourinary infection. Asymmetric, predominantly large joint involvement is typical. The onset is acute and associated with fever and malaise. An associated vasculitis is sometimes found (Fig. 3.6.1).

Investigations

Stool culture or analysis of a genital swab may confirm the causative organism.

Management

Treatment is with NSAIDs and intra-articular steroid injections. In most cases, symptoms are self-limiting and last between 3 months and 2 years. Prognosis is usually good and immunosuppressive agents are rarely required.

Ankylosing spondylitis

Ankylosing spondylitis is the most common spondyloarthritides (inflammation involving the spine). Others include reactive spondyloarthritis, psoriatic spondyloarthritis, spondyloarthropathy associated with inflammatory bowel disease and undifferentiated spondyloarthropathy.

Epidemiology

Prevalence is unknown but is estimated to be between 0.25 and 2% of the population. It occurs more commonly in males in their early twenties, with a male:female ratio of 2:1. The spondyloarthritides are strongly associated with *HLA-B27*.

Pathogenesis

Precise aetiology is unknown but chronic inflammation at the enthesis (the area of tendon and ligament insertion to bone) eventually leads to fibrosis and ossification.

Clinical features

Patients often complain of low-back pain of an insidious onset inflammatory type (pain improves with activity) that radiates to the buttocks (Table 3.6.1). Examination reveals tenderness over the sacroiliac joints; lumbar spinal movements become restricted as the disease progresses. In advanced disease, chest expansion becomes impaired by ossification of costochondral junctions, and neck movements become reduced. Extraspinal features caused by tendonitis and enthesitis include Achilles tendonitis, plantar fasciitis and dactylitis. Asymmetric large-joint arthritis of hips and knees is not uncommon.

Ankylosing spondylitis is a systemic disease associated with anterior uveitis, bilateral apical pulmonary fibrosis, aortic incompetence and myocardial conduction disturbances. Neurological manifestations such as spinal root or cord compression are rare.

Investigations

FBC may show anaemia and CRP and ESR may be raised. Radiography of the sacroiliac joints shows features of sacroiliitis. Spine radiography can show squaring of vertebra and, in

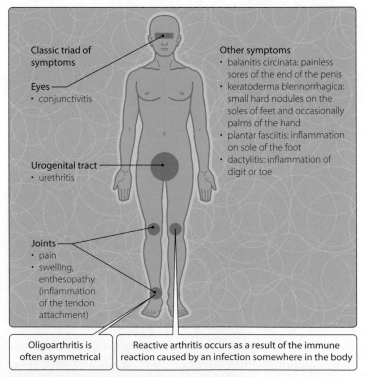

Fig. 3.6.1 Clinical features of reactive arthritis.

Table 3.6.1 DIFFERENCES BETWEEN INFLAMMATORY AND MECHANICAL BACK PAIN

	Inflammatory back pain	Mechanical back pain
Onset	Insidious	Acute
Morning stiffness	+++	+
Sleep disturbance	++	+ or −
Effect of exercise	Better	Worse
Effect of rest	Worse	Better
Involvement of other systems	+	−
Family history	+	−
Radiological signs	+	−

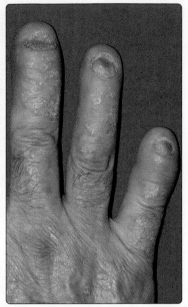

Fig. 3.6.2 Bamboo spine in a patient with advanced ankylosing spondylitis.

Fig. 3.6.3 Distal interphalangeal joint involvement, psoriatic plaques and nail dystrophy in psoriatic arthritis.

advanced disease, syndesmophytes, which are caused by ossification of the intervertebral ligaments and give a typical 'bamboo spine' (Fig. 3.6.2) appearance.

Management

Management until recently was conservative, in the form of education, physiotherapy and NSAIDs. Recently anti-tumour necrosis factor drugs (e.g. infliximab) have revolutionized the lives of some individuals. Surgery is occasionally useful to correct spinal deformities. Most patients have mild to moderate disease only, but early hip involvement, onset below 16 years of age and elevated ESR at time of diagnosis suggest a poorer prognosis.

Psoriatic arthritis

Psoriasis is an autoimmune disease of the skin that affects 2% of whites, of whom 10–20% develop chronic inflammation of joints. Patients with nail lesions (Fig. 3.6.3) are more likely to develop arthritis. It has some similarities to rheumatoid arthritis (Table 3.6.2) but is genetically and clinically different.

Epidemiology

The incidence of psoriatic arthritis is 5/100 000 and prevalence is 1/10 000 of the UK population. Males and females are equally affected. Most patients have mild disease but approximately 20% of patients have chronic, progressive disease.

Clinical features

Patients typically present with symptoms of inflammatory arthritis affecting two to four joints (oligoarthritis), which may be associated with dactylitis, enthesitis or tendonitis. Other patterns

of psoriatic arthritis are recognized but are less common. The most common extra-articular feature of psoriatic arthritis is uveitis, especially in those with spine involvement.

Investigations

Radiography may show marginal erosion, with proliferative new bone formation, joint fusion, acro-osteolysis (lysis of terminal phalanges), 'pencil-in-cup' deformity and periostitis.

Management

Many patients can be managed with NSAIDs and local intra-articular steroid injections. In progressive disease, second-line disease-modifying drugs such as methotrexate, leflunomide and anti-tumour necrosis factor may be required. Significant disability is unusual with psoriatic arthritis.

Table 3.6.2 DIFFERENCES BETWEEN PSORIATIC AND RHEUMATOID ARTHRITIS

	Psoriatic arthritis	Rheumatoid arthritis
Sex ratio	F = M	F > M
Symmetry of joint involvement	Less common	Very common
DIP joint involvement	Common	Uncommon
Spondylitis	+	−
Psoriasis/nail changes	+	−
Enthesitis	+	−

7. Pseudogout and gout

Questions
- How does pseudogout differ from gout?
- What factors predispose to gout?
- What is the management of acute and chronic gout?

Pseudogout

Pseudogout is the most common cause of acute monoarthritis in the elderly and is caused by deposition of calcium pyrophosphate crystals.

Pathogenesis

The exact mechanism remains elusive but excess production of pyrophosphate in the cartilage may lead to formation and deposition of calcium pyrophosphate crystals, causing acute inflammation.

Epidemiology

Incidence of acute attacks varies between 1 and 1.5 per 1000 adults. In those > 85 years, nearly 50% have radiological evidence of calcium pyrophosphate deposition. Only large joints are affected in most patients, with the knee being the most common site, followed by the wrist, shoulder, ankle and elbow.

Clinical features

Pseudogout usually presents as rapidly developing severe pain, stiffness, swelling and overlying erythema. Examination reveals tenderness over the joint and an effusion may be present. Fever is common and the patient can appear unwell and mildly confused.

Trauma, intercurrent illness, institution of thyroid-replacement therapy and dehydration may be implicated in its development. Most cases are idiopathic but it is associated with haemachromatosis, hyperparathyroidism, hypomagnesaemia and hypophosphataemia.

Investigations

Any acutely swollen joint should be aspirated to exclude septic arthritis. In pseudogout, the fluid is often turbid with low viscosity. Plain polarizing microscopy shows small rhomboid or rod-shaped calcium pyrophosphate dihydrate crystals with weak birefringence. Electron microscopy is more sensitive but is not widely available. Radiography of the affected joint may show calcification of cartilage (Fig. 3.7.1). It is not uncommon to see chondrocalcinosis without features of acute arthritis.

Management

Treatment involves identifying triggering factors and reducing pain with simple analgesics and NSAIDs. Joint aspiration and intra-articular steroids may reduce inflammation. Acute episodes are usually self-limiting and resolve within 1–2 weeks.

Gout

Gout occurs as a result of deposition of uric acid crystals in the synovium of joints, causing acute inflammation.

Epidemiology

Gout is more common in whites and affects approximately 1% of the general population. It is more common in males than females (10:1) and is uncommon before the menopause. The peak incidence in males is between the fourth and sixth decades but in females it more often occurs in the sixth and seventh decades.

Pathogenesis

Hyperuricaemia is a prerequisite for gout, although gout develops in only 10–20% of individuals with hyperuricaemia (Fig. 3.7.2). Uric acid in serum is increased in a number of conditions:

- obesity
- high alcohol intake
- hypertension
- renal impairment
- chronic diuretic use (e.g. bendroflumethiazide).

Levels of uric acid may decrease during an acute episode. Trauma, dehydration, some drugs and foodstuffs and binge drinking may precipitate an acute attack. Gout may also occur secondarily in a number of conditions:

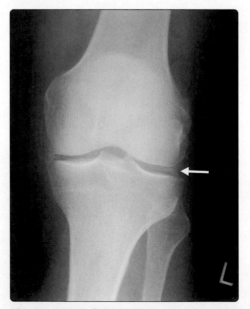

Fig. 3.7.1 Calcification of the articular cartilage in a patient with pseudogout (arrow).

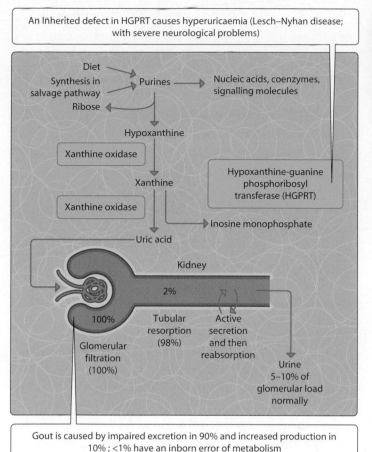

An Inherited defect in HGPRT causes hyperuricaemia (Lesch–Nyhan disease; with severe neurological problems)

Diet
Synthesis in salvage pathway
Ribose
Purines → Nucleic acids, coenzymes, signalling molecules

Hypoxanthine

Xanthine oxidase

Xanthine

Xanthine oxidase

Hypoxanthine-guanine phosphoribosyl transferase (HGPRT)

Inosine monophosphate

Uric acid

Kidney

2%

100%
Glomerular filtration (100%)
Tubular resorption (98%)
Active secretion and then reabsorption
Urine 5–10% of glomerular load normally

Gout is caused by impaired excretion in 90% and increased production in 10% ; <1% have an inborn error of metabolism

Fig. 3.7.2 Uric acid production and excretion.

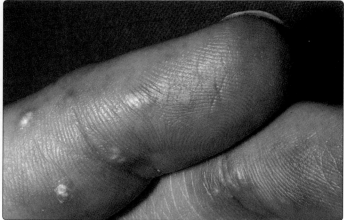

Fig. 3.7.3 Gouty tophi.

in soft tissues can be found in ear pinnae, hands and elbows. The interaction between uric acid and the kidney is complex, but urate nephropathy and urate renal stones are well recognized.

Investigations

Clinical features are often sufficient to make the diagnosis. Serum urate is usually elevated. Blood urea and creatinine should be checked to exclude renal impairment.

Negatively birefringent, needle-shaped uric acid crystals are found on polarizing microscopy in the synovial fluid or in the discharge from tophi.

Management

Management essentially has three targets: the acute attack, reducing uric acid levels to prevent deposition of urate crystals into tissues and prophylactic hypouricaemic therapy. Acute episodes respond well to NSAIDs. In patients with renal or heart failure or a history of peptic ulceration, colchicine or steroids (intra-articular or oral) are useful. In order to help to prevent recurrent episodes, patients should be advised to lose weight if obese and limit dietary intake of alcohol. Drugs to reduce serum uric acid should be considered following the second episode of acute gout (once symptoms have settled). Allopurinol, which blocks xanthine oxidase, is the most commonly used drug, although uricosuric drugs such as probenicid and sulfinpyrazone are useful in patients who are intolerant of allopurinol. Since these drugs are associated with the risk of flare up of gout, NSAIDs should be given as these drugs are started.

■ overproduction of uric acid: myeloproliferative disease, haemolysis, psoriasis, tumour lysis syndrome (renal failure from rapid lysis of malignant cells), excessive alcohol consumption
■ underexcretion of uric acid: renal impairment, lead exposure, high alcohol intake, chronic diuretic use
■ drugs, e.g. ciclosporin, pyrazinamide (interferes with uric acid excretion).

Clinical features

Gout typically causes an acute monoarthritis, with the first metatarsophalangeal joint most commonly affected. Swelling, redness, heat and extreme tenderness usually occur, and in large joints there may be a detectable effusion. In chronic gout, acute attacks are polyarticular and tophi (deposits of urate; Fig. 3.7.3)

8. Septic arthritis

Question
■ What are the clinical features of septic arthritis?

Septic arthritis is caused by direct bacterial infection of a joint and results in inflammation and the development of an effusion (Fig. 3.8.1). There is no difference in incidence between sexes but it is more common in the elderly and in those with damaged or prosthetic joints. Polyarticular involvement occurs in up to 15% of patients (Fig. 3.8.2), particularly in the immunocompromised and in those with gonococcal septic arthritis (Table 3.8.1).

Staphylococcus is the most commonly isolated organism followed by *Streptococcus* but virtually every bacterial organism has been reported to cause septic arthritis. Degenerative joint disease, rheumatoid arthritis and oral steroids may increase the risk of septic arthritis.

Septic arthritis presents with acute pain, swelling, erythema, warmth and tenderness. The severity of pain and tenderness is usually greater than in any other acute arthritis. Patients usually have a fever and appear unwell.

Joint aspiration should be carried out prior to starting antibiotics. Synovial fluid and blood should be sent for culture.

Table 3.8.1 DIFFERENCES BETWEEN GONOCOCCAL AND NON-GONOCOCCAL ARTHRITIS

	Gonococcal infection	Non-gonococcal infection
Age group	Healthy young adults	Very old or young
Sex ratio	F > M	M > F
Arthralgia	Migratory polyarthralgia common	Uncommon
Extra-articular features	Rash and tenosynovitis common	Uncommon
Outcome	Rapid, usually full recovery	Slow response, joint damage; 10% mortality

Delay in antibiotic treatment leads to joint destruction and is associated with a high mortality rate particularly in the elderly. It is important to differentiate from other forms of acute monoarthritis as management is entirely different. Non-gonococcal arthritis is usually treated for 4 weeks with i.v. antibiotics. Infection of a prosthetic joint requires much longer treatment. The septic joint should also be aspirated repeatedly or considered for joint lavage.

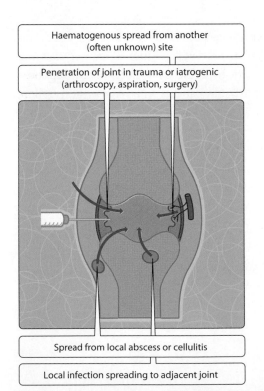

Haematogenous spread from another (often unknown) site

Penetration of joint in trauma or iatrogenic (arthroscopy, aspiration, surgery)

Spread from local abscess or cellulitis

Local infection spreading to adjacent joint

Fig. 3.8.1 Common routes by which pathogens infect joints and bones.

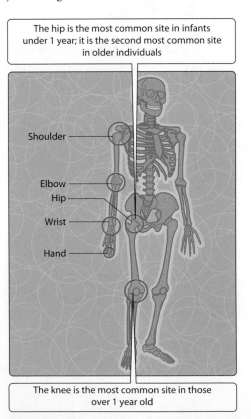

The hip is the most common site in infants under 1 year; it is the second most common site in older individuals

Shoulder

Elbow

Hip

Wrist

Hand

The knee is the most common site in those over 1 year old

Fig. 3.8.2 Common sites of infection in septic arthritis.

9. Fibromyalgia

Questions
- What are the clinical features of fibromyalgia?
- What conditions are associated with fibromyalgia?

Fibromyalgia is the most common cause of widespread musculoskeletal pain. Until recently, many physicians failed to recognize the condition and regarded it as a psychological problem.

Epidemiology
In Western countries, it is estimated that the prevalence at any time is approximately 2%. It is more common in those aged 25–60 years. It is at least eight times more common in females than males.

Pathogenesis
The cause of fibromyalgia is unknown. Symptoms often follow a traumatic event, which can be either physical or emotional. There may be increased pain sensitization, changes in sleep pattern with reduced REM sleep, and dysregulation of the autonomic nervous system.

Clinical features
The main features are widespread musculoskeletal pain, unrefreshing sleep, tiredness and low mood. The patient may already have consulted a number of specialists before a diagnosis is made.

Conditions associated with fibromyalgia include irritable bowel syndrome, tension/migraine headaches, temporal mandibular joint dysfunction, restless leg syndrome and depression.

Fibromyalgia is mainly a clinical diagnosis associated with widespread body pain for at least 3 months and a painful response in at least 11 'trigger' points out of a maximum of 18 using a force of approximately 4 kg (the pressure required to blanch the thumb nail edge) (Fig. 3.9.1). Polymyalgia rheumatica, hypothyroidism, systemic lupus erythematosus, Sjögren's syndrome, depression

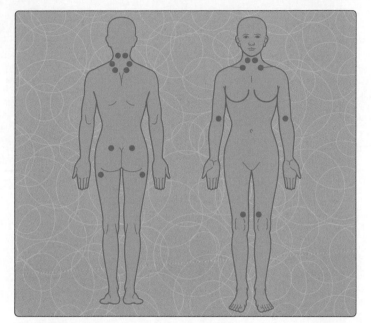

Fig. 3.9.1 Tender 'trigger' points in fibromyalgia.

and hypocalcaemia should be excluded as these may mimic early stages of fibromyalgia.

Investigations
Blood and imaging investigations are unhelpful, although they can exclude other conditions.

Management
An approach involving reassurance, education, medication, graded exercise and cognitive–behavioural therapy is usually required. Reassurance that the illness is not factitious may be the single most important step, and it is also useful to inform patients that it is neither life threatening nor deforming. Antidepressants may have a role. Tramadol alone or in combination with paracetamol is more effective than anti-inflammatory drugs; low-dose tricyclic antidepressants (e.g. amitriptyline) may improve the duration and quality of sleep.

10. Osteoporosis

Questions
- What is a DEXA scan for?
- What is the management of osteoporosis?

Osteoporosis is a skeletal disease characterized by low bone mass and micro-architectural deterioration of bone tissue (Fig. 3.10.1). This results in increased bone fragility and susceptibility to fracture. It carries significant mortality and morbidity from fractures and associated complications, although osteoporosis is potentially treatable and preventable.

Epidemiology

It is estimated that 1 in 3 females and 1 in 8 males develop osteoporosis. Although the risk of fracture mainly depends on bone mineral density, factors such as age and risk of falls determine the absolute risk in any given individual. Risk factors for falls are increased in those with poor balance, postural hypotension, muscle weakness, poor vision or cognitive impairment, or using sedative drugs.

The most common fracture sites are hip, spine and wrist. The incidence of fracture increases with age and is greater in females. The impact of a fracture is significant, since the mortality rate approaches 20% in the elderly with hip fracture, while 60% may remain incapacitated and 20% require residential care.

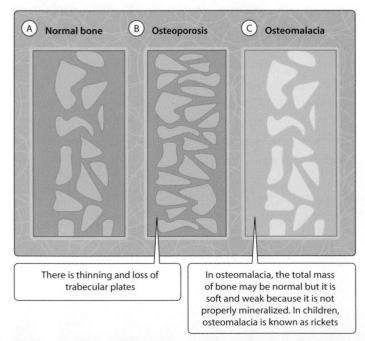

| A | Normal bone | B | Osteoporosis | C | Osteomalacia |

There is thinning and loss of trabecular plates

In osteomalacia, the total mass of bone may be normal but it is soft and weak because it is not properly mineralized. In children, osteomalacia is known as rickets

Fig. 3.10.1 Bone changes in osteoporosis and osteomalacia.

Pathogenesis

Bone is a dynamic structure, with bone formation dominating over bone resorption until peak bone mass is achieved between 25 and 30 years of age. Peak bone mass is determined by genetic factors and environmental factors such as nutrition and exercise. Other factors that influence bone mass include sex and lifestyle. Bone resorption dominates over bone formation in postmenopausal women because of loss of oestrogen. The exact mechanism is not known but oestrogen loss enhances osteoclast function.

Secondary causes of osteoporosis include:
- liver disease
- malabsorption
- rheumatoid arthritis
- excess alcohol
- hyperthyroidism or hyperparathyroidism
- smoking
- oral or systemic steroids
- prolonged bed-rest
- low body mass index.

Bone resorption is more pronounced in hyperthyroidism, hyperparathyroidism and malnutrition, leading to osteoporosis. However, bone formation is impaired to a greater extent in liver disease, and glucocorticoids decrease bone formation and increase bone resorption equally.

Clinical features

Osteoporosis is asymptomatic until a fracture occurs. Hip and spine fractures are common in osteoporosis. Individuals may have acute back pain from vertebral fractures but many are asymptomatic and vertebral fracture may be an incidental finding on radiography. Vertebral fractures result in loss of height, dorsal kyphosis, contact between the pelvis and ribs and a change in posture. Rib fractures following minor trauma are relatively common.

Investigations

Blood tests are aimed at excluding secondary causes of osteoporosis and may include renal and liver function, calcium, phosphate, alkaline phosphatase, immunoglobulins, ESR, thyroid function and endomysial antibodies (for coeliac disease).

Radiography may show reduced bone density (Fig. 3.10.2). DEXA (dual energy X-ray absorptiometry) scans assess bone mineral density. The result is reported as a difference in standard deviations from adult mean scores (T-scores); a T-score of less than -2.5 is consistent with osteoporosis.

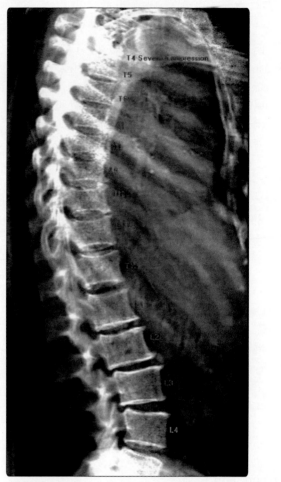

Fig. 3.10.2 Radiograph showing generalized osteopenia and a wedge fracture of an upper thoracic vertebra (T4).

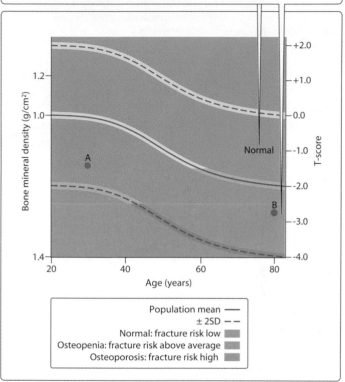

T-score measures the departure from the mean for a young healthy population (units of population SD)

Z-score uses a healthy age- and sex-matched population and so is not used for osteoporosis. Patients A and B both have z-scores of 1.0, in normal range for age, but only patient B has osteoporosis

Population mean ——
± 2SD – –
Normal: fracture risk low
Osteopenia: fracture risk above average
Osteoporosis: fracture risk high

Fig. 3.10.3 Changing bone mineral density with age.

Management

Absolute fracture risk in any individual depends on age, bone density (Fig. 3.10.3) and risk for falls; management depends on assessing these.

Normal bone density (T-score of less than −1.0): fracture risk low, give lifestyle advice

Osteopenia (T-score −1.5 to −2.5): fracture risk above average, give lifestyle advice plus consider calcium and vitamin D supplements

Osteoporosis (T-score less than −2.5): high risk of fractures, manage as for osteopenia but also consider giving drugs to improve bone density.

Once osteoporosis is diagnosed, a number of management strategies may be required. Lifestyle changes such as nutritional improvement, increasing physical activity, smoking cessation and avoiding heavy alcohol consumption are recommended, particularly in at-risk groups such as postmenopausal women and those on long-term steroids. A diet high in calcium or calcium supplements should be used as an adjunct to other treatments if estimated daily calcium intake is low. Secondary causes of osteoporosis should be identified and managed appropriately.

Additional drugs may be required if the future fracture risk is high. Bisphosphonates are a group of synthetic analogues that inhibit bone resorption; alendronate and risedronate taken weekly or ibandronate taken monthly are widely used. Hormone replacement therapy should be considered in postmenopausal women and testosterone in hypogonadal men. Pulsed parathormone injection may also improve bone density.

11. Other disorders of bone

Questions
- What are the complications of Paget's disease?
- What are the features of osteogenesis imperfecta?
- What is the cause of osteomyelitis?

Paget's disease

Paget's disease is a localized bone disorder characterized by increased osteoclastic and osteoblastic activity. This abnormal remodelling leads to structurally disorganized bone, which is mechanically weak and susceptible to deformity and fracture despite apparent thickening of the bone.

Epidemiology

Paget's disease is more common in whites, particularly those living in Europe, USA, Australia and New Zealand, and less commonly found in Asians and Africans. A positive family history is found in over 10% of those affected.

Although it usually begins in the fifth decade of life, the diagnosis is often delayed because of the asymptomatic nature of the disease. The male to female ratio is 3:2. Many patients have more than one bone affected. Morbidity from Paget's disease is common, but death is extremely rare.

Pathogenesis

The cause of Paget's disease is not known. The characteristic features include bone resorption, bone formation, increased blood flow through the affected bone, and fibrous tissue deposition in bone marrow.

Clinical features

Most individuals are asymptomatic, although approximately 5% report symptoms; deep and boring bone pain is the most common feature. Characteristic findings include bowing deformity in long bones, erythema and increased warmth over the affected area (Fig. 3.11.1), but examination may be normal. Sarcomatous change of the bone is an uncommon feature.

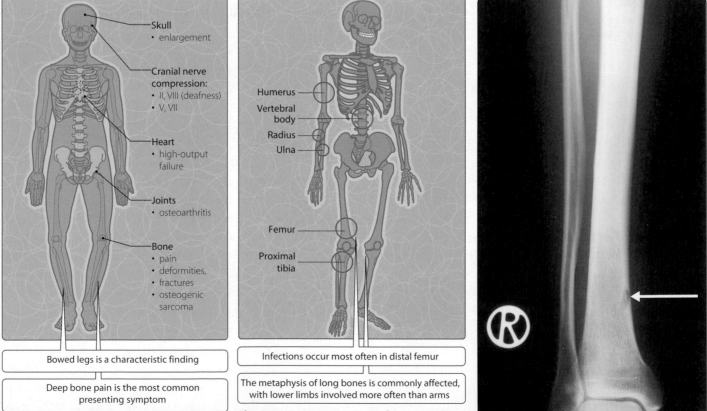

Fig. 3.11.1 Clinical features of Paget's disease.

Fig. 3.11.2 Common sites of osteomyelitis.

Fig. 3.11.3 An area of osteomyelitis of the distal tibia.

Investigations

Alkaline phosphatase of bony origin is raised and calcium is usually normal, except in patients who are immobile. Urine hydroxyproline levels are increased. Radiographs of bones may show lytic areas in the early stages of disease and sclerosis later. Isotope bone scans are useful to identify the extent of skeletal involvement. Bone biopsy is occasionally required.

Management

Most asymptomatic patients do not require treatment. Indications for treatment are bone pain; progressive skeletal deformity; compression of spinal cord, nerve roots or cranial nerves; and fracture. In such circumstances, bisphosphonates are used. Biochemical parameters should be monitored during treatment to assess response. Surgery is sometimes required in patients with secondary osteoarthritis, long-bone deformities affecting gait, and nerve root compression.

Osteogenesis imperfecta

Osteogenesis imperfecta is an inheritable form of connective disease and is principally caused by deficiencies in synthesis of type 1 collagen. The estimated incidence is 1 per 20 000 births.

Pathogenesis

Collagen is an important constituent of bone, tendon, ligament, skin, sclera and dentine. Genetic mutations lead to either decreased collagen production (associated with milder skeletal abnormalities) or structural problems (associated with severe clinical manifestations) in type 1 collagen.

Clinical features

Several different types of osteogenesis imperfecta have been recognized. Features vary but include abnormal dentition, blue sclera, ligament laxity, joint hypermobility and bone fractures.

Management

No effective treatment is available, although bisphosphonates are sometimes tried. Orthopaedic input is required for fractures and prevention or correction of long-bone deformities.

Osteomyelitis

Osteomyelitis is usually caused by bacterial infection of bone and bone marrow, although all types of organism, including viruses, parasites and fungi, can be implicated.

Epidemiology

The prevalence of osteomyelitis is approximately 2/10 000 population, with incidence varying between 1/10 000 and 2/10 000. Incidence is even higher in developing countries because of poor wound care and inadequate use of antibiotics. Osteomyelitis from haematogenous spread is more common in children than adults. For unknown reasons, it is twice as common in males as females. Bones in the spine are more commonly affected in adults, while in children long bones (such as the femur) are more commonly affected. Conditions such as diabetes mellitus, sickle cell disease, HIV, i.v. drug use, alcoholism, chronic steroid use, immunosuppressant therapy and chronic joint disease may increase the risk.

Pathogenesis

Staphylococcus aureus is responsible for up to 90% of osteomyelitis but no organism is isolated in almost 50% of patients. The type of infective organism depends on age, comorbid conditions and the mode of spread.

Infection may reach the bone by haematogenous spread (the most common), contiguous spread or direct implantation. Infection of the bone leads to necrosis and sequestrum formation (dead bone); at the same time, new bone formation called involucrum occurs to circumscribe the sequestrum.

Clinical features

Osteomyelitis may present with throbbing bone pain, fever, malaise and chills. Findings include local swelling, warmth, tenderness and reduction in use of the affected part (Fig. 3.11.2). Chronic osteomyelitis can result in sinus tract drainage, which develops when there is delay in diagnosis, antibiotics or surgical treatment.

Investigations

FBC shows a raised white cell count. CRP and ESR are elevated. Positive blood cultures are found in approximately 50%. Cultures of aspirate in chronic osteomyelitis may be negative.

Radiograph changes are not evident for up to 3 weeks and may show periostial elevation followed by cortical or medullary lucencies (Fig. 3.11.3). Isotope bone scan is sensitive in detecting bone infection before the development of radiological changes. MRI may also be useful for early detection.

Bone biopsy (the gold standard test) is occasionally required.

Management

Initial treatment involves high-dose i.v. antibiotics, usually flucloxacillin and benzylpenicillin, although antibiotics should be tailored according to sensitivities. The optimal duration of antibiotics is uncertain but is normally 4–8 weeks. Occasionally the site of infection requires surgical drainage. In untreated or partially treated patients, complications such as pathological fractures, secondary amyloidosis, endocarditis and rarely sarcoma of the infected bone may arise.

12. Amyloidosis and relapsing polychondritis

Questions
- What is amyloidosis?
- What are the features of relapsing polychondritis?

Amyloidosis

Amyloidosis is characterized by extracellular tissue deposition of various insoluble proteins: 'amyloid' fibrils. These proteins may accumulate locally, causing relatively few symptoms, or widely in multiple organs. The amyloid deposits are metabolically inert but interfere physically with organ structure and function. Amyloid is derived from abnormal proliferation of the proteins of the immune system; these are enzymically altered and then polymerized into fibrils that are deposited in tissues.

Pathogenesis

Amyloid is an insoluble protein formed by abnormal folding of soluble protein that is deposited in various tissues and organs. Although all amyloid deposits have a uniform appearance, each type of amyloid protein is associated with a distinct pattern of organ involvement (Fig. 3.12.1). The kidneys are the most common organ affected but amyloid protein can also be deposited in liver, heart, spleen, adrenal glands, thyroid, tongue and GI tract.

There are three major systemic forms of amyloidosis.

Primary (AL amyloid).   The abnormal protein is an immunoglobulin, usually a light chain fragment (Bence Jones protein) but occasionally a heavy chain fragment (AH amyloidosis). It is caused most often by a plasma cell dyscrasia and can affect any organ.

Secondary (AA amyloid).   The abnormal protein is a degradation product of the acute-phase reactant serum amyloid A (SAA); this accumulates secondary to chronic infections (e.g. bronchiectasis, tuberculosis), inflammatory (e.g. rheumatoid arthritis) and malignant conditions. This is the most common systemic type of amyloidosis and typically involves kidneys, liver and spleen.

Familial autosomal dominant.   Mutations lead to accumulation of a mutated version of a plasma protein (most commonly transthyretin). Nearly all of the abnormal protein is produced by the liver. Familial amyloidoses usual present in middle age.

There are two major localized forms. Intracellular deposition of amyloid fibrils occurs in Alzeimer's disease, where amyloid precursor protein (a normal cell constituent) is converted to Aβ amyloid protein and then to amyloid plaques in the brain. Deposition of an amyloid islet polypeptide occurs in the pancreas of patients with type 2 diabetes. In addition, there are several other forms, such as accumulation of β_2-microglobulin, which is associated with chronic haemodialysis.

Clinical features

There are no specific clinical features as these depend on the organ affected.

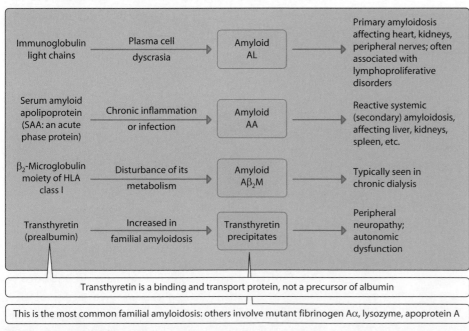

Fig. 3.12.1 Amyloid proteins.

Investigations

Protein electrophoresis and absence of Bence Jones proteinuria (light chains in the urine) exclude underlying plasma cell dyscrasias.

Biopsy, most often of rectum, kidneys or gingival margin, is required to show amyloid deposition on Congo red staining or demonstration of green birefringence within subcutaneous fat.

Prognosis

Prognosis for systemic amyloidosis is poor and is dependent on treatment of the underlying condition.

Relapsing polychondritis

Relapsing polychondritis is a rare condition causing episodic inflammation of multiple cartilaginous structures. It mainly affects the ears, nose and respiratory tract and, less commonly, the eyes, skin and kidneys. It is thought to be an autoimmune condition and is found more often in those > 50 years.

Patients often present with a non-erosive asymmetrical polyarthritis; other features include intermittent red ears, cough, hoarseness and stridor. Clinical examination can reveal synovitis, erythematous tender pinnae with sparing of the lobes and tender nasal bridge; repeated inflammatory episodes result in floppy ears or saddle nose. An associated vasculitis is sometimes found.

The mainstay of treatment is oral steroids, with patients often requiring a low maintenance dose. Prognosis is good, especially in the absence of vasculitic complications.

PART XI

Neurological disorders

Chris Derry

The big picture

Neurology involves the diagnosis and treatment of disorders and diseases of the nervous system. Although recent technological advances (e.g. in imaging and genetics) have revolutionized neurological practice, it remains a highly clinical specialty in which thorough history taking and focused examination are paramount.

Epidemiology

It has been estimated that up to 20% of acute medical admissions arise from neurological conditions. Stroke alone is responsible for approximately 12% of deaths each year in England and Wales, and is the most common cause of acquired disability. The incidence of stroke is approximately 190 per 100 000/year, with approximately 20% of patients becoming dependent on carers for activities of daily living. Other common neurological conditions include epilepsy (present in around 700 people per 100 000 population), multiple sclerosis (affecting around 100 people per 100 000 population in the UK) and migraine, which affects over 10% of the population. However, there are many other neurological conditions that are relatively rare and may be seen only infrequently by GPs and general physicians; such cases tend to require specialist neurological input for diagnosis and management.

Clinical approach to a patient with a neurological complaint

When faced with a patient with neurological complaints, arriving at the correct diagnosis is not always straightforward. In order to maximize the chances of doing so, it is important to take a logical approach, based on the history and examination. The first aim is to make an 'anatomical diagnosis' based on the clinical presentation. In other words, the clinician should try to localize where in the nervous system the pathological process is occurring. If the clinical presentation is consistent with a lesion in the brain, an attempt should be made to establish which hemisphere and region of brains affected (Fig. 1.1.) Second, a mechanism should be considered; for example, sudden onset of symptoms often suggests a vascular event, whereas subacute onset over days to weeks might be more consistent with an inflammatory or infective pathology.

Once a conclusion has been reached about the anatomical site of the pathology and the potential mechanisms involved, specific pathological diagnoses should be considered. At this stage, further investigations should be arranged to confirm or refute these possibilities. These should be used to test specific hypotheses that have been generated by clinical assessment. In many straightforward cases, no investigations are required. Some investigations, such as neuroimaging and neurophysiological studies, can be very difficult to interpret in the absence of an appropriate a priori hypothesis and may lead to erroneous conclusions if used in this way.

The aim of this part of the book is to provide an overview of the major neurological conditions faced in clinical practice. It is not designed to cover the practicalities of neurological history taking and examination, nor does it cover in detail the basic neuroanatomy and neurophysiology that students and clinicians require when assessing a patient with a neurological complaint. Rather, it is a review of those neurological conditions with which the student should be familiar as part of his or her undergraduate medical training.

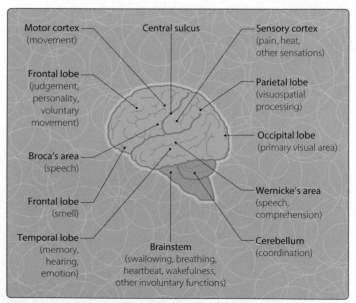

Fig. 1.1 Localization of function within the brain.

Table 1.1 INCIDENCE RATES FOR COMMON NEUROLOGICAL DISORDERS IN THE UK

Neurological disorder	Incidence (new cases per 100 000 population per yer)
Migraine	400
Stroke	200
Epilepsy	50
Dementia (all types)	50
Peripheral neuropathy (all types)	40
Parkinson's disease	20
Subarachnoid haemorrhage	15
Brain tumour (primary)	5
Multiple sclerosis	4
Motor neuron disease	2

1 **Stroke** is the sudden onset of neurological dysfunction of vascular cause lasting > 24 h. The term **transient ischaemic attack** is used if features resolve within 24 h. Approximately 85% of strokes are caused by infarction (ischaemic stroke) and 15% by intracerebral haemorrhage (haemorrhagic stroke). Investigations are aimed at confirming a stroke and identifying an underlying cause. Immediate treatments available for ischaemic stroke include aspirin and thrombolysis. Acute stroke should be managed on a dedicated stroke unit. **Cerebral venous sinus thrombosis** presents with features of raised intracranial pressure (headache, vomiting, drowsiness, papilloedema); seizures and focal neurological deficits may also occur.

2 **Intracerebral haemorrhage** accounts for approximately 15% of all strokes. Intracerebral bleeds are immediately visible on CT. **Subdural haemorrhage** is caused by rupture of bridging veins between the cerebral cortex and venous sinuses. It most commonly affects the elderly and may occur spontaneously or after minimal injury. **Extradural haemorrhage** usually occurs after a significant head injury causing skull fracture; it often results from rupture of the middle meningeal artery. **Subarachnoid haemorrhage** is usually caused by rupture of an intracranial saccular (berry) aneurysm, or less commonly an arteriovenous malformation.

3 **Motor neuron disease** is a progressive degenerative disease of upper and lower motor neurons. It is characterized by progressive limb, bulbar and respiratory muscle weakness, leading to severe disability and death. In **myasthenia gravis**, antibodies to postsynaptic acetylcholine receptors block neurotransmission at the neuromuscular junction. This causes a fatiguable weakness in ocular, bulbar and limb muscles, which usually responds to treatment. **Lambert–Eaton myasthenic syndrome** is a non-metastatic (paraneoplastic) manifestation of cancer. **Muscular dystrophies** are inherited disorders characterized by progressive degeneration of specific muscle groups.

Myotonic dystrophy is an autosomal dominant disorder with a number of characteristic features such as progressive muscle wasting, cardiac arrythmias and myotonia (difficulty in relaxing the muscles).

4 **Mononeuropathy** is an abnormality of a single peripheral nerve, and may result from compression, ischaemia or systemic disease (e.g. diabetes); the median, ulnar and common peroneal nerves are most commonly affected. In **polyneuropathy,** multiple nerves are affected. The most common type is a peripheral neuropathy, which causes 'glove and stocking' sensory loss. Diabetes mellitus, chronic alcoholic abuse and drugs (such as amiodarone and metronidazole) are the most common causes. **Guillain–Barré syndrome** is an acute autoimmune (often post-infective) polyneuropathy causing ascending paralysis.

5 **Cranial nerve** palsies may be caused by lesions in the brain (cerebrovascular disease, multiple sclerosis) or by lesions of the peripheral nerve. **Bell's palsy** (an acute idiopathic lower motor neuron facial weakness) is the most common cranial nerve palsy. Lesions of cranial nerves III and IV (controlling eye movements) are also common and have a variety of possible causes.

6 **Multiple sclerosis** is an inflammatory demyelinating disease of the CNS. It has a variety of forms but most commonly presents in early adulthood with relapsing and remitting neurological symptoms. Common presentations include optic neuritis and brainstem or spinal cord features. Demonstration of lesions on MRI brain and oligoclonal bands in CSF support the diagnosis. Disease-modifying drugs (e.g. interferon beta) may reduce the rate of relapse.

7 **Migraine** is characterized by throbbing, severe and often unilateral headache, associated with nausea and photophobia. Some patients experience an 'aura' (most commonly visual disturbance) prior to headache. **Cluster headache** is characterized by recurrent episodes of severe unilateral periorbital pain, often associated with nasal congestion and a red eye. **Trigeminal neuralgia** is severe, unilateral, lancinating facial pain in the distribution of the trigeminal nerve. It may be caused by vascular anomalies compressing the trigeminal nerve.

8 **Hydrocephalus** describes increased CSF volume with dilation of the cerebral ventricles. It can arise through obstruction of CSF pathways or impaired CSF reabsorption. Presentation is usually with features of raised intracranial pressure. **Normal pressure hydrocephalus** is characterized by gait disorder, dementia and urinary incontinence. Neuroimaging demonstrates enlarged cerebral ventricles, but CSF pressure is typically normal. **Idiopathic intracranial hypertension** is elevated intracranial pressure of unknown cause; it is most common in obese women. It usually present with headache and visual symptoms and papilloedema. Untreated it can result in permanent visual loss.

9 **Spinal cord lesions** present with bilateral limb weakness, sensory disturbance below the level of compression, and bowel and bladder dysfunction. Lesions may be intrinsic (e.g. multiple sclerosis) or extrinsic (e.g. spinal metastases causing cord compression). **Cervical spondylosis** is a degenerative condition of the spine and usually presents with neck pain. Other neurological symptoms may occur from compression of the spinal cord or nerve roots. **Subacute combined degeneration of the cord** is caused by chronic vitamin B_{12} deficiency. It presents with a mixture of spinal cord features and peripheral neuropathy. **Syringomyelia** is an abnormal fluid-filled cystic cavity within the spinal cord. Initial symptoms are pain and sensory loss in the upper limbs.

10 **Epilepsy** is the tendency to recurrent seizures. There are many types of epilepsy, which can be grouped into focal (start in one part of the brain and spread) or generalized (affect most of the brain at onset). Treatment with antiepileptic drugs is usually necessary following two or more seizures. **Status epilepticus** describes continuous or recurrent seizures, without recovery of consciousness, for over 30 min. It is a neurological emergency requiring treatment with i.v. benzodiazepines or phenytoin.

11 **Dementia** is a progressive deterioration of intellect, behaviour and personality that interferes with social and occupational functioning. It should be differentiated from delirium, which is an acute disturbance of brain function often caused by drugs or infection. Personality change, memory loss and difficulties in learning and retaining new information are frequent presentations. Common causes are **Alzheimer's disease** and **vascular dementia** (cerebrovascular disease); rarer causes are dementia with Lewy bodies and frontotemporal dementia. Potentially reversible causes include vitamin B_{12} deficiency, neurosyphilis, tumours and hypothyroidism.

12 The **akinetic-rigid** (or parkinsonian) syndromes are characterized by slow, reduced movements (bradykinesia) and increased muscle tone. **Parkinson's disease** is a progressive condition caused by loss of central dopaminergic neurons. It present with bradykinesia, rigidity and a characteristic tremor. Similar features (parkinsonism) may be seen following treatment with antipsychotic drugs, in cerebrovascular disease, and in the rare 'Parkinson plus' syndromes (multiple system atrophy and progressive supranuclear palsy).

13 **Essential tremor** is a bilateral postural upper limb tremor, which is often familial and not associated with other neurological features. **Huntington's disease** is an autosomal dominant neurodegenerative disease characterized by progressive chorea and dementia. **Wilson's disease** is a rare autosomal recessive disorder of copper metabolism, causing progressive chorea, cognitive imparment and deranged liver function.

14 The **cerebellum** controls motor coordination and balance. Midline cerebellar lesions cause an unsteady broad-based ataxic gait and truncal ataxia. Lateralized cerebellar lesions cause limb ataxia, dysdiadochokinesis, intention tremor and nystagmus. Dysarthria is also characteristic. Common causes of cerebellar damage include cerebrovascular disease, drugs (alcohol and phenytoin), multiple sclerosis, stroke and tumours.

15 Primary **tumours** of the CNS may be benign or malignant. They typically present with seizures, progressive focal neurological deficits or features of raised intracranial pressure. Brain CT or MRI usually confirms the presence of a mass lesion. Cerebral metastases arise from a primary at a distant site but have a similar neurological presentation. Treatment is aimed at the primary cancer and may involve surgery, chemotherapy and/or radiotherapy.

1. Cerebrovascular disease I: thromboembolic stroke

Questions
- What are the main causes of stroke?
- What is the management of patients with acute stroke?

A stroke is the sudden onset of neurological dysfunction lasting for over 24 h, caused by a disruption of blood supply. The term transient ischaemic attack (TIA) is used when symptoms and signs fully resolve within 24 h. Most strokes (approximately 85%) result from infarction, while the remainder (approximately 15%) are caused by intracerebral haemorrhage.

Ischaemic stroke

Epidemiology
Stroke accounts for 12% of all deaths in the UK and is the leading cause of long-term disability. Although more common with increasing age, approximately a quarter of strokes occur in individuals aged under 65.

Pathogenesis
The brain's blood supply can be divided into the anterior and posterior circulations (Fig. 3.1.1). The anterior circulation originates from the carotid arteries, which divide to form the middle and anterior cerebral arteries. These supply the frontal, parietal and part of the temporal lobes. The posterior circulation arises from the vertebral arteries, which join to form the basilar artery; this itself then divides to form the posterior cerebral arteries. The posterior circulation supplies the occipital and medial temporal lobes, thalamus, brainstem and cerebellum. In health, the anterior and posterior circulations are joined via the circle of Willis (although this system may be damaged by atherosclerosis) (Fig. 3.1.2).

Ischaemic strokes arise from occlusion of a blood vessel, causing infarction of brain tissue. This can arise through a variety of mechanisms, the most common of which include:
- *arterial atherosclerosis* : thrombus forms on arterial atherosclerotic plaques in the internal carotid artery or intracranial vessels
- *cardioembolism* : cardiac thrombus (arising in atrial fibrillation or recent myocardial infarction) travels to the cerebral circulation
- *small-vessel occlusion* ('lacunar stroke') : thrombosis forms in small penetrating arteries that have been damaged by long-standing hypertension
- *non-atheromatous disease* : thrombus develops in arteries damaged by vasculitis or arterial dissection.

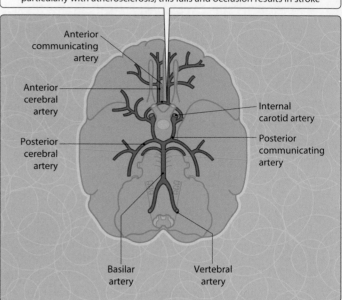

The circle of Willis should preserve cerebral blood supply if one internal carotid artery is occluded. However, in many people, particularly with atherosclerosis, this fails and occlusion results in stroke

Fig. 3.1.1 The arteries supplying the brain.

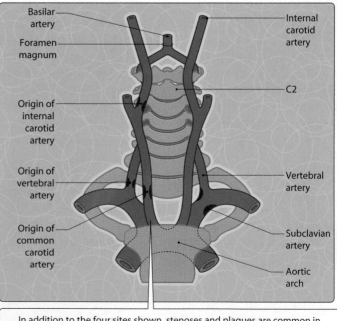

In addition to the four sites shown, stenoses and plaques are common in the carotid artery syphon within the cavernous sinus

Fig. 3.1.2 Principal sites of atheromatous disease in extracerebral arteries.

Clinical features

Patients with stroke present with a combination of symptoms and signs depending on the area of brain affected (see Fig. 1.1, p. 256).

Anterior circulation stroke. Strokes are more common in the anterior than posterior circulation, and most frequently occur in the middle cerebral artery territory. Clinical features include hemiplegia, hemisensory disturbance, dysphasia and sensory neglect.

Posterior circulation stroke. Posterior circulation strokes affect the occipital lobes, cerebellum or brainstem. Damage to the occipital lobes results in a homonymous hemianopia; cerebellar strokes present with vertigo, vomiting and ataxia, and brainstem strokes may present with hemiparesis, coma, cranial nerve palsies, ataxia and vertigo. Basilar artery occlusion may rarely result in the **'locked-in syndrome'**; in this condition, extensive damage to the upper pons results in complete loss of speech and quadriplegia but preserved consciousness and normal eye movements.

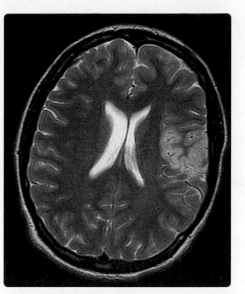

Fig. 3.1.3 MRI showing a left middle cerebral artery infarct.

Investigations

Investigations have two main aims: first, to confirm the diagnosis and distinguish ischaemia from haemorrhage; second, to identify the underlying cause of stroke (e.g. atherosclerosis, atrial fibrillation, etc.).

Investigations to establish the underlying cause of stroke include:

- blood tests (full blood count, renal function, lipids and glucose)
- ECG and Holter monitor (looking for cardiac arrhythmia or recent ischaemia)
- echocardiogram (looking for structural cardiac abnormalities)
- carotid doppler ultrasound (looking for carotid artery stenosis)
- CT brain (used to confirm the diagnosis and distinguish haemorrhage from infarction), required urgently if the patient is a potential candidate for thrombolysis
- MRI (occasionally used in diagnostic difficulty as it is more sensitive than CT in detecting ischaemic strokes, but is slower and less widely available) (Fig. 3.1.3).

Management

Acute management. Patients should be managed in a specialised stroke unit. All patients with ischaemic stroke should receive aspirin within the first 48 hours. Ischaemic stroke presenting within 3 hours of onset should be considered for thrombolysis; this treatment may reduce the disability after stroke but carries a risk of life-threatening haemorrhage.

Secondary prevention. Vascular risk factors (cigarette smoking, hypertension, hyperlipidaemia and diabetes mellitus) should be identified and managed appropriately. Long-term antiplatelet therapy (usually aspirin and often dipyridamole) is generally indicated after ischaemic stroke; clopidogrel may be useful if aspirin is not tolerated. Warfarin is preferred to antiplatelet agents in individuals with atrial fibrillation unless specific contraindications are present. ACE inhibitors and statins have also been shown to be beneficial in secondary prevention studies and are usually prescribed. Individuals with significant carotid artery stenosis (> 70%) should be considered for carotid endarterectomy.

Transient ischaemic attack (TIA)

The term TIA is used to describe episodes in which neurological deficits fully resolve within 24 hours. One well-recognized type of TIA is **amaurosis fugax**, a sudden monocular visual loss arising from temporary occlusion of the ophthalmic artery; this symptom is highly suggestive of a significant ipsilateral carotid stenosis.

A TIA is a strong predictor of subsequent stroke (approximately 30% of individuals with a TIA develop a stroke within the next 5 years). The risk of stroke is greatest soon after the TIA: 5–10% within 1 week and 10–20% within 3 months. Urgent investigation and appropriate management (which may include carotid endarterectomy) are vital.

Venous sinus thrombosis

Thrombosis can occur in cerebral veins as well as arteries, but results from different pathology to arterial stroke. Predisposing factors include hypercoagulable states, the oral contraceptive pill, dehydration, mastoid infection and direct pressure on a venous sinus (e.g. from tumour); however, no cause is found in up to 25%. Patients often present with headache, seizures, nausea and vomiting. Focal neurological deficits and papilloedema occur in some patients. CT or MRI venography is usually required to confirm the diagnosis, as standard CT may be normal in this condition. Management is with anticoagulation and treatment of the underlying cause.

2. Cerebrovascular disease II: intracerebral and intracranial haemorrhage

Questions
- What are the differences between extradural and subdural haemorrhage?
- What are the features of subarachnoid haemorrhage?
- What investigations are used in subarachnoid haemorrhage?

Intracranial haemorrhage describes any haemorrhage occurring inside the skull. Intracerebral haemorrhages (i.e. inside brain tissue) are considered a type of stroke, whereas bleeds within the skull but outside the brain (e.g. subarachnoid haemorrhage, subdural and extradural haematomas) are usually considered separately (Fig 3.2.1).

Intracerebral haemorrhage

Intracerebral haemorrhage accounts for approximately 15% of all strokes. The most common cause is degenerative disease of small perforating vessels deep within the brain (lipohyalinosis) from long-standing hypertension. In elderly patients, degenerative changes may occur in small blood vessels supplying the cerebral cortex (amyloid angiopathy), predisposing to more superficial haemorrhages.

The clinical features of intracerebral haemorrhage are similar to cerebral infarction, but signs of raised intracranial pressure (headache, vomiting or reduced level of consciousness) may occur with larger haemorrhages. In contrast to cerebral infarction, intracerebral haemorrhage shows immediate change on CT.

Patients should be managed on a dedicated stroke unit and treament is largely supportive. Hypertension is common following intracerbral haemorrhage but should be treated with caution as sudden falls in blood pressure may worsen neurological impairment. Neurosurgical intervention is considered when haemorrhage causes life-threatening elevation of intracranial pressure. Long-term treatment for hypertension is usually required.

Cerebellar haemorrhage

Cerebellar haemorrhage causes abrupt onset of headache, vomiting, nausea and vertigo, with features of cerebellar dysfunction (nystagmus, dysarthria and ataxia). Cerebellar haemorrhages are particularly likely to cause dangerous increases in intracranial pressure, as the bleed may compress the cerebral aqueduct (communication between the third and fourth ventricles), blocking CSF flow and causing acute hydrocephalus. This can result in transtentorial herniation ('coning'), which is usually fatal (Chs 8 and 14). Cerebellar haemorrhage is visible on CT or MRI brain.

Immediate management depends on the size of the haemorrhage and clinical features. Patients with normal consciousness are usually treated similarly to those with other intracerebral haemorrhages; those with impaired consciousness or intracranial hypertension may require urgent CT brain scan and neurosurgical intervention.

Subdural haemorrhage

Subdural haemorrhage results from rupture of bridging veins between the cerebral cortex and venous sinuses. This causes an accumulation of blood in the subdural space. It is more common in the elderly and those with a history of head trauma or using warfarin. Symptoms occur through a local mass effect (which may cause focal neurological deficits) and raised intracranial pressure (which causes headache and drowsiness). Symptoms are insidious over weeks. The diagnosis is confirmed by CT. Neurosurgical advice should be obtained as burr holes or craniotomy may be required.

Extradural haemorrhage

Extradural haemorrhage results from arterial rupture, usually of the middle meningeal artery. This causes rapid accumulation of blood between the skull and dura mater. Subsequently (within minutes to hours), patients complain of increasingly severe headache and conscious level falls. Focal neurological signs such as hemiparesis may develop, and the patient may exhibit a Cush-

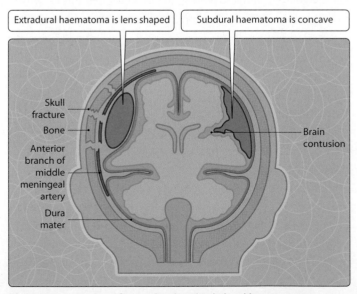

Extradural haematoma is lens shaped | Subdural haematoma is concave

Skull fracture
Bone
Anterior branch of middle meningeal artery
Dura mater
Brain contusion

Fig. 3.2.1 Features of extradural and subdural haematomas.

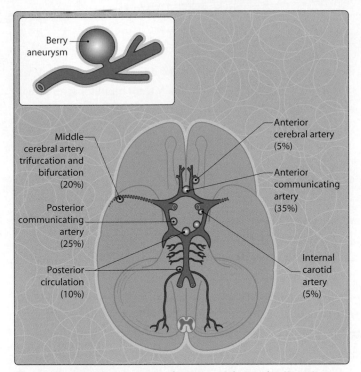

Fig. 3.2.2 The sites of origin of intracranial saccular (Berry) aneurysms on the inferior surface of the brain.

Table 3.2.1 THE HUNT AND HESS GRADING SYSTEM FOR SUBARACHNOID HAEMORRHAGE AND PROGNOSIS

Grade	Clinical features	Outcome (% with long-term survival)
1	Asymptomatic or mild headache	70
2	Moderate to severe headache; nuchal rigidity; no neurological deficit other than possible cranial nerve palsy	60
3	Mild alteration in mental status (confusion, lethargy); mild focal neurological deficit	50
4	Stupor and/or hemiparesis	20
5	Comatose and/or decerebrate posturing	10

ing's response (hypertension, bradycardia and bradypnoea), which indicates rapidly rising intracranial pressure. Diagnosis is confirmed by CT. Urgent neurosurgical input is essential, and craniotomy and evacuation of the haemorrhage is usually required.

Subarachnoid haemorrhage

Subarachnoid haemorrhage (SAH) most commonly results from rupture of a saccular ('berry') aneurysm on the circle of Willis. It tends to affect a younger age group, with the average age being 50 years. It has an annual incidence of 10–15/100 000 population.

Pathogenesis

Approximately 80% of SAH occurs from rupture of a berry aneurysm (Fig. 3.2.2). These usually develop at bifurcations in the circle of Willis; predisposing factors include hypertension and smoking. Less commonly, SAH may be caused by head trauma or rupture of an arteriovenous malformation.

Clinical features

Typically, there is a sudden, severe headache; the patient may describe it as the worst headache of their life. Neck stiffness, photophobia, drowsiness, nausea and vomiting are common. Seizures occur in approximately 10–20%, and focal neurological deficits may be present. Some individuals may have preceding symptoms (caused by aneurysmal expansion or a small leak of blood) such as headache or painful cranial nerve III palsy.

Investigations

CT shows subarachnoid blood in approximately 80–95% (sensitivity is greater if the scan is performed early). Lumbar puncture should be performed if the CT is non-diagnostic. The presence of oxyhaemoglobin and bilirubin (blood breakdown products) in CSF are highly suggestive of SAH. Once SAH is confirmed, cerebral angiography (usisng CT, MRI or digital subtraction angiography) is needed to identify the causal aneurysm.

Management

Management is aimed at preventing the complications of SAH (vasospasm, rebleeding and hydrocephalus) and treating the causal aneurysm to prevent further bleeds. Untreated vasospasm may result in ischaemic stroke and permanent neurological deficit; nimodipine, a calcium channel blocker, is given to prevent this. Bed-rest, analgesia and adequate fluids are also essential to prevent changes in cerebral perfusion, which may result in rebleeding or cerebral ischaemia. Definitive treatment involves either surgical clipping or endovascular coiling of the aneurysm.

Prognosis

The most important predictor of prognosis is the severity of the initial neurological deficit (Table 3.2.1). Overall, approximately 10–15% of patients with subarachnoid haemorrhage die before they reach hospital. The mortality rate at 1 week may be as high as 40%, while over one-third of survivors have significant neurological deficits.

3. Neuromuscular disorders

Questions
- What are the clinical features of motor neuron disease?
- How is myasthenia gravis diagnosed?

Motor neuron disease

Motor neuron disease (MND) is a progressive degenerative disease of upper and lower motor neurons resulting in progressive disability and death (Fig. 3.3.1). MND occurs in 2/100 000 adults per year, with a mean age of onset around 65 years. The male to female ratio is 3:2 and 10% of cases are familial.

Clinical features

Presentation is variable; patients typically develop either progressive weakness of one or more limbs over months or progressive bulbar weakness, with dysarthria, dysphagia, tongue weakness and wasting. On examination, muscle wasting and fasciculation, with brisk reflexes and extensor plantar responses (i.e. mixed lower and upper motor neuron features), are characteristic. There is no sensory involvement. In advanced disease, respiratory muscle weakness causes breathlessness when lying flat (orthopnoea) and eventually respiratory failure. A minority also develop frontotemporal dementia. Death usually occurs 3–5 years after the onset of first symptoms.

Investigation and management

MND is a clinical diagnosis. Investigations are aimed at excluding differential diagnoses and identifying supportive changes of denervation and reinnervation on electromyography (EMG). Riluzole

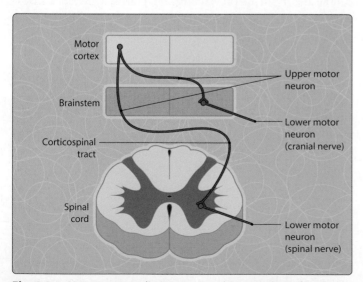

Fig. 3.3.1 Motor neuron disease causes degeneration of both upper and lower motor neurons.

is the only treatment known to slow disease progression but has only modest benefit. Multidisciplinary team input for symptomatic and supportive management is essential. Patients may require percutaneous endoscopic gastrostomy feeding for dysphagia and non-invasive ventilation in chronic ventilatory failure.

Myasthenia gravis

Myasthenia gravis (MG) is an acquired autoimmune disease in which antibodies to the postsynaptic acetylcholine receptor (Fig. 3.3.2) impair neuromuscular transmission. The condition is associated with hyperplasia of the thymus gland in approximately 70%; in up to 10% a malignant thymoma is present. There is also a strong association with other autoimmune conditions. The female to male ratio is 2:1. The overall annual incidence is 0.2–0.4/100 000 per year; the condition preferentially affects young women (second and third decades), with a second peak in older men (sixth and seventh decades).

Clinical features

MG causes fatigable muscle weakness, which fluctuates but typically worsens late in the day and following exertion. Most commonly, MG tends to affect the eyes (causing fatigable ptosis and diplopia) facial and bulbar muscles (dysphagia and dysarthria), and upper limb muscles. On examination, fatigable weakness can be demonstrated by repeated or sustained movement of an affected muscle group.

Investigations

Anti-acetylcholine receptor antibodies are present in 80–90% and are diagnostic. Nerve conduction studies and EMG may show characteristic features. Chest CT is required to exclude an underlying thymoma. The tensilon test (an intravenous bolus of the anticholinesterase edrophonium) may result in dramatic temporary improvement in weakness (Fig. 3.3.3), but this test is unreliable and associated with risks of cardiac arrhythmia.

Management

Symptomatic treatment with pyridostigmine (an oral anticholinesterase) is first-line therapy. Immunosuppression with oral steroids (prednisolone) and azathioprine is often required. Thymectomy may improve myasthenia in selected patients. In some patients, MG may worsen rapidly, particularly in the context of infection, and involvement of respiratory muscles can cause acute respiratory failure. Such patients often require ventilation and additional treatment such as plasma exchange.

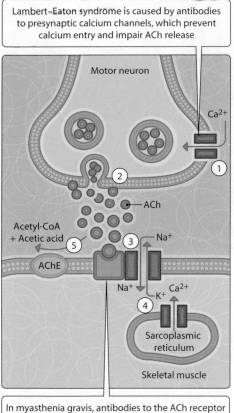

Lambert–Eaton syndrome is caused by antibodies to presynaptic calcium channels, which prevent calcium entry and impair ACh release

Motor neuron

Ca^{2+}

ACh

Acetyl-CoA + Acetic acid

Na^+

AChE

Na^+ K^+ Ca^{2+}

Sarcoplasmic reticulum

Skeletal muscle

In myasthenia gravis, antibodies to the ACh receptor inactivate it, thus preventing activation of the muscle

Fig. 3.3.2 Transmission at the neuromuscular junction. 1, Calcium ions enter the neuron in response to the nerve impulse arriving at the motor end-plate. 2, This stimulates release of acetylcholine (ACh) from storage vesicles in 'packets' into the neuromuscular junction. 3, Binding of ACh to its receptor on the muscle causes depolarization. 4, Depolarization initiates muscle contraction. 5, Acetylcholinesterase (AChE) removes ACh from the neuromuscular junction and terminates its action.

Lambert–Eaton myasthenic syndrome

Lambert-Eaton myasthenic syndrome (LEMS) is a rare auto-immune syndrome characterized by antibodies against calcium channels of the presynaptic motor nerve terminal (Fig. 3.3.2). This results in a myasthenia-like illness with fluctuating weakness. LEMS typically affects the lower limbs. It is associated with an underlying malignancy in 40–70% (typically small-cell lung cancer). Treatment is that of the underlying malignancy and sometimes with 3,4-diaminopyridine.

Muscular dystrophies

Muscular dystrophies are inherited disorders characterized by progressive muscle weakness and wasting. **Duchenne muscular dystrophy** is the most common and is caused by a mutation in the gene coding for the protein dystrophin. It is an X-linked recessive disorder affecting males alone and presenting early in life, often with delayed motor milestones. Proximal muscles are predominantly affected, but calf enlargement (pseudohypertrophy)

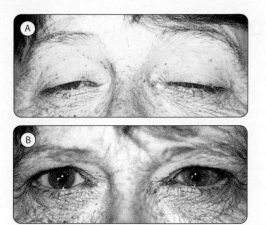

Fig. 3.3.3 The edrophonium (Tensilon) test: before (A) and after (B) injection of edrophonium (short-acting acetylcholinesterase inhibitor), which gives an immediate increase in muscle strength.

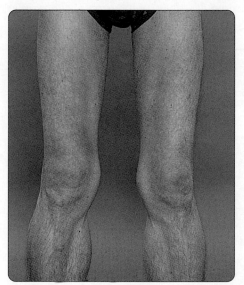

Fig. 3.3.4 An adult with Becker's muscular dystrophy; note the wasting of the quadriceps and apparent calf hypertrophy.

is commonly seen. Mild learning disability and cardiac arrhythmias are also features. Individuals are usually confined to a wheelchair by the second decade and death occurs before the age of 30.

Becker muscular dystrophy is also an X-linked condition of the gene for dystrophin; it presents in a similar fashion to Duchenne muscular dystrophy but is less severe (Fig. 3.3.4). Onset is usually in childhood but may be later. Cardiomyopathy may develop in the third decade.

Myotonic dystrophy is an autosomal dominant condition demonstrating genetic anticipation (subsequent generations are increasingly severely affected, with earlier disease onset). Individuals typically present in early adulthood with distal limb weakness, stiffness and myotonia (delayed muscle relaxation following contraction). Other features include mild cognitive impairment, early prefrontal balding, cataract formation, bilateral ptosis, testicular atrophy, cardiomyopathy with conduction defects, pituitary dysfunction and diabetes mellitus.

4. Neuropathies

Questions
■ What is Guillain–Barré syndrome?
■ What are mononeuropathy, peripheral neuropathy and autonomic neuropathy?

Mononeuropathy

A mononeuropathy is a disorder of a single peripheral nerve. It usually results from trauma or compression of the nerve, but infection or systemic inflammatory conditions such as vasculitis may sometimes be the cause. Certain nerves are particularly prone to damage because of their anatomical course (Fig. 3.4.1). **Carpal tunnel syndrome** describes compression of the median nerve at the wrist (Fig. 3.4.2). Any process that causes narrowing of the carpal tunnel by affecting bones or ligaments (such as pregnancy, obesity, hypothyroidism, acromegaly, rheumatoid arthritis or diabetes mellitus) can predispose. Patients complain of pain and tingling in the hand, which is usually worse at night,

and develop altered sensation in the median nerve distribution (Fig. 3.4.1). There may be weakness of thumb abduction and wasting of the thenar eminence; symptoms can be reproduced by wrist flexion (Phalen's sign) or by tapping over the palmar surface of the wrist (Tinel's sign). The diagnosis is confirmed by nerve conductionstudies. Symptoms may be relieved by splinting or local steroid injections, but definitive treatment usually involves surgical decompression.

Mononeuritis multiplex

Mononeuritis multiplex is damage to two or more individual peripheral nerves, and is often painful. It usually results from nerve infarction and occurs in a variety of underlying systemic conditions, most commonly diabetes mellitus but also rheumatoid arthritis, systemic lupus erythematosus and vasculitis. Nerve conduction studies confirm the diagnosis, but further investigations are required to establish the underlying cause.

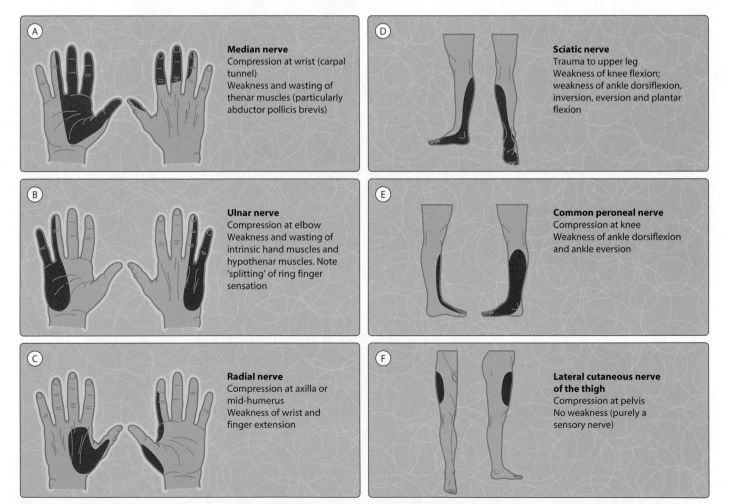

Fig. 3.4.1 Areas of sensory impairment (yellow) found in the most common entrapment neuropathies and the accompanying motor weaknesses.

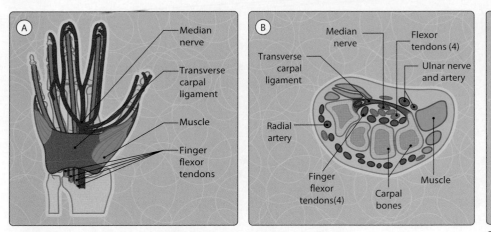

Fig. 3.4.2 Location of the carpal tunnel and surrounding anatomy.

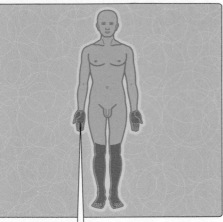

Nerve involvement is 'length dependent' and so the hands are usually not involved until lower limb disturbance reaches at least to the knee

Fig. 3.4.3 Sensory disturbance in a 'glove and stocking' distribution in peripheral neuropathy.

Peripheral neuropathy

Peripheral neuropathy describes a process of 'length-dependent' nerve damage. It begins distally and spreads symmetrically in a 'glove and stocking' pattern (Fig. 3.4.3); the legs are affected before the arms as the peripheral nerves are longer in the lower limbs. Sensory, motor and autonomic functions may all be affected. Diabetes mellitus and chronic alcohol abuse are most often responsible, but drugs (e.g. amiodarone, metronidazole), vitamin B_{12} deficiency, renal failure and thyroid disease are also common causes.

Guillain–Barré syndrome

Guillain–Barré syndrome is an immune-mediated, rapidly progressing ascending polyneuropathy. Its annual incidence is approximately 2–3/100 000. It is usually postinfective, with certain organisms (often *Campylobacter jejuni*, but occasionally Epstein–Barr virus, cytomegalovirus and HIV) being particularly associated. A cell-mediated autoimmune response is triggered against myelin or other components of the peripheral nerve, causing nerve damage.

Clinical features

Clinical features usually appear 2–4 weeks following a diarrhoeal or upper respiratory tract infection. Symptoms include paraesthesiae in the extremities, but weakness in the proximal limb muscles is the dominant feature; facial weakness is also common. Pain often occurs. The neurological deficits progress over hours to days, usually reaching a maximum within 1–3 weeks; sometimes deterioration may be very rapid. Patients with respiratory muscle weakness may require ventilatory support. Autonomic involvement is common and may cause postural hypotension and cardiac arrhythmias.

Investigations

CSF protein is elevated (usually 1–3 g/l) but cell count and glucose are normal. Nerve conduction studies usually show evidence of a demyelinating polyneuropathy.

Management

Intravenous immunoglobulin, and sometimes plasma exchange, are given to arrest the disease process. Both have been shown to reduce the severity of paralysis and speed recovery time. Acute management includes monitoring for cardiac arrhythmias and respiratory muscle weakness (using serial vital capacity measurements), as well as adequate hydration, analgesia and thromboprophylaxis. Physiotherapy should be commenced early. Most patients make a full functional recovery, although this may take up to 18 months. Up to 10% are left with a residual neurological defcit, and the mortality rate is approximately 5% (usually from ventilatory failure, infection or pulmonary embolism).

Autonomic neuropathy

The autonomic system controls non-sensory and non-motor functions such as blood pressure, heart rate, digestion and bowel and bladder emptying. Autonomic neuropathy may occur in combination with a sensorimotor polyneuropathy or may be an isolated finding. The most prominent symptom is syncope from postural hypotension. Constipation, diarrhoea, urinary retention, erectile dysfunction, blurring of vision, dry mouth and lack of sweating (anhydrosis) may also occur. Diabetes mellitus is the most common cause but other causes include amyloidosis, coeliac disease and drugs (vincristine and cisplatin). Management is difficult and usually involves treatment of the underlying cause.

5. Cranial nerve lesions

Questions
- What are the main causes and clinical features of cranial nerve palsies?
- What is Bell's palsy?

Cranial nerve I: olfactory nerve

Cranial nerve (CN)I begins as multiple small branches in the nasal mucosa; these enter the skull via the cribiform plate, synapse in the olfactory bulb and continue as the olfactory tract to the brain. Damage to CNI from a head injury or a space-occupying lesion in the frontal lobe results in anosmia (loss of sense of smell).

Cranial nerve II: optic nerve

CNII originates in the retina and travels, via the optic chiasm and optic tract, to the lateral geniculate nuclei. From here, the optic radiation carries fibres to the occipital cortex (Fig. 3.5.1). Optic nerve damage (i.e. anterior to the optic chiasm) is associated with:

- monocular visual loss (reduced acuity, reduced colour vision, scotoma)
- relative afferent papillary defect (on examination of papillary light reflex)
- papilloedema or optic atrophy (on fundoscopy).

Important causes of CNII damage are demyelination (optic neuritis/retrobulbar neuritis), ischaemia (ischaemic optic neuropathy), compression (e.g. by tumour), vitamin B_{12} deficiency and hereditary optic neuropathies (e.g. Leber's optic atrophy).

Cranial nerves III, IV and VI: oculomotor, trochlear and abducens nerves

CNIII, CNIV and CNVI innervate the extraocular muscles and mediate eye movements. They can be affected in isolation or combination.

CNIII originates in the midbrain, passes through the cavernous sinus and superior orbital fissure and supplies four extraocular muscles (inferior oblique, and superior inferior and medial recti), the levator palpebrae superioris (which lifts the eyelid) and the sphincter pupillae (which constricts the pupil under the control of parasympathetic fibres). Palsy of CNIII results in ptosis, failure of adduction and upward gaze (the eye points 'down and out') and a dilated pupil.

Causes of CNIII palsies can be divided into two main groups: compressive (surgical) and microvascular (medical). Compressive CNIII palsies are often painful; causes include berry aneurysm of the posterior communicating artery and herniation of the

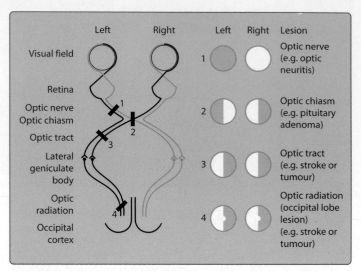

Fig. 3.5.1 Main types of visual disturbance and their anatomical location.

uncus (temporal lobe) across the tentorium cerebelli as a result of raised intracranial pressure. Microvascular CNIII palsies result in infarction of the nerve and may or may not be painful. They classically tend to 'spare' the pupil (i.e. the pupil remains reactive). Causes include diabetes mellitus, hypertension and vasculitis.

CNIV supplies the superior oblique muscle. Isolated lesions are uncommon; patients complain of diplopia, especially on looking down, and may adopt a 'head tilt' away from the side of the lesion.

CNVI supplies the lateral rectus muscle, which is responsible for abduction of the eye. Lesions result in inability to abduct the eye on the affected side and diplopia (Fig. 3.5.2). Causes include raised intracranial pressure (a 'false localizing sign', Ch. 15), multiple sclerosis, hypertension and diabetes mellitus.

Horner's syndrome

Horner's syndrome is the result of a unilateral sympathetic nerve lesion. It is characterized by ptosis, meiosis (constricted pupil), apparent enopthalmus (the eye appears 'sunken') and facial anhydrosis (loss of sweating). It should be distinguished from a CNIII palsy, as both cause ptosis. Important causes include apical lung tumour (Pancoast's tumour), carotid dissection and brainstem stroke.

Cranial nerve V: trigeminal nerve

CNV supplies all facial sensation (but not taste) via its three divisions (ophthalmic, maxillary and mandibular) and motor fibres to muscles of mastication. Patients with trigeminal nerve palsy complain of facial numbness or paraesthesia, which may involve

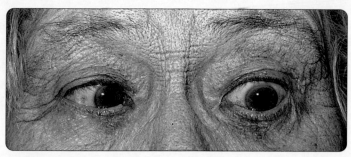

Fig. 3.5.2 Left cranial nerve VI palsy, causing weakness of the lateral rectus muscle. The patient is shown here attempting to look to the left.

the tongue and buccal mucosa. Main causes include brainstem (pontine) lesions (e.g. stroke, multiple sclerosis), or lesions in the cerebellopontine angle (e.g. acoustic neuroma).

Cranial nerve VII: facial nerve

CNVII supplies the muscles of facial expression, taste from the anterior two-thirds of the tongue (via the chorda tympani) and the stapedius (which restricts bony ossicle movement in the ear). Upper motor neuron lesions of CNVII produce weakness of the lower part of the face, sparing the forehead and eye closure, whereas lower motor neuron lesions produce weakness of all muscles of facial expression on the affected side.

Causes of upper motor neuron lesions include stroke, multiple sclerosis and brain tumours. Lower motor neuron lesions are most commonly caused by Bell's palsy but may also result from herpes zoster infection (Ramsay–Hunt syndrome), middle ear infection, sarcoidosis, parotid tumours and Guillain–Barré syndrome.

Bell's palsy is an acute, unilateral, lower motor neuron facial weakness, resulting in pain or discomfort behind the ipsilateral ear, followed by unilateral facial weakness. Full spontaneous recovery occurs in up to 90% but may take 9 months. The cause is uncertain, although viral infection has been postulated. A short course of oral prednisolone increases the likelihood of full recovery. Eye protection is important as weakness of eyelid closure may allow corneal abrasions to occur.

Cranial nerve VIII: vestibulocochlear nerve

CNVIII carries both auditory fibres from the cochlea and vestibular fibres (responsible for balance) from the semicircular canals. Lesions cause sensorineural deafness, tinnitus, vertigo and nystagmus. Common causes include stroke, multiple sclerosis, trauma and cerebellopontine angle tumours (e.g. acoustic neuroma).

Cranial nerves IX and X: glossopharyngeal and vagus nerves

CNIX provides sensation to the pharynx and taste to the posterior third of the tongue; CNX provides the motor supply to the pharynx, larynx and upper oesophagus. CNIX and CNX are

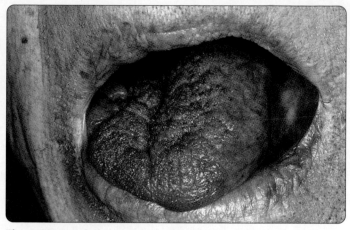

Fig. 3.5.3 A right hypoglossal nerve palsy causing unilateral tongue wasting.

usually affected together, often with other lower cranial nerves as they are closely related anatomically and run through the jugular foramen. The clinical features reflect impairment of pharyngeal control and swallowing:

- bulbar palsy (lower motor neuron): nasal speech, dysphagia with nasal regurgitation, weak 'bovine' cough, wasted tongue, absent gag reflex
- pseudobulbar palsy (upper motor neuron): spastic dysarthria, dysphagia with choking, spastic, immobile tongue, 'emotional lability', brisk jaw jerk, brisk gag reflex.

Bulbar palsy can result from motor neuron disease, myaesthenia gravis, Guillain–Barré syndrome and muscular dystrophy. Causes of pseudobulbar palsy include motor neuron disease, cerebrovascular disease and multiple sclerosis.

Cranial nerve XI: accessory nerve

CNXI supplies the trapezius and sternocleidomastoid muscles. Lesions cause muscle weakness, impaired 'shoulder shrug' and head rotation. Isolated lesions are uncommon.

Cranial nerve XII: hypoglossal nerve

CNXII is the motor supply to the tongue. Lesions cause unilateral weakness, wasting and fasciculation of the tongue (Fig. 3.5.3); on protrusion of the tongue, there is deviation towards the affected side. Causes of CNXII palsy include malignant meningitis and base of skull fracture.

6. Multiple sclerosis

Questions
- What investigations are required in suspected multiple sclerosis?
- What disease modifying treatments are available for multiple sclerosis?

Epidemiology

Multiple sclerosis (MS) is an inflammatory demyelinating disease of the CNS and is one of the leading causes of long-term neurological disability in the UK. MS has an annual incidence of approximately 5/100 000 in the UK and a prevalence of 100/100 000. There is a relationship between latitude and prevalence, with higher rates in northern Scotland than southern England and very low rates near the equator. MS is predominantly a disease of young adults, with age of onset usually between 20 and 45 years. It is more common in females than males, with a ratio of approximately 2:1.

Pathogenesis

The CNS inflammation in MS is mediated by activated T lymphocytes, which cross the blood–brain barrier and initiate an inflammatory cascade resulting in areas (or plaques) of demyelination. These plaques may develop in any part of the CNS, but certain areas such as the optic nerves, brainstem, spinal cord and periventricular white matter are particularly susceptible. Peripheral nerves are not affected.

The aetiology of MS is unknown, but it is likely that genetic and environmental factors both play a part; first-degree relatives of an individual with MS have a 5% risk of developing the disease (compared with 0.1% in the general population).

Clinical features

For a diagnosis of MS, there must be evidence of lesions 'disseminated in time and place'; that is to say, lesions affecting more than one part of the CNS occurring at different times. MS usually presents in one of three patterns: relapsing–remitting, primary progressive or secondary progressive (Fig. 3.6.1). Relapsing–remitting MS reflects recurrent clinical episodes of acute demyelination, wheras primary and secondary progressive disease reflects a progressive degeneration of axons.

Relapsing–remitting form (80–90%). This is characterized by clearly defined relapses caused by the appearance of new areas of demyelination. Symptoms usually develop gradually over days or weeks and resolve over several weeks. Resolution may be complete or incomplete, but there is no disease progression between specific relapses. Clinical features depend on the location of demyelinating plaques. For example:

- brainstem demyelination causes double vision, nystagmus, vertigo, facial numbness, dysarthria and ataxia
- spinal cord demyelination causes weakness and paraesthesiae in the limbs and impaired bladder function
- optic nerve demyelination (optic neuritis; Fig. 3.6.2) causes blurred vision, reduced visual acuity, ocular pain, reduced colour vision and optic disc swelling or atrophy.

Primary progressive form (10–20%). This is characterized by a slow and inexorable progression in neurological symptoms and disability. It tends to present at an older age, most commonly with a paraparesis caused by thoracic spinal cord demyelination.

Secondary progressive form. Approximately 75% of those who present with relapsing–remitting MS will eventually develop secondary progressive disease. This is characterized by slow-

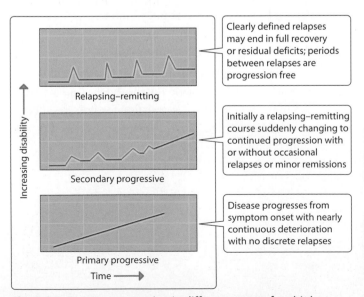

Fig. 3.6.1 Disease progression in different types of multiple sclerosis.

Relapsing–remitting — Clearly defined relapses may end in full recovery or residual deficits; periods between relapses are progression free

Secondary progressive — Initially a relapsing–remitting course suddenly changing to continued progression with or without occasional relapses or minor remissions

Primary progressive — Disease progresses from symptom onset with nearly continuous deterioration with no discrete relapses

Increasing disability / Time

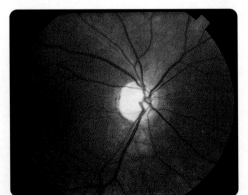

Fig. 3.6.2 Pale optic disc from optic atrophy in a patient with multiple sclerosis.

ly progressive disability unrelated to acute relapses. Patients may develop widespread neurological deficits; spinal cord, cerebellar and brainstem dysfunction are common. Cognitive impairment may occur in advanced disease.

Investigations

The diagnosis is made on the basis of history and examination, although confirmatory investigations are required. MRI of the brain (and sometimes spinal cord) is the most important investigation, showing multiple white matter lesions, particularly in the periventricular region, corpus callosum, brainstem and cervical cord (Fig. 3.6.3).

Lumbar puncture demonstrates CSF oligoclonal IgG bands in up to 90% of patients.

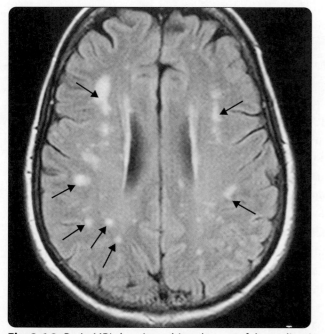

Fig. 3.6.3 Brain MRI showing white plaques of demyelinating lesions (arrowed).

Management

Once the diagnosis has been established, medical management centres around acute relapses, disease-modifying therapy and symptom control.

Relapse management. Acute relapses may be treated with a short course of high-dose steroids (methylprednisolone). This may hasten recovery from an individual relapse but has no effect on the long-term neurological outcome or frequency of subsequent relapses.

Disease-modifying therapies. A number of treatments have been shown to reduce the frequency and severity of relapses in relapsing–remitting MS. These drugs are offered to individuals who have had at least two disabling relapses over the previous 2 years. They tend to be useful only in relapsing–remitting disease and are of no value in primary or secondary progressive disease. The most commonly used drug is interferon-beta, which reduces relapse frequency by approximately 30%. For those with aggressive MS and frequent relapses, natalizumab (a monoclonal antibody with actions against T lymphocytes) is effective. It carries a small risk of inducing progressive multifocal leukoencephalopathy.

Symptom control. Patients with MS develop a variety of transient and chronic symptoms; a multidisciplinary team approach is useful in overall management. Common symptoms and treatments are summarized in Table 3.6.1.

Prognosis

The course of MS is variable and difficult to predict in individual patients. Relatively good prognostic features include initial symptoms of optic neuritis or isolated sensory dysfunction, younger age at onset and little or no disability after 5 years. Relatively poor prognostic features include older age at onset, initial symptoms involving cerebellar, spinal or pyramidal systems, high initial disease activity (e.g. early attack frequency, short first interattack interval, moderate disability reached by 5 years) and a large number of white matter lesions on MRI at time of first clinical attack.

Table 3.6.1 TREATMENTS FOR SYMPTOMATIC RELIEF IN MULTIPLE SCLEROSIS

Symptom	Management
Muscle spasticity	Antispasticity drugs (baclofen, tizanidine, dantrolene); local treatments (e.g. botulinum toxin injections into affected muscles); physiotherapy; orthotic devices such as splints
Bladder dysfunction (urinary urgency/ incontinence)	Anticholinergic drugs (oxybutynin); treatment of urinary tract infections with antibiotics; urinary catheter
Trigeminal neuralgia	Antiepileptic drugs (carbamazepine, phenytoin, gabapentin)
Neuropathic pain and dysaesthesia	Pain-modulating drugs (amitriptyline, gabapentin)
Fatigue	Stimulant drugs (amantadine, modafinil)
Mood disturbance (anxiety and depression)	Psychological therapies, antidepressants

7. Primary headache syndromes

Questions
- What are the differences between tension-type headache and migraine?
- What is trigeminal neuralgia?
- What is cluster headache?

The first priority when assessing a patient with headache is to identify those in whom there may be a structural (and potentially life-threatening) cause such as subarachnoid haemorrhage, meningitis or raised intracranial pressure. In many cases, however, no such cause will be present; such patients have 'primary headache' disorders, such as migraine, tension-type headache and cluster headache.

Migraine

Clinical features

Migraine is a common cause of headache, affecting approximately 8% of males and 20% of females, often with a familial tendency. The underlying pathophysiology is uncertain.

Migraine is usually subdivided into two main types: with aura (20% of patients) and without aura (80% of patients). The headache in both forms is moderate to severe, throbbing, pulsatile and often (but not always) unilateral. It is worsened by activity and associated with photophobia, nausea and vomiting. In migraine with aura, focal neurological symptoms develop over 15–20 min prior to the headache (Fig. 3.7.1). Auras are most commonly visual (flashing lights, scotomata, blurred vision and zig-zag lines), but almost any neurological symptom may be experienced. Precipitating factors for migraine include relaxation after stress ('weekend migraine'), menstruation, bright lights, dyhydration, cheese, red wine or chocolate. Migraine may appear or worsen in females taking the oral contraceptive pill. In this group, there is a small but definite risk of stroke, and the oral contraceptive pill should be discontinued. Examination between attacks of migraine is normal and no investigations are usually required.

Management

Medical treatment of migraine is divided into treatment of the acute attack (rescue therapy) and prevention of attacks (prophylaxis).

Treatment of acute migraine. Patients should be advised to take simple analgesics (high-dose aspirin) at onset, often in combination with an antiemetic. If simple analgesia is insufficient, triptans (5-hydroxytryptamine agonists such as sumatriptan) should be considered. If analgesics (particu-

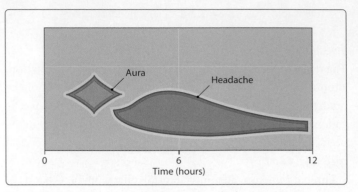

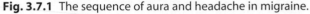

Fig. 3.7.1 The sequence of aura and headache in migraine.

larly opioids) or triptans are taken frequently (more than 3–5 days per month), there is a risk of developing medication-overuse headache. This is a chronic headache largely resistant to analgesia and difficult to treat. Frequent analgesia should be avoided.

Migraine prophylaxis. Avoiding precipitating factors may be sufficient to prevent migraine attacks. Prophylactic treatment should be considered in individuals with two or more episodes a month or if migraine causes significant functional disruption. Drugs used to prevent migraine include beta-blockers, amitriptyline, pizotifen, sodium valproate and topiramate.

Tension-type headache

Tension-type headache is common and may exist in episodic form or as chronic daily headache. It is usually bilateral and may be described as being like a 'tight band' around the head (Fig. 3.7.2). The intensity is variable, but generally mild to moderate, and patients can usually continue with day to day activities; nausea, vomiting and photophobia are not present. Tension headache may be exacerbated by stress or anxiety. Neurological examination is normal, although the scalp and neck may be tender to touch. Investigations are usually unnecessary. Treatment consists of avoidance of trigger factors and relaxation techniques. Simple analgesia may be useful for occasional headaches, but regular use of analgesics (particularly codeine) should be avoided as this may result in medication-overuse headache.

Cluster headache

Cluster headache is an uncommon condition that usually affects middle-aged male smokers. It is characterized by recurrent episodes of intense pain and erythema around one eye, with ipsilateral nasal congestion and a red watering eye. These symptoms often occur on waking and last for around an hour.

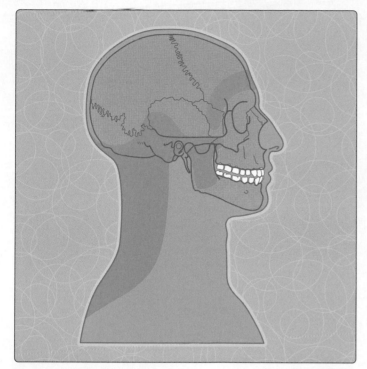

Fig. 3.7.2 Typical areas of pain in tension headache (red); the pain is usually bilateral and 'tight'.

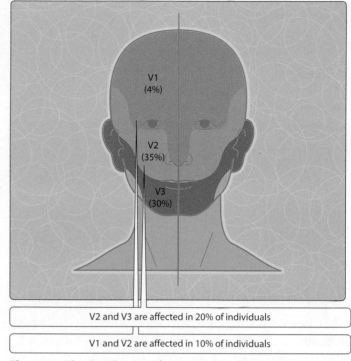

V1
(4%)

V2
(35%)

V3
(30%)

V2 and V3 are affected in 20% of individuals

V1 and V2 are affected in 10% of individuals

Fig. 3.7.3 The distribution of trigeminal neuralgia.

Horner's syndrome may occur during attacks and even persist between attacks. Typically, one or two episodes occur each day for several weeks (a 'cluster'), followed by months with no headaches. Cluster headaches are sometimes associated with an underlying cerebral lesion (such as an arteriovenous malformation or tumour) and neuroimaging with MRI may be necessary. Response to simple analgesia is poor but triptans or high-flow oxygen may be helpful during an acute episode. Prophylaxis with verapamil or lithium may be effective.

Trigeminal neuralgia

Trigeminal neuralgia is a syndrome of facial pain rather than headache (Fig. 3.7.3). It occurs predominantly in the elderly and is characterized by recurrent episodes of sudden, severe, unilat-

eral, lancinating facial pain that lasts from seconds to minutes. The pain occurs in the distribution of the trigeminal nerve and is usually described as sharp or stabbing; there may be some residual ache following attacks. Triggers include eating, talking, brushing teeth and cold wind. Neurological examination between attacks is normal. The cause is not always identified, but it may result from an aberrant blood vessel lying in contact with the trigeminal nerve. Less commonly, trigeminal neuralgia may be a feature of multiple sclerosis or a tumour in the cerebellopontine angle. MRI of the head may be indicated. First-line treatment is usually with carbamazepine; gabapentin or clonazepam may also be useful. In resistant cases, trigeminal nerve ablation or surgical microvascular decompression may be considered.

8. Disorders of cerebrospinal fluid circulation

Questions
- What is hydrocephalus?
- What is idiopathic intracranial hypertension?

The CSF provides mechanical protection to the brain. It is produced by the choroid plexus of the lateral, third and fourth ventricles and circulates around the brain and spinal cord (Fig. 3.8.1). From the subarachnoid space, it is reabsorbed into the venous sinuses through arachnoid granulations.

Hydrocephalus

Hydrocephalus is an increase in CSF volume associated with dilation of the cerebral ventricles. It occurs either from obstruction of CSF flow within the ventricular system, usually at the cerebral aqueduct, causing dilatation of the lateral and third ventricles (obstructive or non-communicating hydrocephalus) or from impaired CSF reabsorption (at the arachnoid villi) causing dilatation of all four ventricles (communicating hydrocephalus).

Pathogenesis

The causes of communicating and non-communicating hydrocephalus differ:

- non-communicating/obstructive: aqueduct stenosis (congenital or acquired), developmental hind brain abnormalities (spina bifida), intraventricular tumours, posterior fossa tumours, haemorrhage or infarct

- communicating: meningitis (infective, inflammatory, malignant), subarachnoid haemorrhage, venous sinus thrombosis.

Clinical features

In adults, hydrocephalus often presents with features of raised intracranial pressure (headache worse in the early morning or on lying flat, nausea and vomiting). In obstructive hydrocephalus, increasing intracranial pressure may eventually result in herniation of lower brainstem and cerebellar structures through the foramen magnum; this results in occipital pain, neck stiffness, coma and death (coning).

Investigations

Hydrocephalus is confirmed on CT or MRI, which may also suggest the underlying cause. Lumbar puncture is contraindicated in non-communucating hydrocephalus because of the risk of precipitating coning.

Management

Hydrocephalus can be treated with shunting (Fig. 3.8.2).

Normal pressure hydrocephalus

Normal pressure hydrocephalus is an uncommon disorder of uncertain aetiology. It is a condition of the elderly, characterized by a gait disorder (gait apraxia), dementia and urinary incontinence. CT brain shows enlargement of the cerebral ventricles suggestive of a communicating hydrocephalus, but CSF pressure on lumbar puncture (Fig. 3.8.3) is normal. Diagnosis is

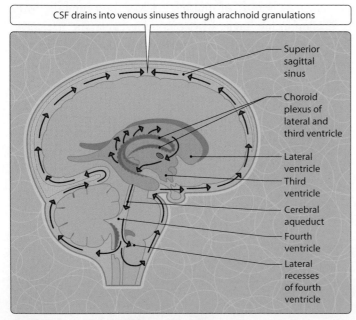

CSF drains into venous sinuses through arachnoid granulations

Superior sagittal sinus

Choroid plexus of lateral and third ventricle

Lateral ventricle

Third ventricle

Cerebral aqueduct

Fourth ventricle

Lateral recesses of fourth ventricle

Fig. 3.8.1 Cerebrospinal fluid circulation.

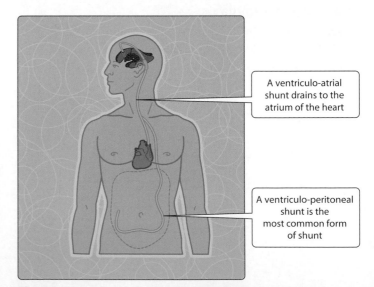

A ventriculo-atrial shunt drains to the atrium of the heart

A ventriculo-peritoneal shunt is the most common form of shunt

Fig. 3.8.2 Ventriculo-atrial and ventriculo-peritoneal shunts.

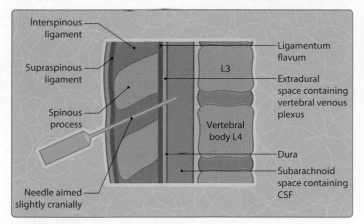

Fig. 3.8.3 The anatomy encountered when performing a lumbar puncture. CSF, cerebrospinal fluid.

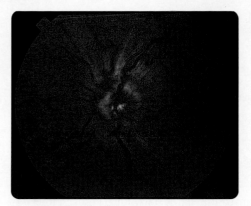

Fig. 3.8.4 Papilloedema in a patient with raised intracranial pressure.

difficult, as distinguishing hydrocephalus from age-related cerebral atrophy on neuroimaging can be unreliable. Ventriculo-peritoneal shunting of CSF is sometimes carried out, but results are variable.

Idiopathic intracranial hypertension

Idiopathic intracranial hypertension usually occurs in females aged between 15 and 45 years. The cause is unclear, although it is associated with obesity and recent weight gain. In some cases an underlying cause, such as venous sinus thrombosis or drugs (particularly steroids), may be identified. Recognition is important, as untreated it can lead to permanent visual loss.

Clinical features

Presentation is typically with generalized headache, worse early in the morning, exacerbated by lying flat or coughing and relieved by upright posture. Transient episodes of visual loss or blurring (visual obscurations) with change in posture or coughing may occur (caused by pressure on the optic nerves). Papilloedema (swelling of the optic disc; Fig. 3.8.4) and an enlarged blind spot may be identified. Permanent visual loss may develop.

Investigations

Neuroimaging is required to exclude other causes of increased intracranial pressure. Diagnosis is confirmed by an elevated CSF pressure on lumbar puncture.

Management

Treatment includes weight loss, repeated therapeutic lumbar puncture and acetazolamide. Regular monitoring of visual fields is required; if vision is threatened, optic nerve fenestration or lumbo-peritoneal shunting may be needed.

Intracranial hypotension

Intracranial hypotension, caused by reduced CSF pressure, is an under-recognized cause of headache. The headache usually starts within seconds or minutes of assuming an erect posture and resolves on lying down. It may be associated with neck stiffness, nausea, double vision, a 'whooshing' sound in the ears and photophobia. It is usually caused by a CSF leak; the most common cause is iatrogenic following lumbar puncture. However, spontaneous, post-traumatic and postsurgical CSF leaks can cause a similar presentation. Treatment includes bed-rest, analgesia, caffeine and rehydration. Following lumbar puncture, an epidural blood patch may be useful.

9. Spinal cord disorders

Questions
- What are the clinical features of spinal cord compression?
- What are the causes of spinal cord compression?

Spinal cord damage (myelopathy) may occur from intrinsic disease (e.g. multiple sclerosis) or through external compression from pathology in other structures, particularly the meninges, intervertebral discs or vertebral bodies (Fig 3.9.1). Clinically, myelopathy is associated (paraparesis or tetraparesis), sensory deficits below the level of the lesion and bladder and bowel dysfunction; the precise features depend on the level of compression and extent of damage (Fig 3.9.2).

Spinal cord compression
Spinal cord compression can be caused by lesions in the vertebral column (e.g. prolapsed intervertebral discs, vertebral metastases, epidural abcess) or the meninges (e.g. meningioma, meningeal metastasis), producing physical pressure upon the spinal cord. The most common causes are trauma and vertebral metastases.

The presentation can be acute or insidious depending on the underlying mechanism. Pain and evidence of local nerve root damage at the level of the lesion are often features.

MRI is urgently required in suspected spinal cord compression.

Urgent surgical decompression of the cord is usually required, although bony metastases causing compression may be treated with radiotherapy. Early treatment maximizes neurological recovery.

In **cauda equina syndrome**, a compressive lesion is located below the end of the spinal cord; rather than causing cord compression, multiple lumbosacral nerve roots are compressed. This typically presents with severe lower back pain, leg weakness, numbness over the buttocks and perineum ('saddle area') and urinary retention.On examination, there is a lower motor neuron pattern of weakness with loss of reflexes, reduced anal sphincter tone and sensory disturbance in a saddle distribution. Urgent MRI and surgical decompression are required.

Cervical spondylosis
Cervical spondylosis describes degenerative changes of the cervical vertebrae, intervertebral joints and ligaments. These changes may narrow the vertebral canal, causing cord compression, and the nerve exit foramina, compressing cervical nerve roots (radiculopathy) (Fig. 3.9.3). Neck pain is often present; arm pain, tingling and weakness may occur in a nerve root distribution (most commonly C_7), and features of spinal cord compression may be present. Diagnosis is confirmed on MRI. In mild radiculopathy, physiotherapy and analgesia may be helpful. If there is cord compression, or conservative measures are unsuccessful, decompressive surgery is required.

Subacute combined degeneration of the cord
In this condition, myelopathy and peripheral neuropathy develop as a result of vitamin B_{12} deficiency. Pernicious anaemia is the most common cause of B_{12} deficiency, but other causes include Crohn's disease, gastrectomy or dietary exclusion in vegans. Patients complain of tingling in the fingers and toes that gradually spreads proximally; limb weakness and gait disturbance may develop. There is evidence of a peripheral sensory neuropathy in a 'glove and stocking' distribution, particularly affecting proprioception, with absent ankle jerks. Diagnosis is confirmed by low vitamin B_{12} levels, and MRI may show hyperintensity in the posterior part of the cord. Management is with long-term vitamin B_{12} supplementation; this may improve the peripheral neuropathy but often has little effect on spinal cord features.

Syringomyelia and syringobulbia
Syringomyelia is the presence of a fluid-filled cystic cavity (syrinx) within the central canal of the spinal cord; syringobulbia describes the same process in the brainstem. Syringomyelia is often associated with an Arnold–Chiari malformation, a

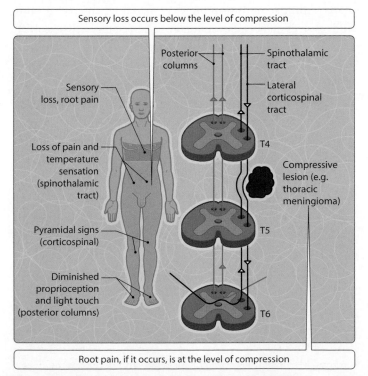

Sensory loss occurs below the level of compression

Posterior columns — Spinothalamic tract

Sensory loss, root pain

Lateral corticospinal tract

Loss of pain and temperature sensation (spinothalamic tract)

T4

Compressive lesion (e.g. thoracic meningioma)

Pyramidal signs (corticospinal)

T5

Diminished proprioception and light touch (posterior columns)

T6

Root pain, if it occurs, is at the level of compression

Fig. 3.9.1 Clinical features of spinal cord compression.

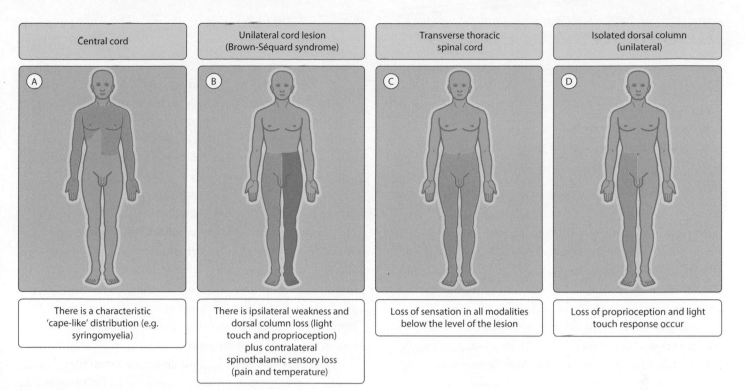

Central cord	Unilateral cord lesion (Brown-Séquard syndrome)	Transverse thoracic spinal cord	Isolated dorsal column (unilateral)
There is a characteristic 'cape-like' distribution (e.g. syringomyelia)	There is ipsilateral weakness and dorsal column loss (light touch and proprioception) plus contralateral spinothalamic sensory loss (pain and temperature)	Loss of sensation in all modalities below the level of the lesion	Loss of proprioception and light touch response occur

Fig. 3.9.2 Patterns of sensory deficit in different spinal cord lesions.

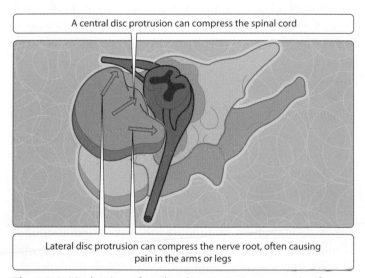

A central disc protrusion can compress the spinal cord

Lateral disc protrusion can compress the nerve root, often causing pain in the arms or legs

Fig. 3.9.3 Mechanism of cord and nerve root compression from intervertebral disc prolapse; this can occur in isolation or in the context of cervical spondylosis.

developmental abnormality in which the cerebellar tonsils extend through the foramen magnum. Patients usually present aged 20–40 years with upper limb pain and tingling worsened by coughing. Loss of pain and temperature sensation (from selective impairment of spinothalamic tracts) in the upper limbs and trunk leads to risk of painless burns, with relative sparing of proprioception and light touch. This 'dissociated' sensory loss typically has a 'cape' distribution (Fig. 3.9.2). Other features include lower motor neuron weakness in the arms and a spastic paraparesis. When extension into the brainstem occurs, individuals may develop Horner's syndrome(see p.265), bulbar palsy, tongue wasting and fasciculation. The diagnosis is confirmed by MRI; management is usually conservative, although surgical treatment of the syrinx is sometimes undertaken.

Transverse myelitis

Transverse myelitis describes acute inflammation of the spinal cord. Patients develop paraplegia or tetraplegia over several days, with bowel and bladder dysfunction and sensory loss below the level of the lesion. It may be an isolated event, but it also occurs in multiple sclerosis, viral infections or systemic inflammatory conditions. MRI of the spine is required to exclude cord compression. Treatment depends on the underlying cause, but high-dose steroids may reduce inflammation. Prognosis is variable.

Anterior spinal artery occlusion

The anterior spinal artery provides the blood supply to most of the spinal cord; occlusion results in a 'spinal stroke', with sudden paraplegia, urinary retention and loss of spinothalamic sensation. Relative sparing of dorsal column sensation (light touch, proprioception and vibration) occurs as this is supplied by the posterior spinal artery. Anterior spinal artery occlusion is associated with vascular risk factors (smoking, hypertension, hyperlipidaemia), atrial fibrillation and vasculitis; it may also occur during aortic surgery. MRI excludes cord compression and may show evidence of an infarct. Neurological recovery is usually limited.

10. Seizures and epilepsy

Questions
- How is epilepsy classified?
- What is the management of status epilepticus?

A seizure is the clinical manifestation of a paroxysmal disturbance of CNS function associated with excessive neuronal discharge; epilepsy is the tendency to recurrent, unprovoked seizures. The annual incidence of epilepsy in the developed world is approximately 50/100 000 and is higher in developing countries. In the UK, up to 5% of the population will experience at least one seizure during their lifetime.

Focal (partial) epilepsy occurs when seizures arise from a particular region of the brain (Fig. 3.10.1). Focal seizures may be:

- simple partial: no impairment of consciousness
- complex partial: impairment of consciousness
- secondary generalized tonic–clonic: seizure spreads from its region of orgin to affect the whole brain.

In **generalized epilepsy**, the whole brain is involved from seizure onset. There are several types of generalized seizure, the most common being absence, myoclonic and generalized tonic–clonic seizures.

Pathogenesis
Focal epilepsy may be caused by an underlying lesion such as cerebral gliosis (scarring following intracranial infection, trauma or stroke), congenital abnormalities or tumours. A common abnormality causing temporal lobe epilepsy is hippocampal sclerosis (atrophy and degenerative change in the hippocampus). Often, no causal lesion is found. Generalized epilepsies are usually idiopathic, although many have a genetic component.

Clinical features
The history must be obtained from both the patient and a witness. Seizures should be differentiated from other causes of altered consciousness such as a vasovagal syncope (simple faint), cardiac syncope (arrhythmia or structural abnormality) and psychogenic non-epileptic attacks (pseudoseizures). Short-lived jerky or twitching movements are common in syncope and may lead to misdiagnosis of seizures.

In **focal seizures**, individuals may describe symptoms in clear consciousness — this is an 'aura' (or simple partial seizure). The symptoms experienced will depend on where in the brain the seizure is occurring; in temporal lobe epilepsy, they may take the form of a smell, taste, a 'rising' sensation in the stomach or déja-vu. If consciousness becomes impaired, the seizure is known as a complex partial seizure; the individual becomes less responsive, stares and may have automatic behaviours such as chewing, lip smacking and fumbling with clothes or nearby objects. In secondary generalized tonic–clonic seizures, the body becomes rigid (tonic phase) followed by rhythmic jerking of the limbs (clonic phase). Patients often bite their tongue and may be incontinent of urine. Seizures usually last for 90–180 seconds (although observers may significantly overestimate this duration). Postictally, the patient is usually very drowsy and confused. Some patients with focal epilepsy will develop transient signs in the postictal period, which resolve over a period of hours (Todd's paresis). Examination between seizures is often normal, although some patients (e.g. with cerebrovascular disease) will have permanent focal signs reflecting an underlying structural abnormality

There are various types of **generalized seizure**. Absence seizures are brief episodes of loss of awareness, with minimal motor manifestations, that typically occur in early childhood. Events usually last for up to 15 seconds and occur many times per day. Myoclonic jerks are brief, shock-like jerks of the limbs with minimal impairment of consciousness. Generalized tonic–clonic seizures are clinically indistinguishable from secondary generalized tonic–clonic seizures (described above) but are not associated with an aura or other focal features.

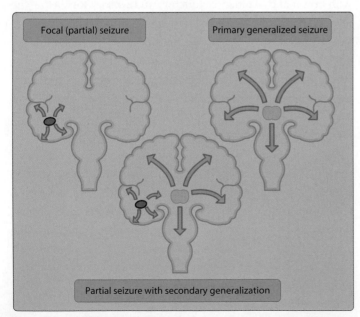

Focal (partial) seizure

Primary generalized seizure

Partial seizure with secondary generalization

Fig. 3.10.1 Different types of seizure.

Table 3.10.1 SOME OF THE MOST COMMONLY USED ANTIEPILEPTIC DRUGS AND THEIR MAIN ADVERSE EFFECTS

Drug	Indications (epilepsy subtypes)	Main adverse effects
Carbamazepine	Focal epilepsy	Dizziness; nausea; ataxia; rash
Sodium valproate	Generalized or focal epilepsy	Weight gain; hair loss; tremor; highly teratogenic
Lamotrigine	Generalized or focal epilepsy	Rash
Phenytoin	Focal epilepsy	Skin changes; gum hypertrophy; facial coarsening; osteoporosis; cerebellar atrophy
Topiramate	Generalized or focal epilepsy	Paraesthesias; cognitive impairment; speech disturbance; kidney stones
Levetiracetam	Generalized or focal epilepsy	Behavioural change; irritability

Investigations

MRI or CT brain scan should be performed following a first seizure to exclude structural intracranial pathology. Electroencephalography (EEG) shows specific epileptiform discharges in approximately 30% of individuals with epilepsy. This can be combined with video monitoring (video-EEG). Cardiac investigations (ECG, echocardiogram or 24 h Holter) may be needed if cardiac syncope is suspected.

Management

Seizure control

Factors such as sleep deprivation, alcohol excess and certain drugs (e.g. opioids and recreational drugs) may lower the seizure threshold. Antiepileptic drugs are usually recommended after at least two unprovoked seizures. The first-line treatment for focal epilepsy (with or without secondary generalized tonic–clonic seizures) is lamotrigine or carbamazepine. For generalized epilepsy, sodium valproate or lamotrigine are usually the drugs of choice. Approximately 70% of people with epilepsy will have seizures fully controlled by a single drug. If treatment is unsuccessful, an alternative agent or combination of drugs should be tried (Table 3.10.1). Monotherapy is generally preferred. Many antiepileptic drugs (e.g. valproate) are potentially teratogenic and some (e.g. carbamazepine) can reduce the effectiveness of the oral contraceptive pill. Epilepsy surgery is considered only in individuals with focal epilepsy that is refractory to multiple antiepileptic drugs and where a clear region of seizure onset can be identified.

Driving

In the UK, any individual having had a seizure is required by law to inform the Driver and Vehicle Licensing Agency (DVLA). The driving licence is usually suspended until the patient has

BOX 3.10.1 MANAGEMENT OF STATUS EPILEPTICUS

1. The airway should be secured, oxygen administered, cardiac and respiratory function assessed and intravenous access obtained.
2. Blood should be taken to check plasma sodium, calcium, magnesium and glucose levels. Anticonvulsant levels, alcohol and drug screen should be performed where necessary.
3. Intravenous lorazepam (4 mg) should be given immediately (without waiting for blood results); this dose can be repeated once if necessary.
4. If seizures continue, i.v. phenytoin (15 mg/kg) with cardiac monitoring should be considered.
5. If seizures persist, anaesthesia with propofol or thiopental is usually required.

been free of seizures for a year (on or off treatment), after which a full licence will be restored. Patients with epilepsy should not drive if medication is being withdrawn and for 6 months after drug withdrawal. Drivers of heavy goods vehicle must be seizure-free for 10 years before their licence is restored.

Prognosis

Most patients with epilepsy (up to 80%) will go into remission at some point, allowing medication to be discontinued. Epilepsy may be more difficult to control in individuals with underlying structural pathology. Mortality rates are 2.5–3 times higher in individuals with epilepsy than in the general population.

Status epilepticus is defined as continuous seizure activity, or recurrent seizures without recovery of consciousness in between, for more than 30 min. It is a neurological emergency carrying a mortality of approximately 10%. Management is given in Box 3.10.1.

11. Dementia

Questions
- What are the differences between delirium and dementia?
- What are the most common causes of dementia?
- What is the management of dementia?

Dementia is as an acquired progressive deterioration of intellect, behaviour and personality of sufficient severity to interfere with social and occupational functioning. It can be caused by a variety of underlying conditions and should not be thought of as a definitive diagnosis in its own right.

Dementia should be distinguished from depression as this may also cause personality change, memory disturbance and intellectual decline. It is also necessary to exclude delirium (acute confusional state caused by infection, drug intoxication or withdrawal, metabolic disturbance or other systemic illness) as a cause of altered cerebral function (Table 3.11.1).

Epidemiology
Dementia affects approximately 5–10% of the population over the age of 65 and approximately 20% of those over 80 years.

Pathogenesis and clinical features
The most common causes of dementia (Fig. 3.11.1) are:
- Alzheimer's disease
- vascular dementia
- dementia with Lewy bodies.

Alzheimer's disease
The incidence of Alzheimer's disease increases markedly with age, being rare under the age of 50 but affecting around 20% of those over 85. Most cases are sporadic, but familial forms may account for 10–15%. Pathologically, it is characterized by neuronal loss and the presence of amyloid plaques and neurofibrillary tangles in the cerebral cortex.

The main clinical features are:
- memory loss, which is usually the earliest, and dominant, feature; patients have a progressive loss of ability to retain and recall new information
- apathy (the patient may appear depressed)
- in advanced disease, dysphasia, apraxia (difficulty using tools and implements) and visuospatial difficulties often develop.

Vascular dementia
Vascular dementia may occur in isolation or coexist with Alzheimer's disease (mixed dementia). It typically occurs in individuals with significant vascular risk factors. It is usually characterized by a stepwise deterioration in cognitive function. Neuropsychological assessment reveals patchy cognitive impairment, and there may be evidence of previous strokes on history, physical examination and/or cerebral imaging.

Dementia with Lewy bodies
Pathologically, dementia with Lewy bodies is characterized by Lewy bodies (aggregates of protein within nerve cells) in the cerebral cortex. Clinically there is overlap with idiopathic Parkinson's disease, as many patients exhibit similar parkinsonian motor features. The main feature is fluctuating cognitive impairment with visual hallucinations, which are often clearly formed

Table 3.11.1 DIFFERENCES BETWEEN DELIRIUM AND DEMENTIA

Characteristics	Delirium	Dementia
Onset	Acute	Insidious
Course	Fluctuating	Stable
Duration	Hours to weeks	Months to years
Attention	Fluctuates	Normal
Perception	Hallucinations	Usually normal
Sleep/wake	Disrupted	Fragmented

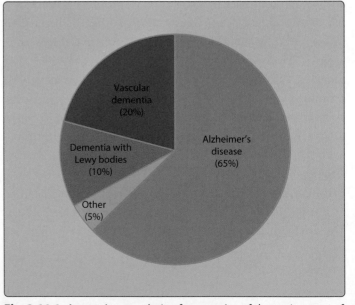

Fig. 3.11.1 Approximate relative frequencies of the main types of dementia in adults aged over 65 years the UK.

and stereotyped in nature. It may mimic delirium because of its fluctuating nature.

Other causes of dementia

Rarer causes of dementia include Creutzfeldt–Jakob disease (CJD, a rapidly progressive of dementia caused by accumulation of an abnormal, transmissible prion protein isoform) and frontotemporal dementia (presenting with marked personality change or dysphasia, but with relatively preserved memory).

Dementia is also a feature of a number of degenerative neurological disorders, including Huntington's disease, Wilson's disease, corticobasal degeneration and progressive supranuclear palsy; it also occurs in about a third of individuals with Parkinson's disease.

Dementia may occur in advanced multiple sclerosis and can be a feature of HIV/AIDS. Alcohol-related dementia is not uncommon in individuals with a long history of chronic alcohol abuse.

Investigations

The diagnosis of dementia is largely clinical, and extensive investigations are not usually required; however, reversible causes (Table 3.11.2) should be excluded. In some patients, particularly those who are young or have an atypical presentation, more extensive investigations may be indicated. These include:

- vitamin B_{12}, syphilis, thyroid function, calcium, glucose
- cerebral imaging (CT or MRI) to exclude a space-occupying lesion or hydrocephalus; this usually shows cerebral atrophy in dementia but may provide additional diagnostic information (such as ischaemic changes in vascular dementia)

Table 3.11.2 POTENTIALLY REVERSIBLE CAUSES OF DEMENTIA

Cause	Investigation
Tumour	CT brain
Normal pressure hydrocephalus	CT brain and lumbar puncture
Vitamin B_{12} deficiency	FBC; B_{12} and folate levels
Hypothyroidism	Thyroid function tests
Neurosyphilis	Syphilis serology
Hypocalcaemia	Serum calcium
Depression ('pseudodementia')	Mental state examination

- neuropsychology assessment to document the pattern of cognitive impairment
- electroencephalography may show diagnostic periodic complexes in CJD.
- lumbar puncture may provide evidence of raised intracranial pressure in inflammation, infection or CJD.

Management

The treatment of dementia is largely supportive, although cholinesterase inhibitors (such as rivastigmine and galantamine) modestly reduce cognitive deterioration in Alzheimer's disease. Treatment of vascular risk factors is important in vascular dementia and may reduce the rate of progression. In most individuals, long-term care is eventually required.

12. Movement disorders I: akinetic-rigid syndromes

Questions
- What are the clinical features of Parkinson's disease?
- What drugs are used in the management of Parkinson's disease?

Movement disorders reflect dysfunction of the extrapyramidal system, which is involved in the initiation and automatic maintenance of movements. The basal ganglia, substantia nigra and parts of the thalamus are key structures in this system.

Movement disorders are relatively common and can be divided into two main groups:

- akinetic-rigid or 'parkinsonian' syndromes, which are characterized by slow, reduced movements (bradykinesia) and increased muscle tone
- dyskinesias, which are characterized by unwanted involuntary movements (Ch. 13).

Parkinson's disease

Epidemiology

Idiopathic Parkinson's disease is the most common akinetic-rigid syndrome, with a prevalence of approximately 120/100 000 population. This increases with age, and median onset is approximately 60 years. It is slightly more common in males with a male to female ratio of 1.5:1.

Pathogenesis

The main pathological finding in Parkinson's disease is degeneration of the pigmented dopaminergic neurons that project from the substantia nigra in the midbrain to the basal ganglia (Fig. 3.12.1). Approximately 70% of these neurons are lost before Parkinson's disease becomes clinically evident; at postmortem, surviving neurons are found to contain characteristic abnormalities known as Lewy bodies. Insufficient dopamine formation leads to the symptoms of Parkinson's disease. Most cases are sporadic, but rare familial forms are recognized.

Clinical features

The classical features of Parkinson's disease are bradykinesia, rigidity and tremor (Fig. 3.12.2). These features are typically asymmetrical and affect one side earlier and more severely than the other.

Bradykinesia. Slowness and difficulty in initiating movement results in a characteristic fixed facial expression, reduced eye blinking and slow soft speech. When combined with rigidity and tremor, bradykinesia significantly affects the ability to

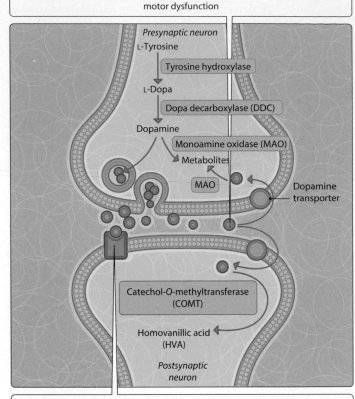

Fig. 3.12.1 Dopamine synthesis and dopaminergic transmission in the basal ganglia.

perform fine motor tasks such as writing, which typically becomes small and 'spidery'.

Rigidity. Increased muscle tone is sustained throughout the range of passive movement of a limb ('lead pipe rigidity'). Tremor superimposed on rigidity is referred to as 'cogwheel rigidity'.

Tremor. This is often the presenting feature in Parkinson's disease. It is most obvious at rest and relatively suppressed by movement and posture. It often affects the hands, causing a characteristic 'pill-rolling' movement.

In addition to these features, patients develop a characteristic gait with small shuffling steps, reduced arm swing and flexed posture ('festinant' gait); loss of postural righting reflexes result in a tendency to fall. Dementia and behavioural problems may develop later in the illness.

Investigations

The diagnosis of Parkinson's disease is clinical, but it is important to consider other akinetic-rigid syndromes (such as drug-induced parkinsonism, cerebrovascular disease or a 'Parkinson plus' syndrome; see below).

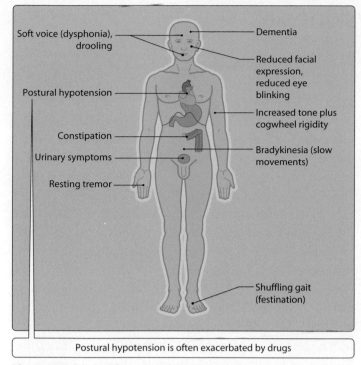

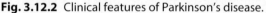

Postural hypotension is often exacerbated by drugs

Fig. 3.12.2 Clinical features of Parkinson's disease.

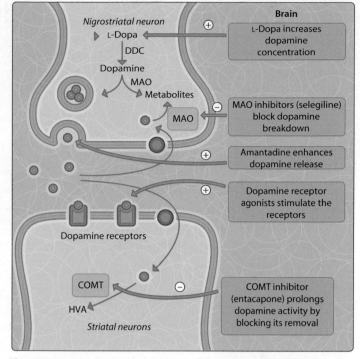

Fig. 3.12.3 The action in the brain of drugs used in Parkinson's disease. Abbreviations are as shown in Fig. 3.12.1.

Management

In the early stages, treatment is often unnecessary. Once symptoms have progressed, dopamine replacement therapy is usually required. Dopamine agonists (e.g. ropinirole and pramipexole) may be useful, particularly early in the disease. Levodopa, a precursor of dopamine, is the most effective treatment (Fig 3.12.3). It is given in combination with a decarboxylase inhibitor (e.g. carbidopa) to minimize its conversion into dopamine outside the brain, which causes unwanted side-effects (particularly nausea). Prolonged use of levodopa is associated with various problems such as a gradual shortening of the duration of benefit, fluctuations in motor function and development of abnormal, involuntary movements (dyskinesias) with increasing doses. Catechol-O-methyltransferase (COMT) inhibitors (e.g. entacapone) may be added to levodopa to reduce motor fluctuations. Amantidine is sometimes helpful in reducing levodopa-associated dyskinesias. In advanced Parkinson's disease, s.c. apomorphine can be used in place of levodopa.

Anticholinergic drugs may be used in patients with tremor although they are associated with adverse effects such as dry mouth, blurred vision, urinary retention, constipation and confusion.

Stereotactic neurosurgery (thalamotomy or pallidotomy) can be useful in the relief of severe tremor or dyskinesias, but it is considered in only a minority of patients.

Other akinetic-rigid syndromes

Other akinetic-rigid syndromes include drug-induced parkinsonism, the 'Parkinson plus' syndromes and vascular parkinsonism.

Drug-induced parkinsonism is a relatively common adverse effect of neuroleptic drugs used for schizophrenia and other psychotic disorders. These drugs block dopamine receptors in the brain and result in clinical features resembling Parkinson's disease. Symptoms may improve if the responsible drug is discontinued.

Parkinson plus syndromes are uncommon disorders resulting in features of parkinsonism and other progressive neurological deficits. Examples include progressive supranuclear palsy (eye movement abnormalities, axial rigidity and early cognitive impairment) and multiple system atrophy (cerebellar ataxia and/or autonomic dysfunction). These syndromes respond poorly to levodopa therapy and have a worse prognosis than Parkinson's disease.

Patients with **diffuse cerebrovascular disease** may present with features similar to those of Parkinson's disease. Individuals present with physical and mental slowing, and a shuffling gait. In contrast to Parkinson's disease, features tend to be symmetrical and a resting tremor is unusual. Other features of cerebrovascular disease such as brisk reflexes, extensor plantar responses and a history of vascular risk factors are often evident. Vascular parkinsonism responds poorly to levodopa.

13. Movement disorders II: dyskinesias

Questions
- In what way does the tremor of Parkinson's disease differ from essential tremor?
- What are the clinical features of Huntington's disease?

The term dyskinesia means abnormal involuntary movements. Dyskinesias can be categorized as follows:

- **tremor**: rhythmic sinusoidal oscillations of a body part; it may be most prominent at rest (resting tremor), with limbs outstretched (postural tremor) or on movement (intention tremor) depending on the underlying cause
- **dystonia**: involuntary sustained muscle contraction, causing twisting movements or abnormal postures
- **chorea**: continuous, irregular, jerky or fidgety movements that move from one part of the body to another in an unpredictable fashion
- **myoclonus**: brief, shock-like jerks
- **tics**: brief, repetitive, stereotyped behaviours that can be transiently controlled by the patient, although doing so causes a build up of inner tension until the tic is allowed to occur.

These terms are descriptions of clinical phenomena and are not specific diseases or diagnoses in their own right. Once the type (or types) of dyskinesia has been characterized, the underlying cause must be established.

Essential tremor is characterized by tremor on holding the arms outstretched or on maintaining certain postures (postural tremor). In contrast to Parkinson's disease, the tremor is minimal or absent at rest, and not associated with any other neurological dysfunction. The underlying cause is unknown, although a family history is present in 50%. The usual presentation is with upper limb tremor provoked by certain activities such as holding or pouring drinks. The tremor is usually bilateral and may also affect the head (titubation). It may be localized, generalized, constant or intermittent. It is exacerbated by anxiety, and patients may notice an improvement after small amounts of alcohol. Treatment is often unnecessary, but in individuals with disabling tremor, beta-blockers and primidone may be helpful.

Huntington's disease is a progressive neurodegenerative disease inherited in an autosomal dominant fashion (Fig. 3.13.1). Affected individuals typically present between 30 and 50 years of age with personality change (irritability, aggression and loss of interest) and chorea. Chorea may be very subtle at onset, and patients may simply appear 'fidgety'. As the disease relentlessly progresses, chorea becomes more florid and dementia becomes more severe. Death occurs 10–20 years after symptom onset. Genetic testing can diagnose Huntington's disease in symptomatic individuals and can identify whether unaffected relatives carry the gene. Further investigations are required in individuals with no family history, and in whom genetic testing is negative. There is no treatment for Huntington's disease. In view of its devastating nature, testing raises many difficult issues for families, and genetic counselling is vital.

Wilson's disease is a rare autosomal recessive disorder of copper metabolism. It results in the accumulation of copper in the liver, brain (particularly the basal ganglia) and other organs. Individuals usually present with impaired liver function and neurological features (dystonia, parkinsonism, tremor or neuropsychiatric disturbance). Kayser–Fleischer rings (copper deposits around the cornea) are seen on eye examination. Investigations show low serum caeruloplasmin and elevated urinary copper; elevated hepatic copper concentration on liver biopsy confirms the diagnosis. Treatment is with chelating agents such as penicillamine.

Sydenham's chorea is a unilateral, postinfective chorea that affects children or adolescents. Onset is usually within several weeks of a group A streptococcal infection; it settles spontaneously over weeks to months.

Gilles de la Tourette's syndrome comprises multiple motor and vocal tics such as grunting, barking or uttering obscenities. It is often associated with behavioural disturbance, particularly obsessive–compulsive disorder or attention-deficit hyperactivity disorder. Neurological examination is normal and there are no diagnostic tests. Clonidine or haloperidol may provide some symptomatic benefit.

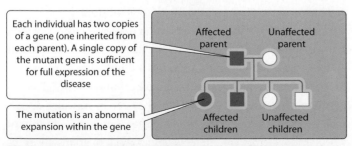

Each individual has two copies of a gene (one inherited from each parent). A single copy of the mutant gene is sufficient for full expression of the disease

The mutation is an abnormal expansion within the gene

Affected parent Unaffected parent

Affected children Unaffected children

Fig. 3.13.1 Autosomal dominant inheritance of Huntington's disease. If one parent is affected, there is a 50% chance that offspring (irrespective of sex) will be affected.

14. Cerebellar disease

Questions
- What are the causes of cerebellar dysfunction?
- What investigations are used in suspected cerebellar dysfunction?

The cerebellum plays a key role in accuracy and coordination of movement. The cerebellar hemispheres (Fig. 3.14.1) coordinate movement in the ipsilateral limbs, while the midline vermis is important in balance and posture. The blood supply is from the posterior circulation (Ch. 1).

Causes of cerebellar disturbance include:
- inherited (spinocerebellar ataxia)
- vascular (haemorrhage, infarction, arteriovenous malformation)
- tumours/malignancy (medulloblastoma, metastatic cancer, acoustic neuroma, paraneoplastic cerebellar degeneration)
- inflammatory/demyelination (multiple sclerosis, coeliac disease)
- toxic (chronic alcohol abuse, drugs such as phenytoin)
- infection (cerebellar abscess, HIV infection).

Clinical features

The cardinal feature of cerebellar dysfunction is ataxia.
Midline cerebellar lesions are associated with:
- an unsteady broad-based ataxic gait
- vertigo and vomiting
- truncal ataxia (difficulty in sitting or standing).

Hemispheric cerebellar lesions are associated with:
- limb ataxia (incoordination of ipsilateral limb movements)
- intention tremor
- dysarthria
- horizontal gaze-invoked nystagmus, with the fast phase towards the abnormal side
- hypotonia and hyporeflexia.

Cerebellar mass lesions (such as tumour, abscess or stroke with oedema) may cause compression of the cerebral aqueduct, obstructing CSF flow. This may result in hydrocephalus, causing raised intracranial pressure. If untreated, the cerebellar tonsils can herniate through the foramen magnum (coning) compressing the brainstem and resulting in coma and death.

Investigations

Blood tests include thyroid function, markers of alcohol abuse (mean corpuscular volume, liver enzymes) and coeliac (endomysial) antibodies.

Chest radiograph may suggest an underlying lung tumour (with cerebellar metastases or paraneoplastic cerebellar degeneration). CT or MRI is almost always required (Fig. 3.14.2). Lumbar puncture may suggest CNS inflammation in multiple sclerosis.

Management

In patients with a cerebellar mass lesion or acute cerebellar stroke, close monitoring for evidence of hydrocephalus is vital; decompressive surgery or insertion of a ventriculo-peritoneal shunt may be required if the patient is at risk of coning.

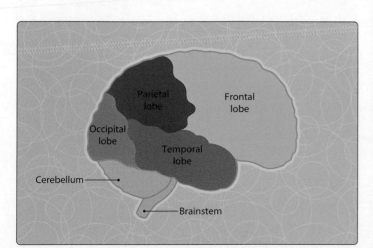

Fig. 3.14.1 The location of the cerebellum in relation to the brain.

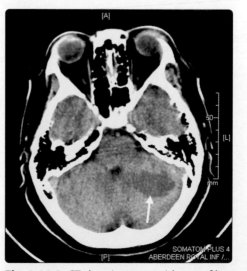

Fig. 3.14.2 CT showing an ovoid area of low attenuation consistent with a left cerebellar infarct (arrow).

15. Brain tumours

Questions
- What are the main clinical features of brain tumours?
- What cancers most commonly cause brain metastases?

Tumours of the CNS may be primary (arising from CNS tissue) or secondary (metastatic tumours arising from elsewhere). Specific types of tumour include:

- **primary benign** (20%): meningioma, neurofibroma (e.g. acoustic neuroma), pituitary adenoma, craniopharyngioma
- **primary malignant** (30%): most commonly gliomas (astrocytoma, glioblastoma multiforme, oligodendroglioma), ependymoma, cerebral lymphoma, medulloblastoma
- **secondary metastatic** (50%): most commonly from breast, lung, thyroid, prostate and kidney cancer, and melanoma.

Clinical features

Brain tumours cause neurological symptoms through local effects of the tumour or effects of raised intracranial pressure (Fig. 3.15.1). Local effects, in which brain function is impaired at the tumour site, occur through infiltration or compression of normal brain tissue (e.g. a tumour in the left temporal lobe may result in dysphasia). Focal seizures arising from the site of the tumour are common.

The expansion of a mass within the skull leads to increased intracranial pressure. This causes headache (typically worse in the morning and exacerbated by coughing), nausea and vomiting, and papilloedema (swelling of the optic disc). Herniation of the lobes of the brain, either laterally (under the falx cerebri) or caudally (across the tentorium cerebelli), can result in focal abnormalities that are not specific to the location of the mass lesion ('false localizing signs'; Fig. 3.15.2). The most common false localizing signs are palsies of cranial nerves VI or III.

Clinical features, therefore, depend on the location, size and speed of growth of the tumour. The most common presenting features include seizures, headache and progressive focal neurological deficits (Fig. 3.15.1).

Investigations

Imaging with CT (Fig. 3.15.3) or MRI is the most useful investigation. Biopsy is sometimes performed to confirm the type and grade of tumour. If cerebral metastases are suspected, investigations to identify a primary source are usually required.

Management

Management depends upon the type of tumour, its location and the fitness of the patient. High-dose steroids are often given to provide short-term symptomatic benefit by reducing local oedema. Anticonvulsants should be given if the patient has had seizures.

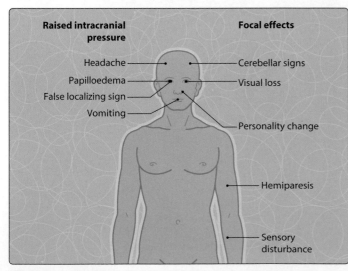

Fig. 3.15.1 Common presenting features of brain tumours.

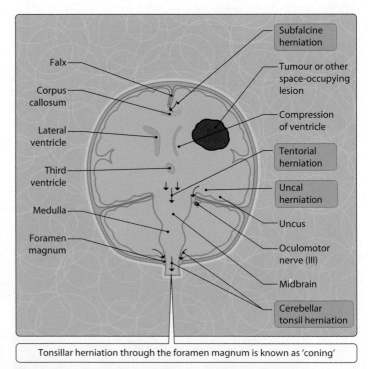

Tonsillar herniation through the foramen magnum is known as 'coning'

Fig. 3.15.2 Coronal representation of the shifts and herniations that occur in the presence of a large space-occupying lesion.

In low-grade benign tumours, observation and serial imaging may be appropriate. However, if there is significant neurological impairment, excision may be possible depending upon the location of the tumour. In malignant tumours, including cerebral metastases, complete surgical removal of the tumour may not be possible, although palliative 'debulking' procedures are occasionally performed. Radiotherapy may be helpful in both primary and secondary brain tumours, although its use is primarily palliative.

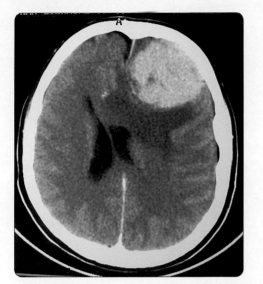

Fig. 3.15.3 CT scan with contrast showing large frontal meningioma. Note the surrounding oedema and midline shift.

PART XII

Blood disorders

Henry Watson and Sajjan Mittal

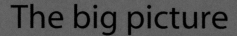

SECTION ONE

The big picture

Haematology encompasses the provision of laboratory and clinical services. Developments in diagnostic tools and new therapies have resulted in a sharp increase in the cost of providing such services.

Blood cells develop from pluripotent stem cells in bone marrow (Figs 1.1–1.3) under the influence of growth factors, many of which have been synthesized.

Haematological disorders vary between, and even within, countries depending on the population. In southern Europe, haemoglobinopathies (e.g. thalassaemias) are common while in northern Europe they are rare.

Malignant haematology

Haematological malignancies may arise from any of the cells that are involved in the formation and development of blood

(haematopoiesis). The three main white cell lines that can undergo malignant change are:

- myeloid precursors: myeloid leukaemia
- lymphoid precursors: leukaemias and the lymphomas
- plasma cells: myeloma.

Incidence and typical age at presentation varies (Table 1.1), for example acute myeloid leukaemia has a median age at diagnosis of 67 years (6%, 6.4% and 7.1%, respectively, at < 20 years, 20–34 years and 35–44 years), whereas acute lymphoblastic leukaemia has a median age at diagnosis of 13 years and 61% present before 20 years. Chronic lymphocytic leukaemia is the commonest haematological malignancy. The median age at diagnosis is 72 years and more than 70% are > 65 years. Chronic myeloid leukaemia is a myeloproliferative

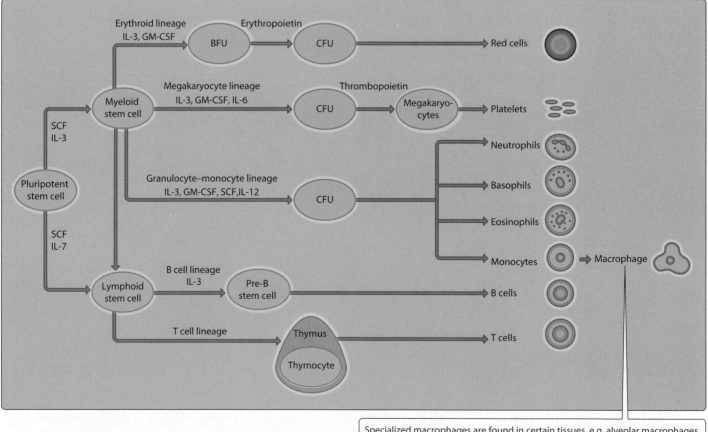

Fig. 1.1 The development of blood cells. BFU, blast-forming unit; CFU, colony-forming unit; IL, interleukin; G-CSF, granulocyte colony-stimulating factor; GM-CSF, granulocyte–macrophage colony-stimulating factor; SCF, stem cell factor.

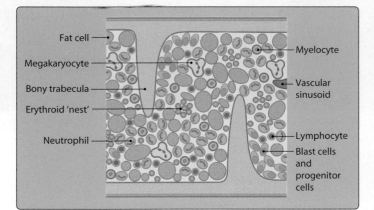

Fig. 1.2 Structure of normal bone marrow.

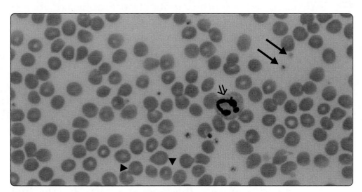

Fig. 1.3 Normal blood film showing red cells (arrowheads), platelets (arrows) and a neutrophil (open arrow).

Table 1.1 INCIDENCE OF DIFFERENT HAEMATOLOGICAL CONDITIONS

	Incidence (per 100 000 per year)
Acute myeloid leukaemia	5
Acute lymphoblastic leukaemia	1.7
Chronic lymphocytic leukaemia	3
Chronic myeloid leukaemia	1.0–1.5
Non-Hodgkin's lymphoma	15–20
Hodgkin's disease	3
Polycythaemia rubra vera	2–3
Essential thrombocythaemia	1.5–2.0
Myeloma	4
Myelodysplasia	4
Aplastic anaemia	0.2–0.3
Pernicious anaemia	100
Idiopathic thrombocytopenic purpura	5.8–6.6
Venous thromboembolism	100

disorder characterized by a specific genetic translocation called the Philadelphia chromosome.

Initial chemotherapy regimens were based on standard combinations of cytotoxic agents. Recent therapies target particular features:

- rituximab, monoclonal antibody targeting CD20-positive cells in B-cell lymphomas
- gemtuzumab, cytotoxic antibody targeting CD33-positive cells in acute myeloid leukaemia
- imatinib, tyrosine kinase inhibitor specifically blocking the kinase activity associated with the *BCR–ABL* translocation in chronic myeloid leukaemia.

The prognosis in some haematological malignancies is now so good that the main emphasis is to identify curative regimens with the least late morbidity. Examples are paediatric leukaemias, good-prognosis acute myeloid leukaemia in adults and Hodgkin's lymphoma.

Transfusion medicine

Transfusion services provide high-quality red cells and platelets for clinical use. Their role has expanded to provide aphaeresis (blood withdrawn from a donor is separated into its compo-

nents and a specific component is removed before returning the blood to the donor by transfusion) services and stem-cell harvesting and storage.

Haemostasis and thrombosis

The concept of thrombophilia, together with media scares about the combined oral contraceptive, hormone replacement therapy and travel-associated thrombosis, has significantly increased the workload for thrombosis and haemostasis services. Plasma-derived concentrates with potential contamination by blood-borne viruses (e.g. hepatitis B and C and HIV) have been replaced by recombinant materials made in mammalian cell lines. The main complication of haemophilia treatment with concentrate is now the development of inhibitory antibodies. The incidence of severe haemophilia A is constant worldwide, at 1/10 000 of the population.

General haematology

The production of quality-assured laboratory results is essential for good clinical care. In addition nutritional deficiencies, iron overload, hyposplenism, haemoglobinopathies, parasitic infections and many reactive changes that are features of other diseases are detected and clarified by a good haematology service.

High-return facts

1 **Hypochromic and microcytic anaemias** have red cells that are pale and small, respectively. Iron-deficiency anaemia can be differentiated from anaemia of chronic disease by finding a low serum ferritin. Blood loss should be sought by appropriate GI investigation except in premenopausal women with no GI symptoms. **Macrocytic anaemias** require assays of serum vitamin B_{12} and folate. Macrocytosis is indicative of a dyspoietic state and diagnoses such as myelodysplastic syndrome and hypoplastic anaemia may present in this way. Pernicious anaemia is diagnosed by finding B_{12} deficiency with positive anti-intrinsic factor antibodies or where a patient has B_{12} malabsorption corrected by giving intrinsic factor in the second part of the Schilling test.

2 **Haemolytic anaemias** may be hereditary or acquired. They are caused by intrinsic (within red cells) or extrinsic (acting upon red cells) factors, resulting in premature destruction of red cells. Hereditary spherocytosis is the commonest hereditary haemolytic anaemia in northern Europeans. Patients usually present with symptoms of anaemia and mild jaundice. **Aplastic anaemia** is almost certainly an immune-mediated form of bone marrow failure. It presents with varying degrees of pancytopenia, does not have a clear malignant phenotype and responds to immunosuppressive therapy with anti-lymphocyte globulin and ciclosporin.

3 **Bleeding disorders** can be congenital (e.g. haemophilia A and B) or acquired (e.g. from drugs such as warfarin). Treatment with plasma-derived coagulation factor carried the risk of viral infection and now treatment is with recombinant coagulation factors. Inherited **thrombophilia** includes deficiencies of antithrombin, protein C, protein S and mutations of factor V Leiden and the prothrombin gene.

4 **Venous thromboembolism** (VTE) has an annual incidence of approximately 1/1000. Risk increases with age and with temporary risk factors known to be associated with a prothrombotic state. Prophylaxis against VTE during high-risk periods is the best way to prevent thrombosis. Unprovoked VTE is associated with a recurrence rate of approximately 35% in the 5 years following 6 months of anticoagulation with warfarin. In general, positive thrombophilia tests do not affect the duration of anticoagulation with the exception of finding antiphospholipid syndrome, myeloproliferative disease and possibly antithrombin deficiency. **Arterial thrombosis** is associated with antiphospholipid syndrome, paroxysmal nocturnal haemoglobinuria, thrombotic thrombocytopenic purpura and heparin-induced thrombocytopenia, but is not strongly associated with inherited thrombophilia.

5 **Haemoglobinopathies** are common in parts of Africa, the Mediterranean, the Middle East, Asia and the Orient. The haemoglobin abnormality is either quantitative (thalassaemic conditions) or qualitative (sickling conditions). **Beta thalassaemia major** presents with transfusion dependency in infanthood. Ethnic origin is often a clue to the diagnosis of thalassaemia, which is confirmed using haemoglobin electrophoresis. **Sickle cell anaemia** is associated with painful bone or visceral crises, acute chest syndrome, stroke and premature death. Hypertransfusion, hydroxycarbamide and allogeneic bone marrow transplant are of value in selected patients.

6 **Myeloproliferative disorders** are associated with hypercellular bone marrow appearances and high peripheral blood counts. Common complications are venous and arterial thromboses; therapy aims to reduce vascular events. Both polycythaemia rubra vera and essential thrombocythaemia may transform to myelofibrosis or acute leukaemia. **Paraproteinaemias** are associated with several diseases including those with a malignant phenotype such as myeloma, plasmacytoma or lymphoma and those classified as monoclonal gammopathy of undetermined significance. **Myeloma** may present with a variety of features such as backache, symptoms of hypercalcaemia or renal failure.

7 **Acute lymphocytic leukaemia** is treated by remission-induction therapy, followed by consolidation therapy, CNS prophylaxis and prolonged maintenance therapy. **Acute myeloid leukaemia** is the most common acute leukaemia in adults. The prognosis is related to age, cytogenetics and response to initial chemotherapy. Some translocations are associated with a good prognosis while deletions in chromosomes 5 and 7 are associated with a poor prognosis. Treatment includes four or five courses of pulsed chemotherapy. **Chronic lymphocytic leukaemia** is the most common of all leukaemias. It is often a chance finding and requires treatment only for bulky lymphadenopathy, constitutional symptoms and bone marrow failure. **Chronic myeloid leukaemia** is characterized by a specific translocation called the Philadelphia chromosome. The resulting fusion protein encodes a tyrosine kinase that is responsible for the disease phenotype. Modern therapy specifically inhibits this tyrosine kinase.

8 **Non-Hodgkin's lymphoma** (NHL) is increasing in incidence. Low-grade NHL, including follicular, mantle cell, marginal zone and small cell lymphocytic lymphomas, are incurable but often indolent, with a prognosis of 5–10 years. High-grade NHL arises de novo or in association with immunosuppression (e.g. after transplantation or in AIDS). The most significant advance in the treatment of B cell lymphoma is the development of the therapeutic monoclonal antibody rituximab (anti-CD20). **Hodgkin's lymphoma** is associated with Epstein–Barr virus infection in approximately a third of patients. Even advanced disease has a cure rate of approximately 50%.

1. Anaemia I: hypochromic, microcytic and macrocytic anaemias

Questions
- What are the causes of hypochromic and microcytic anaemia?
- What are the causes of macrocytic anaemia?

Hypochromic and microcytic anaemias

Hypochromic and microcytic anaemias are characterized by red cells that are pale and small, respectively (Fig. 3.1.1). Red cell indices are reduced: mean corpuscular volume (MCV), mean corpuscular haemoglobin (MCH) and mean corpuscular haemoglobin concentration (MCHC). The clinical presentation and ethnic origin of the patient are important in making a diagnosis.

Pathogenesis

Disorders that result in a lack of usable iron (iron deficiency and anaemia of chronic disease) and disorders of haemoglobin synthesis (congenital sideroblastic anaemia and thalassaemias) present with hypochromic anaemia. Anaemia of chronic disease may be normocytic while the others are microcytic.

Clinical features

Iron-deficiency anaemia may result from poor dietary intake or malabsorption. A history of blood loss or of conditions associated with GI bleeding should be sought. Menorrhagia and pregnancy may result in iron deficiency. Examination may reveal pallor, koilonychia (spoon-shaped nails) and angular cheilosis (Fig. 3.1.2) or features of the underlying cause (e.g. uterine fibroids, abdominal or rectal mass).

Anaemia of chronic disease is associated with chronic infection, inflammatory disorders and malignancy.

Thalassaemia is often evident from family history and ethnicity. Patients have typical facial features and may have splenomegaly.

Investigations

Table 3.1.1 gives features of various anaemias.

In iron-deficiency anaemia, further investigations include endomysial antibodies for coeliac disease, endoscopy and/or colonoscopy for GI bleeding and angiography for small intestine bleeding. Premenopausal women with no GI symptoms do not require further investigation.

In thalassaemias, further investigations include haemoglobin electrophoresis, disease phenotyping in family members and DNA studies for specific mutations.

Bone marrow examination and DNA studies are helpful in suspected sideroblastic anaemia.

Management

In iron deficiency, replacement is best achieved orally with ferrous sulphate. Iron is best absorbed in the fasting state and should be given for 3 months to replenish stores. Side-effects

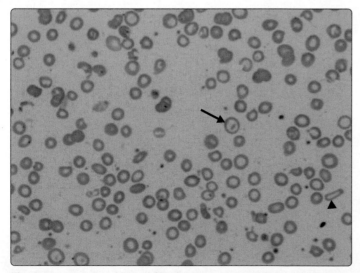

Fig. 3.1.1 Peripheral blood film from a patient with iron-deficiency anaemia in which hypochromic microcytic red cells including target cells (arrow) and rod forms (arrowhead) can be seen.

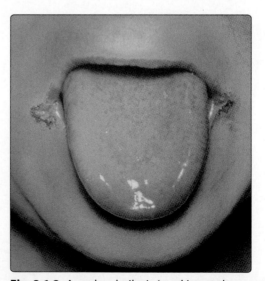

Fig. 3.1.2 Angular cheilosis (cracking at the corner of the mouth) and glossitis (smooth, shiny tongue) in a patient with megaloblastic anaemia.

Table 3.1.1 INVESTIGATIONS IN ANAEMIAS

	Iron deficiency	Chronic disease	Thalassaemia	Congenital sideroblastic anaemia
Cell indices[a]	All low and in relation to anaemia	Low or normal	Very low in relation to anaemia	All low
Ferritin	Low	Normal or high	Normal or high	High
Serum iron	Low	Low	Normal	High
Total iron-binding capacity	High	Low	Normal	Normal
Blood film	Target cells, pencil cells, ± thrombocytosis	Variable upon primary diagnosis	Target cells, poikilocytes, basophilic stippling, 'H' bodies	Diamorphic, basophilic stippling

[a]Mean corpuscular volume, mean corpuscular haemoglobin and haemoglobin concentration.

are common and include nausea, constipation and diarrhoea. Intravenous iron is indicated for severe intolerance of oral iron and in malabsorption. Any underlying cause of iron deficiency should be treated. There is no specific management for congenital sideroblastic anaemia.

Macrocytic anaemias

Macrocytic anaemias are characterized by large red cells and a high MCV. The upper limit of normal for MCV is approximately 100 fl (100 µm²).

Pathogenesis

Macrocytic anaemias can be divided into two groups.

Megaloblastic anaemias. Abnormal marrow appearances are characterized by delayed nuclear maturation relative to the cytoplasm and involvement of all three developing cell lines. Defective DNA synthesis accounts for megaloblastic change and is most often caused by vitamin B_{12} or folate deficiency.

Non-megaloblastic macrocytic anaemias. Abnormalities are typically confined to circulating macrocytes.

Clinical features

Causes of macrocytic anaemia:

- megaloblastic: B_{12} deficiency, folate deficiency, transcobalamin deficiency, anti-folate drugs, hydroxycarbamide therapy, cytarabine therapy
- non-megaloblastic: alcohol and other drugs, liver disease, hypothyroidism, pregnancy, myelodysplastic syndromes, aplastic anaemia, reticulocytosis.

Vitamin B_{12} deficiency presents with symptoms of anaemia, mild jaundice (from haemolysis), peripheral neuropathy, subacute combined degeneration of spinal cord, glossitis (Fig. 3.1.2), thrombocytopenia or sterility. Causes include partial gastrectomy, malabsorption from the terminal ileum (e.g. Crohn's disease) and dietary deficiency is strict vegans.

Pernicious anaemia also causes vitamin B_{12} deficiency. It is an autoimmune disorder in which the gastric mucosa is atrophic with loss of parietal cells, causing intrinsic factor deficiency. There is often a personal or family history of organ-specific autoimmune disease (e.g. thyroid disease).

Folate deficiency presents with symptoms of anaemia. Causes include dietary deficiency, malabsorption (e.g. coeliac disease or previous small-bowel surgery), anticonvulsant and sulfasalazine therapy or pregnancy.

Investigations

Macrocytosis is assessed with FBC, reticulocytes and blood film, liver function tests, thyroid function tests, vitamin B_{12} and red cell folate assays. Bone marrow examination is carried out in suspected myelodysplastic syndrome and aplastic anaemia.

Anti-intrinsic factor antibody measurement (specific for pernicious anaemia) and the Schilling test, assess vitamin B_{12} absorption in the absence and presence of intrinsic factor. Pernicious anaemia is confirmed if giving oral intrinsic factor corrects vitamin B_{12} malabsorption. Malabsorption at the terminal ileum is likely if intrinsic factor has no effect.

Management

In severe pernicious anaemia, vitamin B_{12} and folic acid are started simultaneously. Hydroxocobalamin is given i.m. 1000 µg weekly for 3 weeks followed by long-term therapy with 1000 µg every 3 months. Prevention is required following gastric and illeal resection.

The underlying disorder is treated in folate deficiency. Prophylaxis is required in pregnancy, renal dialysis and chronic haemolytic anaemias.

2. Anaemia II: haemolytic and aplastic anaemias

Questions
- What is the pathogenesis of haemolytic anaemia?
- What are the causes of aplastic anaemia?

Haemolytic anaemias

Haemolytic anaemia may be hereditary or acquired. Hereditary conditions involve abnormalities of the membrane, haemoglobin molecule or red cell enzymes.

Epidemiology

Hereditary spherocytosis is the commonest hereditary haemolytic anaemia, with an incidence of 1/5000 in Caucasians. Autoimmune haemolytic anaemia is slightly more common in females and increases in incidence with age.

Pathogenesis

These normochromic and normocytic anaemias are caused by intrinsic (acting from within the red cells) or extrinsic (acting upon red cells) factors that result in premature destruction of red cells. In compensated haemolytic anaemia, the bone marrow can maintain normal red cell numbers in the circulation by increasing its activity. Classification is into three major types based on whether the disease is hereditary or acquired, immune (alloimmune or autoimmune) or non-immune, and extravascular or intravascular.

Hereditary haemolytic anaemias include red cell membrane defects (e.g. hereditary spherocytosis), red cell enzymopathies (e.g. glucose-6-phosphate dehydrogenase deficiency) and abnormal haemoglobin (e.g. thalassaemias and sickle cell disease).

The **non-immune acquired haemolytic anaemias** include microangiopathic haemolytic anaemia, haemolytic uraemic syndrome (caused by *Escherichia coli* O157H), thrombotic thrombocytopenic purpura, paroxysmal nocturnal haemoglobinuria (PNH) and March haemoglobinuria; haemolysis can also occur in sepsis, malaria and with prosthetic heart valves.

Alloimmune haemolytic anaemia is associated with antibodies against red blood cells from another source: haemolytic transfusion reaction and haemolytic disease of the newborn. There are two main types of **autoimmune haemolytic anaemia**; in both, autoantibodies attach to and destroy red blood cells. In the warm antibody type, autoantibodies attack at temperatures equal to or in excess of normal body temperature whereas in the cold antibody type, autoantibodies become active at temperatures below body temperature. The warm type can be primary or secondary to disease (e.g. lymphoma, systemic lupus erythematosus) or drugs. The cold type can be idiopathic (cold haemagglutinin disease), caused by paroxysmal cold haemoglobinuria or secondary to infection (Epstein–Barr virus or mycoplasma) or lymphoproliferative diseases.

Clinical features

Patients usually present with symptoms of anaemia and mild jaundice. Brown/red urine occurs in haemoglobinuria. A hereditary cause is suspected if symptoms develop in infancy or if there is a family history. Splenomegaly and lymphadenopathy may be present.

Investigations

Diagnosis is established by finding reticulocytosis (FBC shows anaemia, mild macrocytosis and reticulocytosis), increased unconjugated bilirubin and lactate dehydrogenase, decreased haptoglobin and peripheral blood smear findings (spherocytes, polychromasia or fragments; Fig. 3.2.1). Haemagglutination is found at room temperature in cold autoimmune haemolysis.

Urinary haemosiderin indicates chronic intravascular haemolysis. The direct antiglobulin test (Coombs' test) detects antibodies or complement on the surface of red blood cells, the hallmark of autoimmune haemolysis.

Management

Any underlying cause should be treated and precipitating factors (e.g. drugs, cold) avoided. Folic acid supplements and transfusions may be required.

Immune haemolytic anaemia is treated with immunosuppressive therapies: steroids, splenectomy and monoclonal antibodies (e.g. rituximab, an anti-CD20 monoclonal antibody). Splenectomy is also considered for severe transfusion-dependent red cell membrane disorders.

Aplastic anaemias

While anaemia typically refers to low red blood cell counts, in aplastic anaemia the bone marrow fails to produce blood cells in all three lineages (**pancytopenia**).

Epidemiology

Aplastic anaemia is a rare disease with an annual incidence of 2–3/1 000 000 in the Western world. In Asia and the Orient, the incidence is 5–10 times higher. Typical acquired aplastic anaemia is a disease of young adults, but a second peak occurs in the fifth or sixth decade.

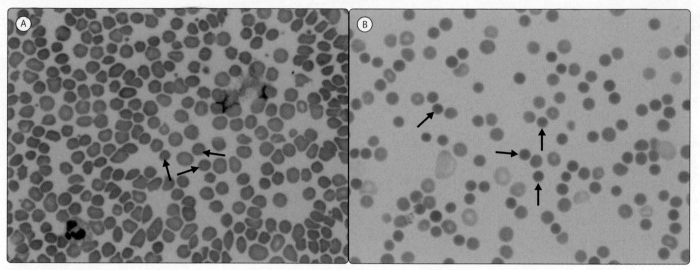

Fig. 3.2.1 Peripheral blood films. A, From a neonate with haemolytic disease showing polychromatic (pinkish blue) red cells and spherocytes (spherical red cells with no central pallor (arrows)). B, From a patient with autoimmune haemolytic anaemia, showing numerous spherocytes (arrows).

Pathogenesis

The cause of acquired aplastic anaemia is usually unknown. There is some association with *HLA-DR2*. Several rare inherited syndromes (e.g. Fanconi anaemia and dyskeratosis congenita) can present as or evolve into aplastic anaemia. Common associations with acquired aplastic anaemia include exposure to drugs (e.g. gold, chloramphenicol, carbamazepine, phenytoin, NSAIDs and cytotoxic agents), environmental toxins or viral infections. Pancytopenia also occurs in megaloblastic anaemia (e.g. pernicious anaemia), bone marrow infiltration (e.g. lymphoma, secondary cancer, acute leukaemia, myeloma, myelofibrosis), hypersplenism, systemic lupus erythematosus, disseminated tuberculosis, PNH and overwhelming sepsis.

Clinical features

History and examination reveal features of pancytopenia: mucosal bleeding, purpura and bruising. There may be symptoms of anaemia and of bacterial or fungal infection as a result of neutropenia. Severe aplastic anaemia has two out of the three following criteria:

- neutrophils $< 0.5 \times 10^9$ cells/l
- reticulocyte count $< 20 \times 10^9$ cells/l in anaemic/transfusion-dependent patient
- platelets $< 20 \times 10^9$ cells/l.

Investigations

FBC shows pancytopenia, mild macrocytosis and reticulocytopenia. Bone marrow aspirate and trephine biopsy (Fig. 3.2.2) show reduction in haematopoietic cells with replacement by fat spaces.

There may be an associated PNH clone. Cytogenetics and specific gene mutation tests are also helpful in inherited syndromes.

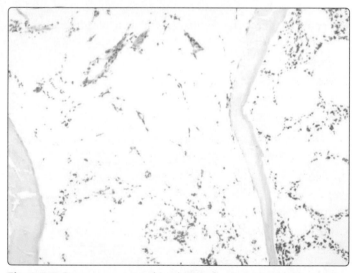

Fig. 3.2.2 Bone marrow trephine biopsy from a patient with severe aplastic anaemia: very scanty normal haematopoietic cells are present.

Management

Mild aplastic anaemia requires careful observation only. Severe forms need supportive treatment with packed red cells, platelets and antibiotics as required. Specific treatment options include immunosuppression (e.g. anti-lymphocyte globulin ± ciclosporin) in older patients and allogeneic bone marrow transplant in patients < 50 years. Androgens and danazol may be useful in refractory disease. Inherited syndromes are also treated with immunosuppressive drugs ± bone marrow transplantation.

Prognosis

Prognosis depends on age, cause and severity. Aplastic anaemia secondary to certain drugs, pregnancy, low-dose radiation or infectious mononucleosis is usually short term. The prognosis is worse in those where there is no obvious precipitating cause.

3. Bleeding disorders and thrombophilia

Questions
- What treatments are available for bleeding disorders?
- What are the causes of thrombophilia?

Normal haemostasis requires blood coagulation (fibrin formation; Fig. 3.3.1), platelet function and fibrin removal.

Bleeding disorders

Bleeding disorders are congenital or acquired. Acquired disorders are becoming more common because of widespread use of drugs, particularly warfarin, antiplatelet agents, chemotherapy and immunosuppressants.

Pathogenesis

Deficiency or lack of function of platelets, von Willebrand factor or coagulation factors may result in a bleeding diathesis.

An inhibitor of coagulation (e.g. heparin) or vascular defect (e.g. hereditary haemorrhagic telangiectasia, Henoch–Schönlein purpura, scurvy, Ehlers–Danlos syndrome and amyloidosis) may also cause haemorrhage.

Thrombocytopenia (low platelet count) can be caused by:

- decreased production: malignancy involving bone marrow, hypoplastic anaemia, myelodysplastic syndrome, chemotherapy or other drug-induced marrow failure
- increased consumption: disseminated intravascular coagulation (DIC), immune thrombocytopenias, hypersplenism, dilutional coagulopathy.

Clinical features

Signs of bleeding include petechiae, bruising, wound haematoma and excessive blood in surgical drains. Important features are site of bleeding, severity, nature (i.e. spontaneous or provoked bleeding), age, previous episodes or bleeding following surgery, and family and drug histories. Surgical bleeding is typified by bleeding from a single site while a general bleeding diathesis involves multiple sites (e.g. drains, lines, wounds, endotracheal tubes).

Coagulation factor deficiency. Typical features are recurrent joint haemorrhage (haemarthroses), muscular haematomas, retroperitoneal haemorrhage, intracranial haemorrhage and postsurgical bleeding.

Platelet and von Willebrand factor abnormalities. These are characterized by recurrent mucosal bleeding (e.g. prolonged epistaxis), easy bruising, oral blood blisters, menorrhagia, postpartum and postsurgical haemorrhage.

Inherited bleeding disorders. Children with severe haemophilia A or B (VIII:c or IX:c deficiency) and rare autosomal disorders (X, V and XIII deficiency) have an increased risk of intracranial haemorrhage and umbilical stump bleeding in the neonatal period (Table 3.3.1).

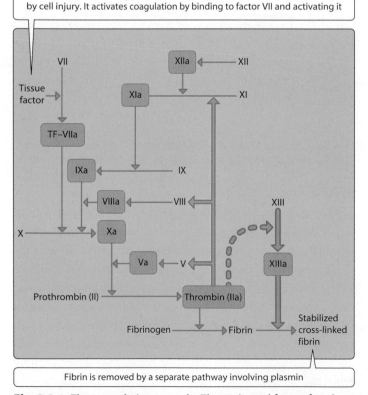

Tissue factor (TF) is a glycoprotein on the surface of cells that is exposed by cell injury. It activates coagulation by binding to factor VII and activating it

Fibrin is removed by a separate pathway involving plasmin

Fig. 3.3.1 The coagulation cascade. The activated form of each factor (in brown boxes) acts as an enzyme to convert the next factor in the sequence to its active form. Pathways shown in red are part of the amplification sequence; those in green are involved in clot stabilization.

Table 3.3.1 FACTOR DEFICIENCY AND PRESENTATION OF THE HAEMOPHILIAS

Disease severity	Circulating factor VIII or IX (%)	Presentation
Severe	< 1	Spontaneous bleeding
Moderate	1–4	Bleeding following minor trauma or surgery
Mild	5–30	Bleeding following major trauma or surgery

Investigations

Platelet count, morphology on blood film and platelet function tests may detect specific abnormalities. Bleeding time may provide non-specific information.

Screening tests for coagulation factors include prothrombin time (PT), activated partial thromboplastin time (APTT) and fibrinogen (Table 3.3.2). A prolonged test time should be followed by repeat test with the patient sample mixed 1:1 with normal pooled plasma. Correction suggests coagulation factor deficiency. Failure to correct suggests presence of an inhibitor of coagulation (e.g. heparin or lupus anticoagulant).

Management

Thrombocytopenia. Platelet transfusion is required for bone marrow failure, DIC, and dilutional coagulopathy. Idiopathic thrombocytopenic purpura is treated with steroids, immunoglobulin and splenectomy.

Disseminated intravascular coagulation. The underlying cause must be treated. Platelets, fresh frozen plasma (FFP) and cryoprecipitate may be necessary.

Warfarin excess. Oral vitamin K is used for minor bleeding and i.v. vitamin K and prothrombin complex concentrate for major bleeding.

Heparins. Bleeding on heparin should be treated by discontinuing therapy and administering protamine sulphate.

Haemophilia A. Those with mild haemophilia can be treated with desmopressin acetate (DDAVP) and tranexamic acid. Severe forms are treated using recombinant factor VIII.

Haemophilia B. All bleeding is treated using recombinant factor IX concentrate.

Von Willebrand disease. DDAVP and tranexamic acid are used in mild disease; factor VIII and vW factor-containing concentrate for bleeding in severely affected patients.

Table 3.3.2 COAGULATION TESTS IN INVESTIGATION OF BLEEDING

Test	Disorders
PT prolonged	Deficiencies of FVII
APTT prolonged	Deficiencies of FVIII, FIX, FXI, FXII; unfractionated heparin, vWD[a]
APTT and PT prolonged	Deficiencies of FX, FV, FII, vitamin K; hypofibrinogenaemia, warfarin
Fibrinogen reduced	Hypofibrinogenaemia, dysfibrinogenaemia
Coagulation tests normal	Platelet disorders, vascular purpura, deficiency of FXIII, low-molecular-weight heparin, fibrinolytic bleeding, vWD[a]

F, factor; PT, prothrombin time; APTT, activated partial thromboplastin time; vWD, von Willebrand disease.
[a]Associated with normal APTT if FVIII levels normal.

Rare congenital deficiencies. Factor XIII deficiency is treated with concentrate; factors X and II with prothrombin complex concentrate; factor XI with factor XI concentrate, or FFP if required; factor V with FFP; and factor VII with recombinant VIIa.

Previous recipients of pooled plasma products made from UK plasma. Special precautions are required during medical and surgical procedures where lymphoid or neural tissue is breached because of the theoretical risk of infection with the agent responsible for variant Creutzfeldt–Jakob disease.

Thrombophilia

Thrombophilia refers to a group of inherited and acquired disorders that may result in thrombosis.

Inherited thrombophilia includes heterozygous deficiencies of anticoagulation proteins; all increase the risk of venous thromboembolism (VTE):

- **antithrombin III deficiency**: incidence 1/10 000; homozygous form is lethal in utero; relative risk for VTE is 20.
- **protein C deficiency**: incidence 1/500–1000; homozygous form is associated with neonatal purpura fulminans and deficiency is associated with warfarin-induced skin necrosis; relative risk for VTE is 5
- **protein S deficiency**: incidence 1/2000; relative risk for VTE 5
- **factor V Leiden mutation**: the most common inherited prothrombotic abnormality in northern Europeans; incidence of heterozygosity of 5–7%; relative risk for VTE of 5–7 in heterozygous state, with a 50-fold increased risk in homozygotes
- **prothrombin *20210A* mutation**: 2–3% of northern Europeans; heterozygotes have a relative risk for VTE of 3.

Among unselected northern Europeans, 10% will have one of these abnormalities, while 50% of patients with unprovoked deep vein thrombosis (DVT) do not have any of them. None of these disorders is associated with an increased risk of arterial thrombosis. Inherited thrombophilia does not influence the intensity of anticoagulation, duration of treatment after a first event or recurrence in most cases.

Testing for thrombophilia may be useful in unusual venous thrombosis (e.g. axillary, cerebral and intra-abdominal venous thrombosis), in unprovoked VTE in young patients and in those with a strongly positive family history. Female relatives considering use of the combined contraceptive pill or hormone replacement therapy should be counselled.

4. Thrombosis

Questions
- How should venous thromboembolism be managed?
- What are the causes of arterial thrombosis?

Venous thromboembolism

Venous thromboembolism (VTE) usually presents with deep vein thrombosis (DVT) of the leg or pelvis, and/or pulmonary embolism (PE). Venous thrombosis of the upper limb, cerebral veins and intra-abdominal splenic, hepatic, portal and mesenteric circulations is much less common.

Epidemiology

The annual incidence of VTE increases with age, rising from 1/10 000 at age 20 years to 1/1000 at 50 years. The risk of VTE is lower in oriental races.

Pathogenesis

Venous stasis and hypercoagulability are predisposing factors. Thrombosis can develop following exposure to the combined oral contraceptive pill, in malignancy or surgery on the pelvis, hip or lower limb. Thrombophilia also increases the risk (see Ch. 3).

PE originates from a DVT that has extended into the popliteal vein, although on occasion no source is apparent. Silent PE can be found in 30–50% of patients presenting with DVT. Post-thrombotic syndrome caused by venous valve damage occurs in 30% of patients with lower limb DVT, usually within 3 years.

Clinical features

DVT presents with leg swelling, oedema, pain and tenderness, warmth and redness. Discoloration, skin pigmentation and venous ulcers suggest post-thrombotic syndrome. PE presents with breathlessness, chest pain (often pleuritic), haemoptysis and in, massive PE, hypotension and collapse. Signs may include tachypnoea, tachycardia, a small pleural effusion and pleural rub. Risk factors include:

- **surgical**: major surgery in previous 4–6 weeks, lower limb orthopaedic surgery, spinal neurosurgery, surgery for abdominal or pelvic cancer, lower limb plaster cast
- **medical**: >3 days immobility, lower limb paralysis, heart failure, nephrotic syndrome, active cancer, heparin-induced thrombocytopenia, anti-phospholipid syndrome, myeloproliferative disorders
- **hormonal**: pregnancy and puerperium, combined oral contraceptive, hormone replacement therapy, ovarian stimulation therapy
- **other**: previous VTE/family history/thrombophilia, varicose veins, long distance travel.

Investigations

In those with a low pre-test Wells' Score (Table 3.4.1), the diagnosis of DVT or PE can be safely excluded by a negative d-dimer test. DVT can be confirmed by ultrasound or venography (Fig. 3.4.1). PE can be confirmed by isotope ventilation/perfusion and CT pulmonary angiogram. CT, MRI and venography are used to diagnose venous thromboses at other sites. Intra-abdominal thrombosis may be diagnosed at laparotomy or on imaging.

Testing for genetic causes of thrombophilia does not affect initial level or duration of anticoagulation.

Management

Anticoagulation therapy involves the use of heparin and warfarin (Fig. 3.4.2). In all cases of prolonged heparin use, platelet count should be checked from day 4 to 14 to exclude heparin-induced thrombocytopenia. Periods of high risk of thrombosis should be identified and mechanical and/or pharmacological prophylaxis provided.

First episode of VTE. Low-molecular-weight heparin (LMWH) is initiated with the dose adjusted for body weight. This is followed by warfarin to maintain a target international normalized ratio (INR) of 2.5 (range, 2–3) for 6 months.

Further episode of VTE or visceral and life-threatening thrombosis. Long-term anticoagulation is considered with a target of INR of 2.5 (range, 2–3).

Table 3.4.1 WELLS' SCORE RISK OF DEEP VEIN THROMBOSIS

Features	Points[a]
Active cancer	1
Paralysis or plaster	1
Bed-rest >3 days, surgery within 4 weeks	1
Tenderness along vein	1
Entire leg swollen	1
Calf swollen >3 cm	1
Pitting oedema (unilateral)	1
Collateral veins	1
Alternative diagnosis likely	−2

[a]Low, ≤0; moderate, 1–2; high, ≥3.

Recurrent VTE on therapeutic anticoagulation. The target INR is increased to 3.5 (range, 3–4.5).

Massive PE. Embolectomy or fibrinolysis using tissue plasminogen activator (tPA) may be suitable.

VTE in pregnancy. LMWH in therapeutic doses used until 6 weeks after delivery.

Prognosis

Recurrence rates at 5 years are 35% for spontaneous VTE, <5% for postsurgical VTE and 10–15% for contraceptive pill-associated VTE.

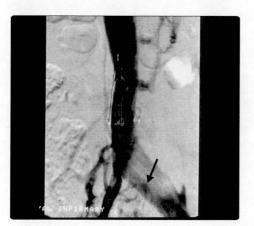

Fig. 3.4.1 Venogram showing left iliac deep vein thrombosis (arrow).

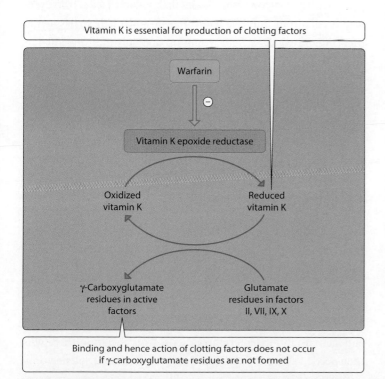

Fig. 3.4.2 Mechanism of action of warfarin in blocking recycling of vitamin K to its active form.

Arterial thrombosis

Arterial thrombosis can present as ischaemic stroke, transient ischaemic attacks (TIAs), acute coronary syndrome and peripheral vascular disease.

Pathogenesis

Most arterial thrombosis is secondary to atherosclerosis and acute plaque rupture. Risk factors for developing atherosclerosis include age, cigarette smoking, diabetes mellitus, systemic hypertension, hyperlipidaemia and a positive family history of precocious arterial thrombosis. Vascular risk is associated with increasing blood fibrinogen and elevated homocysteine levels.

Anti-phospholipid syndrome is associated with persistent anti-phospholipid antibodies. It may be primary or secondary (e.g. to systemic lupus erythematosus). Diagnosis is based on venous or arterial thrombosis or fetal loss during pregnancy, combined with persistent anti-cardiolipin antibodies or lupus anticoagulant. Patients with thrombosis should have long-term anticoagulation with warfarin (INR target 2.5).

Paroxysmal nocturnal haemoglobinuria results from an acquired gene mutation and presents with aplastic anaemia, nocturnal haemoglobinuria or arterial or venous thrombosis. Treatment is usually with long-term anticoagulation with warfarin (INR target, 2.5) for patients with thrombotic events.

Thrombotic thrombocytopenic purpura is caused by an autoantibody directed against von Willebrand factor-cleaving protease. It presents with thrombocytopenia, microangiopathic haemolytic anaemia, renal failure, fever and flitting neurological signs. Treatment is with plasma exchange using fresh frozen plasma, and prednisolone. Patients who have ischaemic strokes should receive aspirin.

Heparin-induced thrombocytopenia is caused by platelet and coagulation activation by antibodies against the complex of anti-platelet factor 4 and heparin. Patients may have venous or arterial thrombosis with moderate thrombocytopenia developing 4–14 days after starting heparin. In patients with exposure to heparin in the previous 100 days, thrombocytopenia may present on day 1 of further heparin exposure. Diagnosis is confirmed by finding anti-platelet factor 4 antibodies. Treatment includes withholding further heparin and achieving anticoagulation with lepirudin or danaparoid until the condition has resolved. Patients with VTE should receive warfarin for 3–6 months.

5. Haemoglobinopathies

Questions
- What is the pathogenesis of the haemoglobinopathies?
- What are the clinical features of thalassaemia and sickle cell anaemia?

The adult haemoglobin (Hb) molecule is made up of four polypeptide chains: two α- and two β-chains. The normal adult form, HbA, comprises $\alpha_2\beta_2$ and makes up 97% of total Hb. Two other types are found in adults: HbA2, containing $\alpha_2\delta_2$ (2.5%), and HbF, containing $\alpha_2\gamma_2$ (0.5%). Abnormalities can occur in the production of the globin chains (thalassaemias), the structure of the chains (e.g. sickle cell (HbS) and HbC diseases) or a combination of these. Other haemoglobinopathies include HbD, HbE and unstable haemoglobins.

Antenatal diagnosis and genetic counselling are important in clinically significant haemoglobinopathies.

Thalassaemias

Thalassaemias are common in parts of Africa, the Mediterranean, the Middle East and Asia (Fig. 3.5.1).

Pathogenesis

Alpha thalassaemia is caused by failure of production of α-chains after deletion of genes for the α-globin chain, which are duplicated on each chromosome. Normally there are four copies, and deletions give rise to different clinical syndromes:

4 genes deleted $(--/--)$: hydrops fetalis (not compatible with life), Hb Barts ($\gamma 4$)

3 genes deleted $(--/-\alpha)$: severe hypochromic microcytic anaemia (HbH disease)

2 genes deleted $(--/\alpha\alpha$ or $-\alpha/-\alpha)$: mild anaemia

1 gene deleted $(\alpha\alpha/\alpha-)$: asymptomatic.

Beta thalassaemia is a group of genetic disorders ranging from beta thalassaemia major to beta thalassaemia trait (minor). It results from reduced rate of synthesis of β-globin. Beta thalassaemia major (Mediterranean or Cooley's anaemia) either has no β-chain ($\beta 0$) or a small amount of β-chain (β^+). There are excess α-chains, which precipitate and shorten red cell lifespan.

Combination of thalassaemia with other haemoglobinopathies may occur: beta thalassaemia with HbE causes severe illness, with HbC causing milder anaemia and with HbS causing severe sickling syndrome.

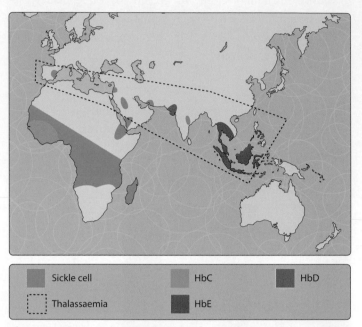

Fig. 3.5.1 Geographic distribution of major haemoglobin (Hb) abnormalities.

Clinical features

Anaemia usually appears between 3 and 6 months after birth in beta thalassaemia major. Hepatosplenomegaly is caused by excess red cell destruction and extra-medullary haemopoiesis. Bony expansion of the marrow cavity causes thalassaemic facies. Iron overload occurs from multiple blood transfusions. Beta thalassaemia trait (minor) usually has no symptoms and only mild anaemia.

Investigations

In beta thalassaemia major, FBC shows moderate to severe hypochromic microcytic anaemia (Hb, 30–90 g/l); mean corpuscular volume and mean corpuscular Hb concentration are reduced. Reticulocytosis is present. Blood film shows marked anisopoikilocytosis (variation in cell size and shape; Fig. 3.5.2) with target cells and nucleated red cells. Hb electrophoresis demonstrates reduced (or absent) HbA ($\alpha_2\beta_2$). In beta thalassaemia trait, red cells are hypochromic and microcytic. Electrophoresis shows raised HbA_2. Skull radiography shows a 'hair on end' appearance in thalassaemia major.

Management

Lifelong blood transfusion will keep Hb elevated and switches off endogenous abnormal erythropoiesis. Iron chelation therapy is then needed along with folic acid supplementation. Splenectomy is necessary in gross splenomegaly. Allogeneic bone marrow transplant is the only curative option.

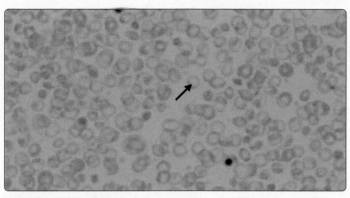

Fig. 3.5.2 Blood film from a patient with β-thalassaemia major, showing red cell anisopoikilocytosis (varying sizes and shapes) including hypochromic microcytic (arrow) and nucleated forms.

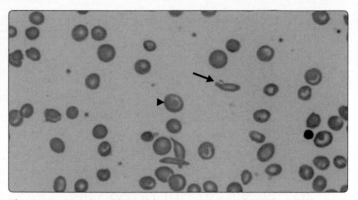

Fig. 3.5.3 Peripheral blood from a patient with sickle cell disease, showing sickle (arrow) and target (arrowhead) cells.

Sickle cell anaemia

In sickle cell anaemia, red blood cells have an abnormal, rigid, sickle shape. This reduces cell flexibility and leads to a tendency to block the microcirculation, causing infarcts.

Sickle cell disease is widespread throughout Africa, the Middle East, parts of India and the Mediterranean. It is common in people (or their descendants) from areas where malaria is common. Those with one or two HbS alleles are resistant to malaria. There are an estimated 30 million sickle cell carriers worldwide.

Pathogenesis

In HbS, substitution of valine for glutamic acid at position 6 of the β-chain produces a molecule that precipitates out as polymerized long fibres (tactoids) at low oxygen tension, which leads to the sickle shape. The homozygous form (HbSS) causes sickle cell anaemia.

Clinical features

Many patients with homozygous disease have few symptoms, while others have severe haemolytic anaemia, with periodic painful crises. Precipitating factors include infection, cold, exercise, dehydration, stress or surgical operations. Crises are characterized by painful infarcts of bone, spleen or other visceral organs, including the lungs (acute chest syndrome) and the brain (stroke). Acute haemolytic crisis can occur and the bone marrow itself may have an 'aplastic crisis' as a result of concomitant folate deficiency or erythrovirus infection. Skin necrosis can occur (usually leg ulcers). The spleen eventually auto-infarcts and becomes small.

Investigations

FBC demonstrates anaemia (Hb, 60–90 g/l usually); mean corpuscular volume is normal. Blood film shows sickle and target cells (Fig. 3.5.3) and features of hyposplenism (e.g. Howell–Jolly bodies). Hb electrophoresis shows no HbA (in HbSS disease) and variable HbF. Liver or renal function may be abnormal. Radiology is required to exclude suspected stroke, acute chest syndrome or avascular necrosis of bone.

Management

Treatment of homozygous disease involves avoiding known precipitating factors, use of folate supplements, prophylactic antibiotics for hyposplenic states and vaccination against *Streptococcus pneumoniae*, *Haemophilus influenzae* and *Neisseria meningitidis*. During crises, patients will need oxygen, hydration with i.v. fluid and pain relief. Infections are treated with antibiotics. Exchange transfusion may be necessary to reduce HbS to < 30%; hypertransfusion will suppress endogenous HbS production. Hydroxycarbamide is indicated for patients experiencing frequent severe painful episodes or chronic pain. Allogeneic bone marrow transplant is the only curative option.

Heterozygotes (HbAS) are asymptomatic with no anaemia (sickle cell 'trait'). Crises can be precipitated by hypoxia. Haemoglobin, mean corpuscular volume and mean corpuscular Hb are normal. HbS plus beta thalassaemia causes severe sickling. HbS plus HbC is associated with thrombotic tendency and severe sickling.

6. Myeloproliferative disorders and paraproteinaemias

Questions
- Which conditions make up the myeloproliferative disorders?
- What are the clinical features of myeloma?

■ MYELOPROLIFERATIVE DISORDERS

The myeloproliferative disorders consist of **polycythaemia rubra vera** (PRV), **essential thrombocythaemia** (ET) and **idiopathic myelofibrosis** (IMF). They are incurable conditions characterized by a prothrombotic state, bone marrow fibrosis and later development of acute leukaemia. Presentation can be at any age but the majority of patients are >50 years at diagnosis.

Pathogenesis

Haematopoietic stem cells acquire a mutation which results in a hypercellular bone marrow and high peripheral blood counts.

Clinical features

Myeloproliferative disorders are often detected incidentally on FBC. All have an increased risk of arterial and venous thrombosis. Arterial events are predominately ischaemic stroke, while venous events include deep vein thrombosis, pulmonary embolism and thrombosis in unusual sites. Small-vessel disease and digital thrombosis are also features. Gout may be a complication. In malignant transformation, bone marrow failure may occur along with sweats and weight loss. ET and PRV are associated with migraine and a burning sensation in the legs. PRV may present with plethoric features and pruritis exacerbated by heat and water. Splenomegaly occurs in 30% of those with PRV, <10% in ET and is often massive in IMF.

Investigations

PRV is diagnosed by raised red cell mass, absence of a cause for secondary polycythaemia, splenomegaly, clonal markers, typically mutations affecting JAK-2 (present in 90%), thrombocytosis (platelets $> 400 \times 10^9$ cells/l), neutrophil leukocytosis, splenomegaly on scan and BFU-E (erythroid burst-forming units) growth or low serum erythropoietin.

In **ET**, peripheral blood film will show thrombocytosis (Fig. 3.6.1). There is a persistent platelet count of $> 600 \times 10^9$ cells/l. Bone marrow examination shows abnormal megakaryocyte morphology and marrow fibrosis. Ferritin assay excludes iron deficiency as a cause. Mutated JAK-2 occurs in 50%.

IMF usually causes anaemia with pancytopenia. Blood film typically shows a leukoerythroblastic reaction with tear-drop poikilocytes. Bone marrow trephine is hypercellular with abnormal megakaryocytes and reticulin fibrosis. Mutated JAK-2 occurs in 50%.

Management

All myeloproliferative disorders require any vascular risk to be addressed (e.g. hypertension and hyperlipidaemia). Patients who have had thrombosis should be treated long term with warfarin or aspirin.

Polycythaemia rubra vera. Venesection to maintain haematocrit < 0.45 and aspirin ± hydroxycarbamide to control platelet counts.

Essential thrombocytosis. For low-risk groups, aspirin only; moderate risk, aspirin ± hydroxycarbamide; high risk, aspirin plus hydroxycarbamide.

Idiopathic myelofibrosis. Transfusions and splenectomy if very symptomatic. Allogeneic bone marrow transplant may be considered in young patients.

Prognosis

For PRV and ET, prognosis depends on comorbidities and transformation to myelofibrosis and acute leukaemia. Stable low-risk disease has a prognosis of 15–20 years. IMF has a poorer prognosis of 5–7 years.

■ PARAPROTEINAEMIAS

Paraproteins are non-functional antibodies, either intact or light chain only, that originate from a clone of plasma cells or B lymphocytes.

Common causes of paraproteinaemia include monoclonal gammopathy of undetermined significance (MGUS), myeloma,

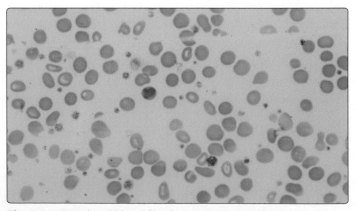

Fig. 3.6.1 Peripheral blood film from a patient with essential thrombocythaemia. Thrombocytosis including large forms can be seen.

solitary plasmacytoma and lymphoproliferative diseases (e.g. lymphoplasmacytoid lymphoma, marginal zone lymphoma). Autoimmune disorders (e.g. rheumatoid arthritis, systemic lupus erythematosus, polymyalgia rheumatica) are less common causes.

Monoclonal gammopathy of undetermined significance

Approximately 50% of patients with MGUS have primary translocations in clonal plasma cells involving the gene for immunoglobulin heavy chain (IgH). Median age of presentation is 66 years. It is more common in Afro-Caribbeans than Caucasians. Patients are asymptomatic and it is often an incidental finding.

FBC and biochemistry are normal. Usually paraproteins are detected with otherwise normal immunoglobulins. Skeletal survey is normal. Bone marrow aspirate shows < 10% plasma cells.

No treatment is required. Progression to myeloma occurs in approximately 1%/year.

Myeloma

Myeloma accounts for 10% of all haematological malignancies. Annual incidence is 4/100 000 and there are 2500 new cases/year in the UK. Median age of presentation is 65 years. A minority arises from MGUS. Radiation, benzene, pesticide exposure and farm working are risk factors.

Pathogenesis

Translocation involving the immunoglobulin heavy chain gene is common. Bone marrow microenvironment is crucial for clonal plasma cell expansion. Activation of the transcription factor NF-κB protects plasma cells from apoptosis (programmed cell death).

Clinical features

Symptoms range from asymptomatic paraproteinaemia to progressive disease with extensive, destructive bony disease and renal failure. Back pain and pathological fractures are common. Patients may have symptoms related to anaemia, hypercalcaemia, symptomatic hyperviscosity, spinal cord compression, amyloidosis and, less frequently, coagulopathy.

Investigations

FBC usually shows normochromic normocytic anaemia with rouleaux. ESR is markedly raised. Urea and creatinine may be raised and there may be hypercalcaemia. Urinalysis shows Bence–Jones protein. Serum paraproteins are detected with suppressed immunoglobulins and abnormal serum free light chain ratio. Skeletal survey identifies osteopenia, lytic lesions (Fig. 3.6.2) or pathological fractures. MRI and CT are used in suspected cord

compression. Bone marrow aspirate will show > 10% plasma cells. Increased β_2-microglobulin and hypoalbuminaemia are markers of poor prognosis.

Management

The 5-year survival is 10–50% depending on disease stage.

General measures:

- pain control with analgesia ± radiotherapy
- correction of renal impairment
- correction of hypercalcaemia with hydration and bisphosphonates
- erythropoetin or packed cell transfusion for anaemia
- hyperviscosity syndrome may require plasmapheresis.

Specific treatment:

- chemotherapeutic agents (e.g. melphalan, VAD (vincristine, doxorubicin and dexamethasone), thalidomide, cyclophosphamide ± autologous transplantation (patient-derived stem cells)
- bisphosphonates reduce skeletal pain and fracture risk
- allogeneic transplant is curative for younger patients
- newer drugs are available to treat patients with relapse.

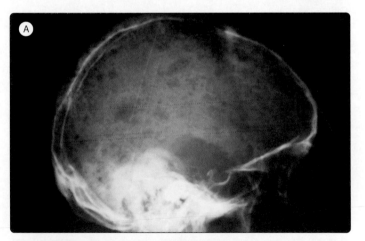

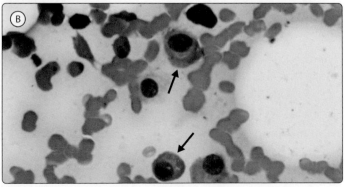

Fig. 3.6.2 Myeloma. A, Skull radiograph showing multiple lytic lesions. B, Bone marrow aspirate showing atypical plasma cells (arrows).

7. Leukaemias

Questions
- What are the different types of leukaemia?
- What is the prognosis for the four major leukaemias?

The leukaemias are neoplastic clonal proliferations of white blood cells; they principally occur in peripheral blood and bone marrow (lymphomas primarily affect lymph nodes). There are four basic types:

- lymphoid (from the lymphoid stem and mature cells):
  - acute: acute lymphoblastic leukaemia (ALL)
  - chronic: chronic lymphocytic leukaemia (CLL)
- myeloid (from the myeloid stem cell and products)
  - acute: acute myeloid leukaemia (AML)
  - chronic: chronic myeloid leukaemia (CML).

Acute leukaemias usually have a fulminant course if untreated, whereas chronic leukaemias are more indolent.

Pathogenesis

A large number of chromosome deletions, balanced translocations and other alterations occur in the leukaemias. (Figs 3.7.1 and 3.7.2).

Epidemiology

ALL occurs at all ages but is frequently diagnosed during childhood. The rare T cell leukaemia-lymphoma is caused by human T cell lymphotropic virus 1.

AML is the most common acute leukaemia in the perinatal period, but most cases occur in adults. Incidence increases with each decade of life. Exposure to radiation, benzene, chemotherapy (e.g. alkylating agents and topoisomerase II) are risk factors.

CLL is the commonest type in those >65 years accounting for 40% of all cases of leukaemia.

CML is a rare disease, with annual incidence of 1.25/100 000 (Fig. 3.7.2). Exposure to radiation and benzene are risk factors.

Acute leukaemias

Clinical features

Symptoms of bone marrow failure include those of anaemia, (weakness, lethargy, breathlessness) and exacerbation of ischaemic phenomena. Bleeding results from thrombocytopenia and infection from neutropenia. There may be symptoms and signs of leukostasis (sluggish flow resulting from the high white cell count), for example confusion, hypoxia, retinal haemorrhage and other mucosal bleeding.

CNS involvement is rare in AML. Widespread lymphadenopathy is rare in AML. Hepatosplenomegaly and orchidomegaly can occur in ALL. Gum hypertrophy and skin infiltration can be found in AML.

Investigations

Investigations include FBC and blood film (Fig. 3.7.3), bone marrow aspirate (20% or more blasts) ± trephine bone biopsy. Cytochemical stains, immunological markers, cytogenetics and

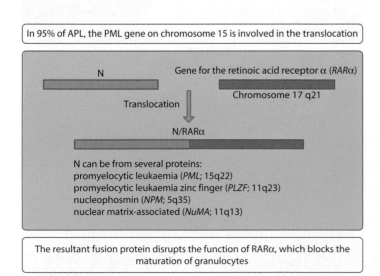

Fig. 3.7.1 Acute promyelocytic leukaemia (APL), a subtype of acute myeloid leukaemia. N indicates the genes coding for the variable N-terminal region.

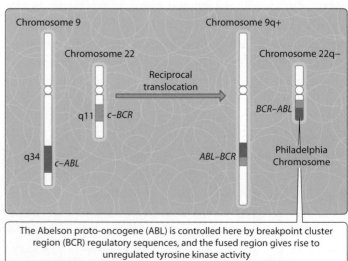

Fig. 3.7.2 Chronic myeloid leukaemia. There is a t(9;22)(q34;q11) reciprocal translocation with formation of the pathognomic 'BCR–ABL' fusion gene on the Philadelphia chromosome.

molecular markers differentiate AML from ALL and further subclassify the disease. CT can identify lymphadenopathy and is used to investigate mediastinal masses (certain subtypes of ALL). Lumbar puncture will detect occult CNS involvement in ALL.

Management

Emergency treatment

Patients with septic shock may require intensive care. Intravenous antibiotics are indicated for neutropenic sepsis. Leukophoresis (separation of white cells from the rest of blood using a cell separator) is required if there are features of leukostasis. Allopurinol or rasburicase and hydration with urinary alkalization prevents tumour lysis syndrome (renal failure caused by rapid lysis of malignant cells) and hyperuricaemia. Supportive packed cell concentrate and platelets are given as required.

Specific treatment for ALL

Remission induction is with combination chemotherapy including vincristine, prednisolone, daunorubicin and asparaginase. CNS prophylaxis combines cranial irradiation and intrathecal chemotherapy. Consolidation therapy is given to reduce tumour burden and further risk of relapse. Allogeneic transplantation is an option for younger patients or those in relapse.

Specific treatment for AML

Patients < 60 years are treated with courses of intensive chemotherapy (usually daunorubicin and cytarabine). In acute promyelocytic leukaemia, all-trans-retinoic acid is used with chemotherapy. Elderly patients receive supportive care. Allogeneic stem cell transplantation from a compatible sibling donor is an option in younger individuals.

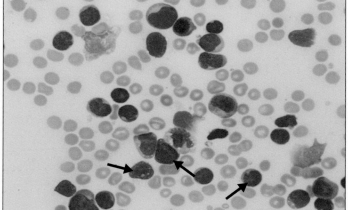

Fig. 3.7.3 Blood film from a patient with acute myeloid leukaemia, showing a large number of pleomorphic myeloblasts (arrows).

Prognosis

ALL. With modern treatment, approximately 90% of children obtain a complete clinical and haematological remission and 60–75% are cured without serious long-term complications. Leukaemia-free survival in adult ALL is < 30% at 5 years.

AML. Relapse rate at 5 years in patients < 60 years with favourable risk cytogenetics is 29–42%, whereas it is 68–90% with unfavourable risk. Current treatment cures 70% of patients with acute promyelocytic leukaemia.

Chronic lymphocytic leukaemia

Clinical features

CLL is often an incidental finding on FBC performed for another reason. It can present with recurrent infections, weight loss and sweats. There may be lymphadenopathy and hepatosplenomegaly and blood film may show immune-mediated haemolysis or thrombocytopenia.

Investigations

FBC and blood film shows lymphocytosis and patients can have anaemia, thrombocytopenia or neutropenia. Immunophenotyping confirms the diagnosis.

The direct antiglobulin test (Coombs' test) may be positive. Fluorescent in-situ hybridization (FISH) identifies abnormalities in chromosomes 11, 12, 13 and 17, which can guide therapy and prognosis in young patients.

Management

Management is the same as for low-grade lymphomas (Ch. 8).

Chronic myeloid leukaemia

Clinical features

At diagnosis, 30% are asymptomatic but most present with fatigue, lethargy, sweats and weight loss. Splenomegaly is common and there are occasionally signs of leukostasis.

Investigations

FBC and blood film show increased white cell count, with prominent neutrophils, myelocytes and basophils. Anaemia and thrombocytosis can occur. There is increased blood urate and lactate dehydrogenase. Myeloid hyperplasia leads to hypercellular bone marrow. Cytogenetics and molecular markers will identify the *BCR–ABL* fusion gene (Fig. 3.7.2).

Management

Imatinib mesylate is the drug of choice. Other options are interferon-alpha plus cytarabine and hydroxycarbamide. Allogeneic transplantation is only considered in young patients with refractory disease or relapse.

8. Lymphomas

Questions
- What is the management of non-Hodgkin's and Hodgkin's lymphomas?
- What is the prognosis of non-Hodgkin's and Hodgkin's lymphoma?

The lymphomas arise from lymphoid cells and primarily affect lymph nodes, spleen and bone marrow. They can be classified into two subgroups depending on histopathology:

- non-Hodgkin's lymphoma (NHL)
- Hodgkin's lymphoma (also known as Hodgkin's disease).

Non-Hodgkin's lymphoma

Epidemiology
The annual incidence in the Western world is 15–20/100 000 (4% of all malignancies). This incidence is increasing because of the increasing age of the population, the HIV pandemic, use of immunosuppressive therapy and improvements in diagnosis.

Pathogenesis
In most cases, the cause is not known. Predisposing factors include chronic antigenic stimulation (e.g. *Helicobacter pylori* infection in gastric mucosa-associated lymphoid tissue (MALT) lymphoma, and viral infections such as Epstein–Barr virus and human T cell leukaemia virus type 1) and exposure to agricultural pesticides, herbicides and fertilizers. There is a two- to three-fold increased risk of NHL in first-degree relatives. Immunoglobulin gene mutations and rearrangements have been characterized in many lymphomas.

Cytogenetic abnormalities (balanced translocations) have been identified in different subtypes of NHL. Major histological subtypes include:

- low-grade mature B cell lymphoma
- high-grade mature B cell lymphoma
- mature T cell and natural killer (NK) cell lymphoma.

Clinical features
Low-grade lymphomas are often widely disseminated at diagnosis but have an indolent course. They are most common in those > 65 years and present with painless lymphadenopathy, effects of bone marrow infiltration and/or constitutional B symptoms (drenching night sweats, weight loss > 10% in 6 months and fever).

High-grade lymphomas often have a short history of localized or disseminated rapidly enlarging lymphadenopathy ± constitutional B symptoms. There may be hepatosplenomegaly and extranodal involvement. Figure 3.8.1 shows mediastinal widening as a result of lymphadenopathy.

Investigations
FBC usually shows normochromic normocytic anaemia with lymphopenia. Blood film may demonstrate a leukoerythroblastic picture or pancytopenia if there is extensive marrow involvement. Occasionally, lymphoma cells are found on blood film, and immunophenotyping is useful. Raised lactate dehydrogenase (LDH) and β_2-microglobulin are markers of poor prognosis. Lymph node or other tissue biopsy gives histological confirmation. Bone marrow biopsy (Fig. 3.8.2) and CT are used for staging. Cytogenetics on blood or bone marrow aspirate may show specific translocations.

Management
Low-grade lymphomas with localized, non-bulky disease are managed with a 'wait and watch' policy or radiotherapy. In advanced disease, a 'wait and watch' strategy can be followed if there is no bulky disease, bone marrow failure or B symptoms.

Treatment includes conventional chemotherapies (e.g. chlorambucil or cyclophosphamide, doxorubicin, vincristine and prednisolone (CHOP)), therapeutic monoclonal antibodies (e.g. rituximab) and purine analogues (e.g. fludarabine) ± radiotherapy. Autologous and allogeneic transplants are considered in younger patients.

In bulky disease, hydration is indicated prior to chemotherapy to avoid tumour lysis syndrome (renal failure from rapid lysis of malignant cells).

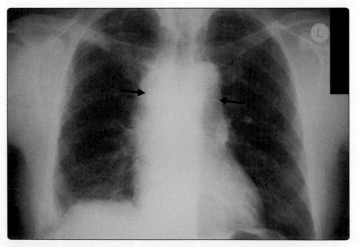

Fig. 3.8.1 Chest radiograph showing mediastinal widening (arrows) in a patient with high-grade non-Hodgkin's lymphoma.

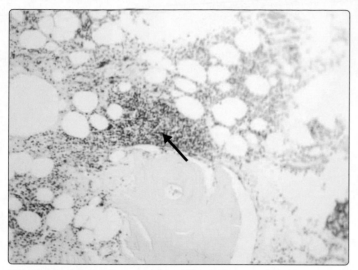

Fig. 3.8.2 Bone marrow trephine biopsy from a patient with low-grade lymphoma (follicular non-Hodgkin's lymphoma), showing a paratrabecular lymphoid infiltrate (arrow).

In **high-grade lymphoma**, many patients are cured by combination chemotherapy (rituximab–CHOP in the UK) or by radiotherapy (localized disease). Stem cell transplantation is used to treat relapsed or refractory high-grade lymphomas.

Prognosis
Median survival of patients with low-grade NHL is 8–10 years while high-grade lymphomas are potentially curable. The 5-year survival ranges from 75% (low-risk group) to 25% in high-risk group. T cell lymphomas have a poorer prognosis.

Hodgkin's lymphoma
Epidemiology
Annual incidence in the Western world is 3/100 000, with a bimodal age incidence including a major peak in the twenties and a minor peak in the sixties. It is associated with high socioeconomic status in childhood.

Pathogenesis
One-third is associated with Epstein–Barr virus infection. In most patients, Hodgkin/Reed–Sternberg cells (derived from B lymphocytes) undergo clonal rearrangement of the immunoglobulin heavy chain gene.

The WHO classifies Hodgkin's lymphoma into:
- classic (Reed–Sternberg cells present); accounts for 95% (subtypes include nodular sclerosing classical, mixed cellularity, lymphocyte-rich, lymphocyte-depleted)
- nodular lymphocytic predominant Hodgkin's lymphoma (atypical lymphocytes and histiocytes are present): accounts for 5%.

Clinical features
There is usually supradiaphragmatic lymphadenopathy (waxing and waning in size and contiguous spread) often with hepatosplenomegaly. Bulky hilar and mediastinal lymphadenopathy may produce local symptoms. In stage A disease, there are no systemic symptoms but in stage B there are drenching night sweats, weight loss and fever.

Investigations
FBC shows normochromic normocytic anaemia, reactive leukocytosis and thrombocytosis ± eosinophilia. ESR and plasma viscosity are increased. Raised LDH reflects disease bulk and hypoalbuminaemia has a poorer prognosis. Biopsies can be taken from lymph nodes, bone marrow (to exclude marrow involvement) and other suspicious sites. Chest, abdomen and pelvis CT or position emission tomography are used for staging.

Management
Patients are stratified according to a variety of factors, each indicating a reduction of the predicted 5-year freedom from progression rate by approximately 8%:
- age > 45 years
- male gender
- serum albumin < 40 g/l
- haemoglobin < 105 g/l
- advanced disease
- leukocytosis (white cell count 15×10^9 cells/l)
- lymphopenia (< 0.6×10^9 cells/l or < 8% white cell count).

Treatment of patients with standard risk is with doxorubicin, bleomycin, vinblastine and dacarbazine (ABVD) ± radiotherapy. Those with poor prognosis should receive bleomycin, etoposide, doxorubicin, cyclophosphamide, vincristine, procarbazine and prednisolone (BEACOPP).

High-dose chemotherapy and stem cell transplantation are reserved for refractory and relapsed Hodgkin's lymphoma.

Prognosis
Hodgkin's lymphoma is a potentially curable disease and approximately 50% presenting with advanced disease will be cured. The 5-year survival from Hodgkin's disease is > 80%.

Index